D0500340

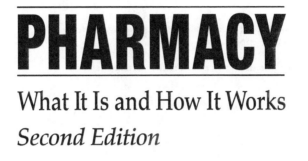

PHARMACY

What It Is and How It Works

Second Edition

CRC PRESS
PHARMACY EDUCATION
SERIES

Pharmacy: What It Is and How It Works, Second Edition
William N. Kelly

Basic Pharmacology: Understanding Drug Actions and Reactions
Maria A. Hernandez and Appu Rathinavelu

Managing Pharmacy Practice: Principles, Strategies, and Systems
Andrew M. Peterson

Essentials of Human Physiology for Pharmacy
Laurie Kelly

Essential Math and Calculations for Pharmacy Technicians
Indra K. Reddy and Mansoor A. Khan

Pharmacoethics: A Problem-Based Approach
David A. Gettman and Dean Arneson

Pharmaceutical Care: Insights from Community Pharmacists
William N. Tindall and Marsha K. Millonig

Essentials of Law and Ethics for Pharmacy Technicians
Kenneth M. Strandberg

Essentials of Pathophysiology for Pharmacy
Martin M. Zdanowicz

Quick Reference to Cardiovascular Pharmacotherapy
Judy W. M. Cheng

Essentials of Pharmacy Law
Douglas J. Pisano

Pharmacokinetic Principles of Dosing Adjustments: Understanding the Basics
Ronald D. Schoenwald

Pharmaceutical and Clinical Calculations, Second Edition
Mansoor A. Khan and Indra K. Reddy

Strauss's Federal Drug Laws and Examination Review, Fifth Edition Revised
Steven Strauss

Inside Pharmacy: Anatomy of a Profession
Raymond A. Gosselin and Jack Robbins

Understanding Medical Terms: A Guide for Pharmacy Practice, Second Edition
Walter F. Stanaszek, Mary J. Stanaszek, Robert J. Holt, and Steven Strauss

Pharmacokinetic Analysis: A Practical Approach
Peter I. D. Lee and Gordon L. Amidon

Guidebook for Patient Counseling
Harvey M. Rappaport, Kelly S. Straker, Tracy S. Hunter, and Joseph F. Roy

PHARMACY

What It Is and How It Works

Second Edition

WILLIAM N. KELLY

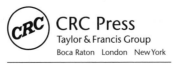

CRC Press
Taylor & Francis Group
Boca Raton   London   New York

CRC Press is an imprint of the
Taylor & Francis Group, an informa business

CRC Press
Taylor & Francis Group
6000 Broken Sound Parkway NW, Suite 300
Boca Raton, FL 33487-2742

International Standard Book Number-10: 0-8493-7246-1 (Hardcover)
International Standard Book Number-13: 978-0-8493-7246-9 (Hardcover)

Library of Congress Cataloging-in-Publication Data

Kelly, William N.
   Pharmacy : what it is and how it works / William N. Kelly. -- 2nd ed.
     p. ; cm. -- (CRC Press pharmacy education series)
   Includes bibliographical references and index.
   ISBN-13: 978-0-8493-7246-9 (alk. paper)
   ISBN-10: 0-8493-7246-1 (alk. paper)
   1. Pharmacy. I. Title. II. Series.
   [DNLM: 1. Pharmacy. QV 704 K29p 2007]

RS91.K36 2007
615'.1--dc22
                                                      2006023249

Visit the Taylor & Francis Web site at
http://www.taylorandfrancis.com

and the CRC Press Web site at
http://www.crcpress.com

DEDICATION

To my mentors: Don Bouchart, Stan Byington, George Phillips, Ted Matthews, Don Rucker, and Bob Chen

FOREWORD

Welcome to Pharmacy

I wish that a book like this had been available when I first considered becoming a pharmacist many years ago. How helpful it would have been to read a systematic overview of the field written by an eminent pharmacist. Later, when I commenced my pharmacy studies, how stimulating it would have been to see, through the eyes of a visionary pharmacist, the exciting opportunities in this profession for helping people improve their lives through safe and appropriate use of medicines. Fortunately, because of this excellent book by Dr. William Kelly, today's seekers of insight into pharmacy will not have to encounter the voids I experienced.

Many dividends await pharmacy students and pharmacy technician trainees who early in their studies acquire an understanding of the breadth and depth of the profession; reading this book is an excellent starting point in making that investment. For high school students who are assessing pharmacy as a career option, this book is a trustworthy guide. Pharmacists and pharmacy technicians should have this book in their personal libraries for ready reference whenever they advise a young person about a career in pharmacy. Practitioners will also find value in this book's documentation of key events in pharmacy and in its coverage of facets of the field with which they are not familiar.

One of this book's strengths is its chapter on pharmaceutical care. This practice philosophy has caused great excitement in recent years because it offers the promise of better alignment between the expertise of pharmacists and the needs that people have for help in making the best use of medicines. Many pharmacists have embraced pharmaceutical care as the ideal model for how the profession should be practiced, and they have committed themselves to shifting the profession in this direction.

Half of the chapters in this book discuss the work of pharmacists in specific sectors of the field — well-known areas such as community pharmacy and hospital pharmacy as well as less common niches such as home health care. When thinking about career choices for pharmacists, it is important to keep in mind what it means to "practice the profession of pharmacy," that is, to provide medications and related services (information or advice) to individual patients. A special relationship, as reflected in the ethics of the profession, exists between the professional (the practicing pharmacist) and the client (the patient).

Most pharmacists are engaged in pharmacy practice. However, others are employed in pursuits in which they use their pharmacy knowledge but do not practice the profession in the sense of serving individual patients in a client–professional relationship. Pharmacists holding such positions tend to be very loyal to the profession and do what they can to nurture the success of pharmacy practice.

Medicines are central to the work of the pharmacist, and Dr. Kelly has wisely included chapters on how drug products are developed, used, and priced. The chapter on pharmacy technicians is very important because of the growing role that this occupation plays in pharmacy practice. Another chapter covers technology and automation, which are having a profound effect on the traditional dispensing role of the pharmacist. Pharmacists have created many organizations to represent their interests, and Dr. Kelly summarizes their vital role. He concludes the book with sound advice on career development for the pharmacist.

For those readers who have already made a commitment to pursue pharmacy education, some bits of advice: first, keep in mind that the information in this book is not the last word on the nature of pharmacy. This is an evolving profession. Only recently, for example, has pharmacy settled on Doctor of Pharmacy degree education as the standard for entry into practice. Changes in the profession are occurring all the time. Prepare yourself for being an active participant in those changes when you become a pharmacist.

Pharmacy will be more fulfilling for you if you go into it feeling that you are part of a movement that is committed to finding better ways to improve its service to the public.

Second, nurture the habit of regularly reading the profession's current periodicals, including scholarly journals. Here you will find information that will expand your knowledge of pharmacy. You will read about the challenges facing health care and pharmacy. You will learn how pharmacists relate with other health professionals.

You will identify pharmacists who are particularly innovative whom you can contact to help you with your own development as a member of the profession.

Finally, get involved in one or more student branches of professional pharmacy organizations. This will help you learn how to get important work done through collective action with your peers. It will help you appreciate what it means to be part of a profession.

Pharmacy is a vibrant, essential health profession that will continue to attract bright, energetic people into its ranks. Current and future pharmacists owe Dr. Kelly a debt of gratitude for expressing his love for the profession through the creation of this book. His well-written and well-organized encapsulation of pharmacy will help ensure that those who enter the field are well-informed and are prepared to become the caring and empathic practitioners that pharmacy treasures.

William A. Zellmer, M.P.H.
Deputy Executive Vice President
American Society of Health-System Pharmacists
Bethesda, Maryland

PREFACE

I was 8 years old when I fell in love with pharmacy. Of course, in the early 1950s, pharmacy was much different than it is today. The corner drugstore was the only place you could go to have your prescription filled. In my case, it was Barber's Drugstore. The large glass window in front of the store framed several "show globes" — large, clear glass containers filled with colored water — a symbol of pharmacy. Some of the show globes sat in ornate stands or hung from the ceiling. The window also had interesting displays of medical items and the latest merchandise to purchase. It was the job of the pharmacy intern to change the displays each month.

The corner drugstore was more than a store and a pharmacy. It was a neighborhood asset. Barber's Drugstore had a soda fountain where you could purchase a Coke — 5¢ for a small one and 10¢ for a large one. For a small boy, the corner drugstore was where you went to buy comic books, bubble gum (with a free baseball card), and maybe see the "yo-yo man," who occasionally came by and performed amazing tricks with a yo-yo. Of course, all of us kids bought yo-yos, but they never performed as well in our hands as they did in the hands of the yo-yo man.

There was no self service at the drugstore. Products were placed behind the counters in glass cases. You had to ask for what you wanted. After purchasing an item, you waited as the the clerk or pharmacist pulled white paper off a roller, cut it to size, and neatly wrapped your package. The packages were always tied with string.

I was intrigued with the pharmacist, Mr. Barber. He wore a crisp, clean, white druggist's jacket, was well respected in the community, and was everyone's friend. He always took time to say hello to everyone who came in the store. I asked Mr. Barber so many questions about pharmacy that he finally invited me behind the counter to watch him work with the medicine. I loved what I saw — all of the chemicals, bottles, and equipment. Mr. Barber compounded most of the medications, measuring and mixing the ingredients, pouring the medicine into tiny colored capsules, and then putting the capsules into small cardboard boxes that measured just 2 or 3 inches wide. He carefully placed a label on top of each box.

Mr. Barber asked me to be the "delivery boy" and to do odd jobs around the pharmacy. I was delighted! I swept the sidewalk, washed the front window, took out the trash, and delivered medicine on my bike each day after school. When I could, I watched Mr. Barber prepare and dispense medication. I could not read the prescriptions, because they were in Latin.

When I reflect on those days and think about what pharmacy is like today, I see tremendous change and progress. Fifty years ago, pharmacists earned a 4-year bachelor of science degree. Today they earn a 6-year doctor of pharmacy degree. Back then, pharmacists filled prescriptions as they were written, unless the prescription reflected an obvious overdose. Pharmacists were not to question the doctor about the patient or the intended use of the prescription. This interfered with the doctor–patient relationship.

Today, pharmacists take responsibility for the patient and for the outcome patients receive from their medication. Some pharmacists are allowed to prescribe medication, monitor a patient's therapy, and recommend initial therapy for patients. Some physicians request pharmacists to perform complex mathematical calculations to dose critically sick patients with powerful drugs.

The respect patients and physicians have for pharmacists has never been higher. Pharmacists in some community pharmacies work with patients, the patients' physicians, and insurance companies to manage the patients' disease states. Some community pharmacists provide immunizations for patients. If Mr. Barber were alive today, he would be thrilled to see how much pharmacy has changed and progressed.

Pharmacy: What It Is and How It Works was written as a primer on pharmacy — the pharmacy I know after being a pharmacy delivery boy, pharmacy student, pharmacist, clinical pharmacist, chief pharmacist, pharmacy academician, and consultant during the past 45 years. This book is intended as an introduction to pharmacy for new pharmacy students, pharmacy technician trainees, and pharmacists who love their profession.

Writing the book has not been easy. There is so much to tell, yet I did not possess the knowledge to discuss every aspect of pharmacy practice. My lack of knowledge has been compensated for by my wife's superb library skills and by a number of colleagues willing to share their knowledge of subjects I knew little about.

This book differs somewhat from other books about pharmacy in that it is broad in scope and extensively referenced. For those interested in knowing when something happened in pharmacy, the information is probably here. For those interested in knowing more about a certain facet of pharmacy, there is adequate referencing and Web sites for this exploration.

The book begins with chapters on pharmacy and pharmacists. For me, these chapters are about the heart and soul of pharmacy. It moves on to discuss how drugs are discovered, the drug-use process, and drug pricing. Next are the important topics of pharmaceutical care and pharmacy technicians. From this point forward, the book covers various areas where pharmacists work. The book ends with chapters on information technology, pharmacy automation, and career planning.

Writing the book has been a wonderful experience. I have learned a great deal and am awed and proud of pharmacy's rich history and accomplishments. Many pharmacists have worked hard to make pharmacy what it is today. After writing the book, I am more in love with pharmacy than ever before.

Whatever wisdom might be gained by reading this book is the result of my own teachers, mentors, and colleagues, my 20 years of experience as a practitioner, 10 years experience as an academician, and much observation, tossed together with a few hopes and dreams.

What has been written was put together with care. There is no doubt, however, that an endeavor of this sort results in a few errors and omissions. For this I apologize in advance and will make corrections in future editions.

When I began writing this book, I planned to title the last chapter "The Future of Pharmacy." After writing about half of the book, it became obvious that the last chapter needed to be on career planning — written for pharmacy students trying to decide on their first job in pharmacy and for pharmacists wanting to explore other career opportunities.

As a result, I did not write "The Future of Pharmacy." However, I often think about pharmacy's future. Will there be one voice — one pharmacy organization that speaks for pharmacy? Will pharmacy require an undergraduate degree before granting a 4-year doctorate degree? Will pharmacists be paid for cognitive services? Finally, will pharmacy become a true clinical profession? Only time will tell, and I hope that I see some of this in my lifetime.

I hope you enjoy the book.

ACKNOWLEDGMENT

I could not have written *Pharmacy: What It Is and How It Works* without the assistance of my wife Trudy, who deserves, but refused, coauthorship. Trudy is a superb reference librarian who performed all of the research for this book, helped edit the contents, and acquired copyright permissions when needed. She also inspired and encouraged me when I most needed it. I would also like to acknowledge the support of T. Donald Rucker, Ph.D., who has mentored me during my career as an academic and in my pursuit of scholarship.

ABOUT THE AUTHOR

William N. Kelly has had a long and varied career in pharmacy. He started his career in pharmacy at 8 years of age as the delivery boy for his neighborhood drug store in Bay City, Michigan. It was during this first pharmacy job that he realized he wanted to be a pharmacist, and he never wavered from that goal. He worked in several community pharmacies while attending pharmacy school at Ferris State College — now Ferris State University in Big Rapids, Michigan.

After graduating with a bachelor of science degree in pharmacy from Ferris in 1968, the author worked for 2 years at White and White Pharmacy in Grand Rapids, Michigan. Here he read about something new — clinical pharmacy. Upon investigating this further, he discovered he needed a new degree in pharmacy — doctor of pharmacy (Pharm.D.) — to practice clinical pharmacy, so back to school he went. This time he attended the University of Michigan in Ann Arbor, Michigan, and while working on the postgraduate degree also completed a residency in hospital pharmacy at the University of Michigan Hospital and Clinics.

After earning his doctorate degree in pharmacy, and completing a hospital pharmacy residency in 1972, Dr. Kelly accepted positions as assistant director of pharmacy and director of drug information at Hamot Medical Center, a 550-bed hospital in Erie, Pennsylvania. At Hamot Medical Center, he and Douglas E. Miller, Pharm.D., Director of Pharmacy, developed and extensively published articles about innovative clinical pharmacy services.

These papers provided helpful road maps for other pharmacists wanting to provide clinical pharmacy services in community hospitals.

Dr. Kelly became director of pharmacy at Hamot in 1982. Over the next 10 years, he further developed pharmacy services at Hamot to include pharmaceutical care and the use of pharmacy automation. He completed a fellowship in executive management at the Leonard Davis Institute of

Health at the University of Pennsylvania in Philadelphia and became an assistant vice-president of the hospital, responsible for pharmacy, the clinical laboratory, home health care, and radiology.

During his time at the University of Pennsylvania, Kelly discovered his enthusiasm for collecting information and data, writing, presenting, and publishing — the functions of an academician. Thus, in 1992 he made a major career change and accepted a position as chairman of pharmacy practice at Mercer University's Southern School of Pharmacy in Atlanta, Georgia. During the next 7 years, Kelly worked with other faculty members to implement an innovative curriculum that incorporated pharmaceutical care, advanced community pharmacy practice, health outcomes, and disease state management.

To pursue his research interests in pharmacoepidemiology, drug safety, and proving the value of pharmaceutical care, Dr. Kelly stepped down as department chair in 1998. Between 1995 and 2000, he enhanced his knowledge of epidemiology and biostatistics by attending graduate classes at the Schools of Public Health at McGill University in Montreal, Canada, and Emory University in Atlanta, Georgia. He further enhanced his skills in pharmacoepidemiology by completing a sabbatical at the Vaccine Safety and Development Branch of the Centers for Disease Control and Prevention (CDC) in Atlanta.

Dr. Kelly was chair and professor of pharmacy in the Departments of Pharmacy Practice and Pharmacy Administration at Mercer University's Southern School of Pharmacy, where he taught the introduction to pharmacy course, a drug misadventures course, and pharmacy law and ethics and helps teach pharmacy management. He also held the position of guest researcher at the National Immunization Program of the CDC.

He currently is president of William N. Kelly Consulting, Inc., a company specializing in providing information, education, and consultation in the areas of medication safety, pharmacoepidemiology, and pharmacy practice.

During his career in pharmacy, Dr. Kelly has been president of the Pennsylvania Society of Hospital Pharmacists (PSHP) and has served on the board of directors of the American Society of Health-System Pharmacists (ASHP). In 1991, he was awarded the Pharmacist of the Year Award by the PSHP, and he is past chair and currently is a member of the United States Pharmacopeia's (USP) Expert Committee on Safe Medication Use.

Dr. Kelly has published extensively throughout his career in professional, peer-reviewed journals and has written several chapters in pharmacy texts. This is the second edition of *Pharmacy: What It Is and How It Works*. His second book, *Prescribed Medication and the Public Health: Laying the Foundation for Risk Reduction* (Haworth Press) was published in 2006. He lives with his wife, Trudy, in Oldsmar, Florida, and enjoys spending time with his two daughters, son-in-law, and three grandsons.

CONTENTS

1

WHAT IS PHARMACY?

When asked about pharmacy, most people will say pharmacy is a drug-store or a place where you buy your medication. Some people may talk about pharmacists (sometimes druggists if the person is over age 50) and drugs. Most people do not think about pharmacy as a profession.

This chapter is a brief introduction to pharmacy. It considers three basic questions:

- What is pharmacy?
- What is pharmacy's purpose?
- What is pharmacy's value?

To address these questions, this chapter begins with information on the nature of pharmacy as a profession. It then examines a brief history of pharmacy, what shapes it, and how it is still evolving as a profession. It ends with a discussion of the value of pharmacy.

LEARNING OBJECTIVES

After reading this chapter, you should be able to:

- Provide at least five reasons pharmacy is a profession.
- State the purpose of pharmacy.
- Provide three factors that control pharmacy.
- State at least three ways the pharmacy profession is shaped.
- Discuss how pharmacy is changing.
- Make a convincing argument that the pharmacy profession provides value.

PHARMACY

Pharmacy is a place, a profession, and sometimes a business. A pharmacy is a place where licensed pharmacists dispense medicine on receiving a valid prescription written by a legal prescriber. A pharmacy is not a drugstore. Some businesses today do not have pharmacies, but do sell medicines bought without a prescription (over-the-counter, or OTC, drugs) along with other nonmedical items such as cosmetics, hardware, and magazines. A pharmacy can be a free-standing building, or it may be found inside other places such as a drugstore, a medical office building, or a hospital.

The word *medicine* in defining pharmacy (as a place) is preferable to the word *drug*, as is the word *pharmacist* over the word *druggist*. In today's society, *drug* usually means an unlawful drug or drug abuse. The word *medicine* is more positive, as its consumption usually improves health. The word *druggist* is derived from the negative word *drug*, and thus *druggist* is a less acceptable term for pharmacist.

Pharmacists are registered by a board of pharmacy and therefore are designated *registered pharmacists*, or R.Ph. However, this title is only conferred after passing rigorous national, state practice, and law examinations. Pharmacists must always be vigilant for bogus prescriptions written by drug abusers who are trying to obtain narcotics and other controlled substances illegally. The last part of defining pharmacy (as a place) includes the words *legal prescriber*. This is someone approved by the state legislature to prescribe drugs — a licensed physician, dentist, or veterinarian and sometimes a physician's assistant or nurse-practitioner depending on the state.

Pharmacy also means the practice of pharmacy as a profession. To discuss this further, we need to explore what it means to be a profession and a member of a profession (a professional).

WHAT IS A PROFESSION?

A profession is a disciplined group of individuals who adhere to ethical standards and uphold themselves to and are accepted by the public as possessing special knowledge and skills in a widely recognized body of learning derived from research, education, and training at a high level and who are prepared to exercise this knowledge and these skills in the interest of others.[1]

There are three widely and commonly recognized characteristics of a profession: study and training, measure of success, and associations.[2]

Study and Training

Instruction and specialized training provided by a professional college over an extended period of time provides professional students with the knowledge and specific skills to practice their profession. In addition, professional students learn the history, attitudes, and ethics of the profession. They also must accept the duties and responsibilities of being a professional. Before being allowed to practice in the profession, the professional student must submit to a comprehensive national and state examination. This is to assure the public that the applicant meets the minimum requirements to practice the profession.

Pharmacists must have 2 to 4 years of college education before being accepted into a doctor of pharmacy program (Pharm.D.) at a college or university. They must then have 1000 to 2000 hours of internship training before being eligible to take licensure examinations on drugs, professional practice, and the law.

Measure of Success

Success in the profession is based on service to the needs of people for which the professional usually receives a fee. However, the primary reward for a true professional is in providing service to the client. Note: In health care, the client is the patient. The focus of a pharmacist's practice should be on the patient and the patient's needs. Counseling and advising patients without financial compensation has been a part of pharmacy practice since its beginning.

Associations

Being a profession means each member of the profession works closely with other members and members of other professions. One of the mechanisms for close association is international, national, state, and local societies composed of members of the profession. Members network with each other, work on developing or improving standards of the profession, and attend educational sessions to improve their skills or learn new methods.

Pharmacists have many professional organizations at the local, state, national, and international level (see Chapter 16: Pharmacy Organizations). Generously sharing information with each other is one of the strengths of the pharmacy profession.

Business of Pharmacy

Pharmacy can also be a business. Pharmacists who own their own pharmacy or are managers of a pharmacy business are business people as well as *practitioners* — patient care providers. Thus, they have two goals: (a) to care for patients and (b) to make enough profit to stay in business.

It is equally important for pharmacists, pharmacy interns, and other pharmacy workers in a pharmacy business to understand the goals of the business and to do all they can to help make the business successful. The more they do this, the more successful the business will be and, in turn, the more successful they will become.

A BRIEF HISTORY OF PHARMACY

Early Development[3]

No one can be sure when pharmacy started. However, early humans most likely discovered that applying water, mud, and some plants soothed the skin. By simple trial and error, humans slowly discovered things in nature that helped them.

The earliest known record of the art of the *apothecary* — the forerunner of the pharmacist — is in Babylon, the jewel of ancient Mesopotamia, now Iran, and previously Persia. Practitioners at this time (ca. 2600 B.C.) were priests, pharmacists, and physicians, all in one. The Chinese also contributed to early pharmacy (ca. 2000 B.C.).

From this point forward in history, the art of crude medicine preparation and pharmacy became more refined by the Egyptians, the Greeks, and the Romans. One Roman in particular, Galen (130 to 200 A.D.), is of special note. He practiced and taught pharmacy and medicine in Rome and is revered by both professions today. His principles of preparing and *compounding* (mixing ingredients) ruled in the Western world for 1500 years.

Separation of pharmacy and medicine took place ca. 300 A.D. and is portrayed by twin brothers of Arabian descent, Damian, the apothecary, and Cosmas, the physician. These twin brothers are considered the "patron saints" of pharmacy and medicine, respectively. The use of the word *apothecary* (meaning pharmacist) is of European origin and is the antecedent of the word *druggist*. There are still apothecaries in the United States today, and they restrict their community practices to prescriptions and specialty medical products.

Plants with medicinal value were cultivated in monasteries by monks during the fifth to twelfth centuries. The Arabs were the first to have privately owned drugstores called apothecary shops. These shops were open street stalls that sold wines, sweets, syrups, perfumes, and medicines.[4] Public pharmacies like these did not appear in Europe until the seventeenth century.

The first official compendium of drugs, or *pharmacopoeia*, originated in Florence, Italy, in 1498 and was compiled by the Guild of Apothecaries and the medical society. The Society of Apothecaries of London was the first organization of pharmacists in the Anglo-Saxon world. It was formed by pharmacists who broke away from the Guild of Grocers, which had jurisdiction over them. Early English apothecaries compounded and dispensed drugs and provided medical advice.[4]

Community Pharmacy in Early America

Apothecary shops first appeared in Boston, New York, and Philadelphia.[5] Some apothecaries prescribed as well as dispensed drugs, as did some physicians. Few of these apothecaries were formally trained as pharmacists.

No one knows for sure who the first apothecary was in America. However, an Irish immigrant, Christopher Marshall, developed a pioneer pharmaceutical enterprise. The Marshall Apothecary in Philadelphia (Figure 1.1) was a leading retail pharmacy, a large-scale chemical manufacturer, a place for training pharmacists, and an important supply depot during the American Revolution. Eventually, the apothecary shop was managed by Christopher Marshall's granddaughter, Elizabeth. She is considered to be America's first female pharmacist.

Most of the early American apothecaries sold various items including crude drugs, chemicals, imported nostrums (secret cures), spices, teas, and coffees. Various European settlements (Dutch, German, Spanish, French, and English) and the American Indians made important contributions to the American colony's unique and developing *materia medica*.[6]

By 1721, there were 14 apothecary shops in Boston, and by 1840 some apothecaries were starting to become wholesalers, importing and buying large quantities of medicinal agents to be sold to other apothecaries. The terms *druggist* and *drugstore* may have had their beginning here.[4]

Patents were first granted in 1790 by the newly founded United States of America. Such patents were granted for so-called secret cures. Patents granted protection of the knowledge of the ingredients for 17 years. The trade in English and American patent medicines became the backbone of American drugstores.[7,8]

Apothecaries made their own private label *patent medicines*, and companies were formed to produce various curious mixtures.[9] Patent medicines flourished, and their popularity moved west with the settlers in the United States. Pioneers often used patent medicines before they went to a doctor for help.

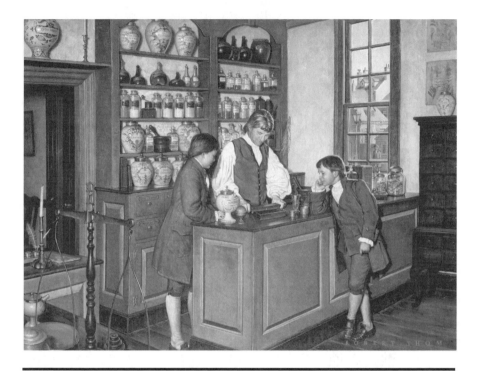

Figure 1.1   The Marshall Apothecary Shop in Philadelphia, 1729. (From Bender, GA and Thom, RA. *Great Moments in Pharmacy; The Stories and Paintings in the Series, A History of Pharmacy in Pictures,* **by Parke Davis & Company. Courtesy of Pfizer, Inc. and Northwood Institute Press, 1965.)**

America's first association of pharmacists, the Philadelphia College of Pharmacy, was founded in 1821 at Carpenter's Hall, the same place that birthed the country's Declaration of Independence. The reasons for forming this association were to improve the practice of pharmacy and the discriminatory classification by the University of Pennsylvania medical faculty in granting an unearned Master of Pharmacy degree to a number of "deserving apothecaries" in Philadelphia. William Proctor, Jr., who served the college for 20 years, is considered by some to be the father of American pharmacy.

The American Pharmaceutical Association (APhA), now the American Pharmacists Association, began in 1852. It was started to improve communication among pharmacists, to develop standards for education and apprenticeship, and to improve the quality control of imported drugs.

The extraordinary financial demands of the Civil War resulted in patent medicines becoming taxed in 1862.[10] Revenue stamps had to be affixed on the patent medicines in such a way that the stamp was torn when the container was opened (see Figure 1.2). Although this helped make patent

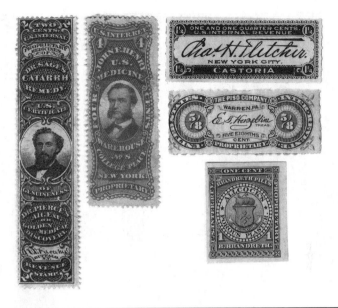

Figure 1.2   Examples of tax stamps used on patent medicines in the late 1800s and early 1900s in the United States.

medicines the domain of large companies, drugstores flourished, and apothecaries (now called druggists) became managers as well as practitioners.

From early 1900 through the early 1940s druggists continued to compound and prepare medicines for patients. However, drug manufacturers were starting to discover the active ingredients of various products derived from nature. Gradually, medicines were made with active ingredients and made available for druggists to dispense directly to patients.[11]

The abundance of drugstores made competing difficult. Shortly after World War II (1945), a young entrepreneur from Erie, Pennsylvania, named Jack Eckerd made his mark by cutting prices and introducing self-service in the pharmacy.[12] Until then, all goods in drugstores were behind the counter in glass cases. Customers had to ask for the items they wished to buy. Eckerd also made sure each employee had a stake in the business. These principles paid off, and Eckerd expanded his business to a chain of drugstores in New York and Delaware. Other chain drugstores following Eckerd's business principles soon sprang up in other parts of the country.

Hospital Pharmacy in Early America

The first hospital pharmacy (Figure 1.3) was established at the Pennsylvania Hospital, started by Benjamin Franklin, in Philadelphia in 1752.[13] The first hospital pharmacist was Jonathan Roberts. However, it was his

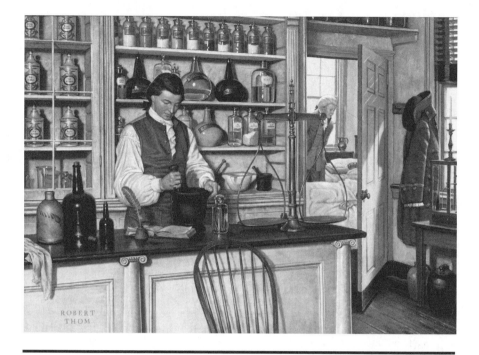

Figure 1.3 The first hospital pharmacy in colonial America at the Pennsylvania Hospital in Philadelphia, 1752. (From Bender, GA and Thom, RA. *Great Moments in Pharmacy; The Stories and Paintings in the Series, A History of Pharmacy in Pictures*, by Parke Davis & Company. Courtesy of Pfizer, Inc. and Northwood Institute Press, 1965.)

successor, John Morgan, who made the biggest impact. Morgan, as a pharmacist, and later as a physician, championed prescription writing and the separation of the two professions. By 1812, the New York Hospital also had a full-time pharmacy practitioner.[13]

Hospital pharmacy practice developed slowly. By 1921, it was estimated that only 500 of the 6000 hospitals in the United States had pharmacists on staff.[14] Most immigrants to the United States were Roman Catholic, and they built Catholic hospitals. The number of pharmacists was increased by the willingness of the Catholic Church to provide training in pharmacy for nuns.[13]

Between 1920 and 1940, an awakening came about because of hospital pharmacists' growing awareness of the problems and the potential of their specialty.[15] The first hospital pharmacy internship program was started by Harvey Whitney in 1927 at the University of Michigan Hospital in Ann Arbor.

A section for hospital pharmacists within the APhA was established in 1936. The American Society of Hospital Pharmacists (ASHP) was formed in 1942 and ended joint membership with the APhA in 1972. In 1995, the organization changed its name to the American Society of Health-System Pharmacists, since many of its members were practicing in organized health care settings rather than exclusively in hospitals.

Pharmacists made many contributions to the American Revolutionary War, World Wars I and II, and the Korean, Vietnam, and Gulf Wars. The contributions of pharmacists during World War II are documented by Worthen.[16,17]

For more information on the history of American pharmacy, consult the American Institute of the History of Pharmacy, located at the University of Wisconsin School of Pharmacy, 777 Highland Avenue, Madison, WI 53705; telephone: (608) 262-5378; Web site: http://www.aihp.org.

WHAT IS THE PURPOSE OF PHARMACY?

Quite a few people, even some pharmacists, answer the above question by saying "to supply medication." However, if this is the primary purpose, why have pharmacists do this? Why not have vending machines? If supplying the medication is pharmacy's primary purpose, is a person with 6 to 8 years of college education needed to do this function?

The purpose of pharmacy practice is to help patients make the best use of their medication. From a public health point of view, pharmacists are needed to ensure the rational and safe use of medication. As a minimum, pharmacists are needed as a double-check in the drug-use process.

WHAT CONTROLS PHARMACY?

To understand pharmacy, one needs to understand what controls and shapes the profession. Some controls for pharmacy are licensure, laws, and rules and regulations. Compliance with pharmacy laws, drug laws, and rules and regulations is checked by announced and unannounced visits to the pharmacy by various agencies. The State Board of Pharmacy, the U.S. Health Department, the Bureau of Narcotics and Dangerous Drugs (BNDD), the Drug Enforcement Agency (DEA), and the Food and Drug Administration (FDA) can show up for an inspection at any time. When this happens, inspectors should be asked to identify themselves.

Pharmacy Licensure

Licensure is a major controlling force in pharmacy. Pharmacists, pharmacy interns, and pharmacies are licensed by a State Board of Pharmacy. It is important to note that a pharmacist is designated as a registered pharmacist (R.Ph.). However, this designation is only provided after passing a State

Board of Pharmacy examination. Thus, all *registered pharmacists* are also *licensed pharmacists.*

State Pharmacy Laws

The regulation of pharmacy practice is the purview of state government, per the U.S. constitution. An example of a pharmacy law would be: "To practice pharmacy in the State of Georgia you must be licensed by the Georgia State Board of Pharmacy." Such laws (also called statutes) are issued by the state legislature and put forth in the State Pharmacy Act. However, other laws concerned with drugs and controlled substances, both state and federal (developed by the U.S. Congress), also affect pharmacists and the practice of pharmacy. An example of a federal drug law would be: "Certain drugs can only be prescribed by a licensed physician." Pharmacists must also know and comply with these laws to practice pharmacy.

State Pharmacy Rules and Regulations

Rules and regulations are written details on how to comply with the law and are developed by an appropriate government agency (such as a State Board of Pharmacy). Rules and regulations carry the weight of the law and usually detail the penalties for not complying with the law. For example, a pharmacy law may say: "Pharmacists must counsel all patients about their medication." A pharmacy rule and regulation under this law might be: "When counseling patients, pharmacists will indicate what the drug is for, how it is to be used, what usual side effects to expect, and what to do if they have any problems or questions."

Federal Laws

Pharmacy is also controlled by federal laws such as the Food, Drug, and Cosmetic Act, the Health Insurance Portability and Accountability Act, and the Medicare Prescription Drug Improvement and Modernization Act. Pharmacists need to know and comply with the details of these acts to help patients and not break the law.

WHAT SHAPES PHARMACY?

In general, society grants pharmacy (and the other health professions) much leeway on how the profession is practiced.[18] In return, society expects pharmacy to help patients in the medication-use process. Thus, outside the law, pharmacists have the power to shape the profession, make changes to improve the practice, and make it better for patients. This is done in organized and interesting ways.

Scope of Practice

Pharmacists operate within their profession by practicing within their *scope of practice*. New roles for pharmacists do not automatically become functions within the profession's scope of practice but must be justified as being "value added" and accepted by other health practitioners. For example, a position paper published by the American College of Physicians discussed new roles for pharmacists such as patient education, rounding with physicians, immunization, and collaborative practice.[19] Innovative practices such as pharmacists prescribing by the use of physician-approved protocols that have been used and accepted within the Veterans Affairs Medical Centers take time to be accepted in all practice settings.[20] Thus, pharmacy's scope of practice is continually evolving.

Organizations

Various pharmacy organizations such as the APhA, the ASHP, the American College of Clinical Pharmacy (ACCP), the American Society of Consultant Pharmacists (ASCP), the American Association of Colleges of Pharmacy (AACP), and the American Managed Care Pharmacy (AMCP) represent the interests of pharmacists practicing in different settings. These organizations are similar in that they improve communication among their members, serve as forums for discussion, help reach consensus on important issues, provide education, and strive to improve the profession and services pharmacists provide to patients. Additionally, there are many state and local pharmacy organizations.

House of Delegates

Many of the pharmacy organizations have delegates elected (usually representing a state or a geographic area) to serve in their house of delegates. This is where the official business of a pharmacy organization takes place. It is also where important issues are discussed, debated, amended, and approved or disapproved. It is the profession's way of reaching consensus on key issues, statements, or standards of practice.

Standards of Practice

A critical role of a pharmacy organization's house of delegates is to approve *standards of practice*. Standards of practice are critical; therefore, they usually are developed slowly and carefully within the organization before coming forward for a vote. Standards of practice are meant to improve practice or keep it safe and to serve as self-policing policies within an organization. However, once standards of practice are in place, they become *quasi-legal* doctrine. Therefore, the organization's standards of practice can be used against a member pharmacist in a court of law for not following the standard. However, if no law applies, the court uses the community standard of practice (how many pharmacists are following the standard) as its best judge of reasonable and prudent behavior. An example of a standard of practice is: "The allergies of patients should be recorded in the patient's pharmacy profile."

Consensus conferences, conference proceedings, white papers, and study commissions are also major mechanisms for improving and moving the profession forward.

Consensus Conferences

Before developing a new, major standard of practice or recommending a major change in practice, pharmacy organizations call a conference and invite leaders in the profession to discuss new directions and reach consensus on a new direction. As shown in Table 1.1, pharmacy has convened several successful, future direction conferences over the past 25 years that have helped shape the profession.

Conference Proceedings and White Papers

Conference proceedings, sometimes called *white papers*, are published for all pharmacists to read and comment on. An example of a white paper is "Automation in Pharmacy," developed by the Automation in Pharmacy Initiative, a coalition of pharmacy associations, members of state boards of pharmacy, and representatives from the pharmacy automation industry.[25] Pharmacists may comment by writing directly to the organization sponsoring the conference or white paper or by writing a letter to the editor of the journal in which the proceedings or white paper was published.

Study Commissions

Sometimes organizations commission expert panels (usually interdisciplinary) to study a major issue or the status or direction of the profession. These expert panels spend long periods of time studying the issue and developing recommendations based on their findings. Examples of some commissioned study reports in pharmacy are shown in Table 1.2.

Table 1.1   Examples of Consensus Conferences Helping Shape Pharmacy over the Last 20 Years[21-24]

Conference	Year	Sponsor	Subject
Pharmacy in the 21st Century	1984	Various	The progress pharmacy could achieve under a variety of different social and economic scenarios
Directions for Clinical Practice	1985	ASHP Foundation	Pharmacy's societal purpose and pharmaceutical care
Pharmacy in the 21st Century	1989	Various	The future impact of changing social, economic, technologic, and health care forces on the profession in the 21st century
Implementing Pharmaceutical Care	1993	ASHP Foundation	Clarifying the concept of pharmaceutical care and developing approaches that can be taken at the practice level to hasten its implementation
Pharmacy in the 21st Century	1994	JCPP	Building on the first two conferences, how can pharmacy survive in the 21st century?
Invitational Conference	2001	NCCMERP	Requiring and standardizing bar codes on all unit-of-use drug packaging

Leadership

The pharmacy profession has been blessed with excellent leadership. Two of the most prominent awards in pharmacy recognize leaders in the profession. The Remington Honor Medal provided by the APhA was started in 1918 to recognize Distinguished Service for American pharmacy during the preceding year. The Harvey A.K. Whitney Award was established in 1950 and is awarded each year by the ASHP to honor outstanding contributions to the practice of hospital (now health-system) pharmacy. Table 1.3 lists the past 20 recipients of these prestigious awards.

Pharmacy is striving to be recognized as a true clinical profession. To accomplish this goal in the shortest period of time will take strong

Table 1.2   Examples of Some Commissioned Study Reports in Pharmacy[25–31]

Report	Year	Sponsor	Contents
The Pharmaceutical Survey (The Elliott Commission)	1946–1949	ACE	Recommended increasing the educational requirements for pharmacists
Mirror to Hospital Pharmacy	1957–1963	ASHP	A comprehensive study of pharmacy in the United States
Communicating the Value of Comprehensive Pharmaceutical Services to Patients (the Dichter Report)	1973	APhA	Identified the value added pharmacy services appreciated by patients
Pharmacists for the Future (The Millis Commission Report)	1973–1975	AACP	Defined pharmacy as a knowledge-based profession
Commission to Implement Change in Pharmaceutical Education	1990–1991	AACP	Recommended the B.S. and Pharm.D. degrees as entry-level degrees for the profession

leadership. As Joe Smith pointed out in his Harvey A.K. Whitney lecture, many leaders in pharmacy are developed through postgraduate residency programs.[32] However, most of these leaders spend their careers in organized health care settings where the pharmacist's clinical role is being accepted. The public's impression of the profession is garnered mostly from what it sees in community pharmacy practice, much of which is commercialized by corporate ownership. Where will leadership be fostered to change the profession's public image?

Peer Review

An important feature in all health professions is *peer review*. The essence of peer review is that someone within the same rank (a peer) reviews the practice procedures of a colleague and cites any major deficiencies. The basis for review is the law, rules and regulations, and practice and ethical standards. Peer review in pharmacy takes place both formally and informally. Formal peer reviews do not take place often, but they are done at the request of a pharmacy manager who would like an outside opinion of the pharmacy to improve and move forward.[33]

Table 1.3   Recipients of the Remington Honor Medal (APhA) and the Harvey A.K. Whitney Award (ASHP), 1980–2006

Year	Remington Honor Medal	Harvey A.K. Whitney Award
1980	Joseph D. Williams	Donald C. Brodie
1981	None	Kenneth N. Barker
1982	None	William E. Smith
1983	Takeru Higuchi	Warren E. McConnell
1984	William M. Heller	Mary Jo Reilly
1985	William L. Blockstein	Fred M. Eckel
1986	Irving Rubin	John W. Webb
1987	Gloria N. Francke	John J. Zugich
1988	Peter P. Lamy	Joe E. Smith
1989	Lawrence C. Weaver	Wendell T. Hill
1990	Joseph A. Oddis	David A. Zilz
1991	George B. Griffenhagen	Harold N. Godwin
1992	Jere E. Goyan	Roger W. Anderson
1993	Robert C. Johnson	Marianne F. Ivey
1994	James T. Deluisio	Kurt Kleinman
1995	Max W. Eggleston	Paul G. Pierpaoli
1996	Maurice Q. Bectel	William A. Zellmer
1997	C. Douglas Hepler	Max D. Ray and Linda M. Strand
1998	Kenneth N. Barker	John A. Gans
1999	Carl F. Emswiller, Jr.	William A. Gouveia
2000	Daniel A. Nona	Neil M. Davis
2001	Jerome A. Halperin	Bernard Mehl
2002	Richard P. Penna	Michael R. Cohen
2003	Mary Louise Anderson	James C. McAllister, III
2004	Lowell J. Anderson	Billy Woodward
2005	Robert J. Osterhaus	Thomas Thielke
2006	Robert D. Gibson	Sara J. White

Informal peer review in pharmacy can take place between two pharmacists, one spotting a failing of the other, and discussion between the two. This can take place in the same pharmacy or between pharmacists working in two different pharmacies. Although these conversations can be delicate, they are necessary, and pharmacy has handled this business well, which is the mark of a truly collegial profession.

Pharmacy Ethics

Another reason pharmacy is a collegial profession is that pharmacists feel the honor of the profession and respect what has been handed down from one generation of pharmacists to the next. In addition, all pharmacists share and subscribe to a code of ethics that has been handed down through decades.

Ethics are standards of conduct. They are also about what a person carries within: attitude, disposition, relationship to self, and relationship to others. Ethics is about style and about adhering to certain principles. For pharmacists, it is about treating others with respect and adhering to the profession's code of ethics.

A code of ethics for a profession does more than spell out rules of conduct for its members. A profession's code of ethics sets it apart from broader groups of occupations or careers. It is the glue that keeps the profession distinctive and together. The constant sense of the profession's ethics is what is distinctive about the *good pharmacist* versus the technically expert pharmacist.

Concern for ethical behavior in pharmacy dates from 1852, when the newly formed APhA obliged its members to subscribe to a strict code of ethics.[34] Five revisions of pharmacy's code of ethics have taken place since 1852.[35,36] The latest revision of pharmacy's code of ethics took place in 1994 and is shown in Table 1.4. The pharmacy code of ethics, like the code of ethics in medicine, has evolved and is less paternalistic than in the past. Today, it provides more respect for patient determination once the patient is properly informed.

At graduation, pharmacy students recite the Oath of a Pharmacist shown in Table 1.5 for all to see and witness the graduating pharmacists' commitment to the patient and the profession.

THE VALUE OF PHARMACY

The pharmacy profession would not exist if it was not needed. Society says there need to be pharmacists in the health care system. Pharmacy's role is to oversee the drug-use process, to make it safe, and to make it efficient. It also exists to help patients make the best use of their medications.

Pharmacists have been consistently rated the most trusted professionals by annual Gallup polls in the United States.[37] However, in the 2000 Gallup poll, nurses were added to the survey, and pharmacists were rated second

Table 1.4 Code of Ethics for Pharmacists[36]

Preamble

Pharmacists are health professionals who assist individuals in making the best use of medication. This Code, prepared and supported by pharmacists, is intended to state publicly the principles that form the fundamental basis of the roles and responsibilities of pharmacists. These principles, based on moral obligations and virtues, are established to guide pharmacists in relationships with patients, health professionals, and society.

Principles

I. A pharmacist respects the covenant relationship between the patient and pharmacist.

Interpretation: Considering the patient–pharmacist relationship as a covenant means that a pharmacist has moral obligations in response to the gift of trust received from society. In return for this gift, a pharmacist promises to help individuals achieve optimal benefit from their medications, to be committed to their welfare, and to maintain their trust.

II. A pharmacist promotes the good of every patient in a caring, compassionate, and confidential manner.

Interpretation: A pharmacist places concern for the welfare of the patient at the center of professional practice. In doing so, a pharmacist considers needs stated by the patient as well as those defined by health science. A pharmacist is dedicated to protecting the dignity of the patient. With a caring attitude and a compassionate spirit, a pharmacist focuses on serving the patient in a private and confidential manner.

III. A pharmacist respects the autonomy and dignity of each patient.

Interpretation: A pharmacist promotes the right of self-determination and recognizes individual self-worth by encouraging patients to participate in decisions about their health. A pharmacist communicates with patients in terms that are understandable. In all cases, a pharmacist respects personal and cultural differences among patients.

IV. A pharmacist acts with honesty and integrity in professional relationships.

Interpretation: A pharmacist has a duty to tell the truth and to act with conviction of conscience. A pharmacist avoids discriminatory practices, behavior or work conditions that impair professional judgment, and actions that compromise dedication to the best interests of patients.

V. A pharmacist maintains professional competence.

Interpretation: A pharmacist has a duty to maintain knowledge and abilities as new medications, devices, and technologies become available and as health information advances.

Table 1.4   Code of Ethics for Pharmacists[36] (Continued)

VI. A pharmacist respects the values and abilities of colleagues and other health professionals.

Interpretation: When appropriate, a pharmacist asks for the consultation of colleagues or other health professionals or refers the patient. A pharmacist acknowledges that colleagues and other health professionals may differ in the beliefs and values they apply to the care of the patient.

VII. A pharmacist serves individual, community, and societal needs.

Interpretation: The primary obligation of the pharmacist is to individual patients. However, the obligations of a pharmacist may at times extend beyond the individual to the community and society. In these situations, the pharmacist recognizes the responsibilities that accompany these obligations and acts accordingly.

VIII. A pharmacist seeks justice in the distribution of health resources.

Interpretation: When health resources are allocated, a pharmacist is fair and equitable, balancing the needs of patients and society.

Table 1.5   The Oath of the Pharmacist

At this time, I vow to devote my professional life to the service of all humankind through the profession of pharmacy.

I will consider the welfare of humanity and relief of human suffering my primary concerns.

I will apply my knowledge, experience, and skills to the best of my ability to assure optimal drug therapy outcomes for the patients I serve.

I will keep abreast of developments and maintain professional competency in my profession of pharmacy.

I will maintain the highest principles of moral, ethical, and legal conduct.

I will embrace and advocate change in the profession of pharmacy that improves patient care.

I take these vows voluntarily with the full realization of the responsibility with which I am entrusted by the public.

only to nurses for honesty and ethical standards.[38] Pharmacy has worked to earn respect from patients, and earns it one pharmacist and one patient at a time.[39]

CHALLENGES

1. One of the greatest challenges facing the profession is raising the profession's public image to that of a true clinical profession. If you are a pharmacy student, with the permission of your professor, write a concise report for extra credit stating the problem and make convincing arguments on how the profession should tackle this important issue.
2. Some innovative thinkers have argued that the profession should try to expand its scope of practice into managing pharmaceutical clinical technology (PCT). Advocates of this expansion feel that it adds a theoretical foundation, something present in medicine and nursing but absent in pharmacy. "PCT adds the use of clinical technologies used in the entire process of care: from diagnostics to devices, instruments, biotech products and single use items."[40] If you are a pharmacy student, with the permission of your professor, write a concise report about PCT and make pro and con arguments for PCT; finally, state your opinion.

SUMMARY

Pharmacists exist because society says there needs to be someone in the health care system to oversee the drug-use process. The profession of pharmacy has a long and proud history. Pharmacy is controlled not only by laws and regulations but also by the profession by approving standards of practice, peer review, a code of ethics, and excellent leadership. Pharmacy has been consistently rated the most trusted profession.

DISCUSSION QUESTIONS AND EXERCISES

Read the first three questions. After reading each one, reflect and record a few answers for each question.

1. What led you to choose pharmacy as a career?
2. What about pharmacy attracts you?
3. What will pharmacy allow you to accomplish?
4. Of the answers provided in questions 1 to 3, circle the two most important answers.
5. As of right now, what do you think your first job will be as a pharmacist?
6. Without consulting anything or anybody, make a list of career opportunities you know are available for pharmacists.

7. Circle two to three opportunities on the list that appeal to you. How do these compare to what you answered in question 5?
8. Do you think there are more opportunities for pharmacists than you listed in question 6?
9. If yes, how will you investigate these opportunities?
10. How does the public form its opinion of pharmacy?

WEB SITES OF INTEREST

American Pharmacists Association: http://www.aphanet.org
National Community Pharmacists Association: http://ncpanet.org
American Society of Health-System Pharmacists: http://ashp.org
American Association of Colleges of Pharmacy: http://www.acp.org
American Institute of the History of Pharmacy: http://www.aihp.org

REFERENCES

1. Australian Council of Professions. The Definition of a Profession. Adopted at the Annual General Meeting, May 26, 1997. Available at http//www.austpro-fessions.com.au/statements/definition.html. Accessed 12/19/00.
2. Deno, RA, Rowe, TD, and Brodie, DC. Pharmacy and other health professions, in *The Profession of Pharmacy*. Lippincott, Philadelphia, 1966, chap. 1.
3. Bender, GA and Thom, RA. *Great Moments in Pharmacy; The Stories and Paintings in the Series, a History of Pharmacy in Pictures*, by Parke Davis & Company. Northwood Institute Press, Detroit, MI, 1965.
4. Devner, K. At the sign of the mortar. *Tombstone Epitaph*, Tucson, AZ, 1970.
5. Deno, RA, Rowe, TD, and Brodie, DC. Roots of community pharmacy, in *The Profession of Pharmacy*. Lippincott, Philadelphia, 1966, chap. 2.
6. Kremers, E, and Urdang, G. The North American colonies, in *History of Pharmacy: A Guide and a Survey,* 2nd ed. Lippincott, Philadelphia, 1951, chap. 10.
7. Kremers, E, and Urdang, G. International trends, in *History of Pharmacy: A Guide and a Survey*, 2nd ed. Lippincott, Philadelphia, 1951, chap. 9.
8. Kremers, E, and Urdang, G. The young republic and pioneer expansion, in *History of Pharmacy: A Guide and a Survey*, 2nd ed. Lippincott, Philadelphia, 1951, chap. 12.
9. Hechtlinger, A. *The Great Patent Medicine Era: Or, Without Benefit of Doctor.* Galahad, New York, 1970.
10. *2006 Specialized Catalogue of U.S. Stamps and Covers.* Scott, Sidney, OH, Fall, 2005.
11. Cowen, DL, and Helfand, WH. The nineteenth century: science and pharmacy, in *Pharmacy: An Illustrated History*. Abrams, New York, 1990, chap. VI.
12. Eckerd, J, and Conn, CP. *Eckerd: Finding the Right Prescription.* Fleming H. Revell, Old Tappan, NJ, 1987.
13. Sonnedecker, G. Antecedents of the American hospital pharmacist. *Am J Hosp Pharm.* 1994;51:2816–2823.

14. Packard, CH. Presidential address. *J Am Pharm Assoc*. 1921;10:655–668.
15. Francke, DE, Latiolais, CJ, and Ho, NFH. Introduction, in *Mirror to Hospital Pharmacy: A Report of the Audit of Pharmaceutical Service in Hospitals*. American Society of Hospital Pharmacists. Washington, DC, 1964.
16. Worthen, DB. Wanted: Memories of pharmacy practice during World War II. *Am J Health-Syst Pharm*. 1996;53:2988.
17. Worthen, DB. Pharmacists in World War II: a brief overview with words and images from the memories project. *JAPhA*. 2001;41(3):479–489.
18. Bezold, C. *Pharmacy in the 21st Century: Planning for an Uncertain Future*. Proceedings from a strategic planning conference for the professional pharmacy community. Institute for Alternative Futures and Project Hope Institute for Health Policy, 1985.
19. American College of Physicians – American Society of Internal Medicine. Pharmacist Scope of Practice. *Ann Intern Med*. 2002;136:79–85.
20. Clause S, Fudin J, Mergner A, et al. Prescribing privileges among pharmacists in Veterans Affairs medical centers. *Am J Health-Syst Pharm*. 2001;58:1143–45.
21. Directions for clinical practice in pharmacy: proceedings of an invitational conference conducted by the ASHP Research and Education Foundation and the American Society of Hospital Pharmacists. *Am J Hosp Pharm*. 1985;42:1287–1342.
22. Conference on Pharmacy in the 21st Century, October 11–14, 1989, Williamsburg, VA. *Am J Pharm Ed*. 1989;53(suppl.):1–53.
23. Implementing pharmaceutical care. Proceedings of an invitational conference conducted by the American Society of Hospital Pharmacists and the ASHP Research and Education Foundation. *Am J Hosp Pharm*. 1993;50:1585–1656.
24. The third strategic planning conference for pharmacy practice: [proceedings of a] conference to understanding and overcoming the obstacles to delivering pharmaceutical care. American Pharmaceutical Association, Washington, DC, 1994.
25. Barker, KN, Felkey, BG, Flynn, EA, and Carper, JL. White paper on automation in pharmacy. *Consult Pharm*. 1998;13;256–293.
26. *The General Report of the Pharmaceutical Survey, 1946–49*. Edward C. Elliott, director. American Council on Education. Committee on the Pharmaceutical Survey, Washington, DC, 1950.
27. Francke, DE, Latiolais, CJ, and Ho, NFH. *Mirror to Hospital Pharmacy*. The American Society of Hospital Pharmacists. Washington, DC, 1964.
28. The Dichter Institute for Motivational Research, Inc. *Communicating the Value of Comprehensive Pharmaceutical Services for the Consumer*. American Pharmaceutical Association, Washington, DC, 1973.
29. *Pharmacists for the Future: The Report of the Study Commission on Pharmacy*. Health Administration Press, Ann Arbor, MI, 1975.
30. Worthen, DB. *A Road Map to a Profession's Future*. The Millis Study Commission on Pharmacy: commissioned by the American Association of Colleges of Pharmacy. Gordon and Breach, Amsterdam, 1999.
31. Commission to Implement Change in Pharmaceutical Education. Entry level education in pharmacy: a commitment to change. *AACP News*. November, 1991.
32. Smith, JE. Leadership in a clinical profession. *Am J Hosp Pharm*. 1988;45:1675–1681.

33. Kelly, WN. Strategic planning for clinical services: Hamot Medical Center. *Am J Hosp Pharm.* 1986;43:2159–2163.

34. Buerki, RA. *The Challenge of Ethics in Pharmacy Practice.* American Institute of the History of Pharmacy, Madison, WI, 1985.

35. Buerki, RA, and Vottero, LD. *Ethical Responsibility in Pharmacy Practice.* American Institute of the History of Pharmacy, Madison, WI, 1994.

36. Vottero, LD. Code of ethics for pharmacists. *Am J Health-Syst Pharm.* 1995;52:2096–2131.

37. Anonymous. Ten in a Row. *America's Pharm.* 1999; 121(Jan):9.

38. Carlson, DK. Honesty/Ethics in Professions. The Gallup Organization, Princeton. November 27, 2000. Available at http://www.gallup.com/poll/releases/Pr001127.asp. Accessed 8/13/01.

39. Raehl, CL. Making a difference for patients, one pharmacist at a time. *Am J Health-Syst Pharm.* 1995;52:1663–1666.

40. Wertheimer AI, and Heller A. Preparing the pharmacist for the future: PCT to the rescue. *Pharm World Sci.* 2003;25(2):39.

2

THE PHARMACIST

All pharmacists, regardless of practice setting or experience, share the same mission: to help patients make the best use of their medication. This chapter introduces you to the pharmacist — one of the public's most trusted professionals.

This chapter will present the general characteristics of pharmacists and how they are educated and trained. Next it will cover information on what pharmacists do, their titles and career paths, how much demand there is for pharmacists, and the rewards of being a pharmacist. The chapter ends with information about job satisfaction, job stress, career development, and the job outlook for pharmacists.

LEARNING OBJECTIVES

After reading this chapter, you should be able to:

- Discuss what pharmacists know
- Discuss how pharmacists are trained
- Explain the characteristics of pharmacists
- Explain the habits of pharmacists
- Explain what pharmacists do
- Discuss the titles and career paths of pharmacists
- Discuss the supply and demand for pharmacists
- Discuss some rewards, stresses, and the job outlook for pharmacists

WHO ARE PHARMACISTS?

In 2004, pharmacists held about 230,000 jobs in the United States (see Table 2.1).[1] This number makes pharmacy the nation's third largest health profession.[2] About three of every five pharmacists work in community

Table 2.1 Active Nurses, Doctors, and Pharmacists in the United States, 1990–2001[2]

Personnel (1000s)	1990	1995	2000	2001
Registered Nurses	1790	2116	2249	2262
MDs/DOs	601	682	783	794
R.Ph.s	168	181	196	206[a]

[a] Estimated

pharmacy. However, pharmacists work in all areas of health care, health care education, and medical research. They are employed in community pharmacies, hospitals, managed care organizations, drug companies, academia, nursing homes, home health care agencies, clinics, physician offices, government, professional pharmacy organizations, and pharmacy software companies and as private consultants.

Pharmacists hold positions as staff members, supervisors, managers, teachers, researchers, and entrepreneurs. Some pharmacists have advanced training in pharmacy and work in specialized areas. Some have added education and training in other fields and combine this knowledge with their background in pharmacy to distinguish themselves.

WHAT PHARMACISTS KNOW

Pharmacy is a knowledge-based profession. Earning this knowledge takes study and training. Pharmacists, and those choosing to be pharmacists, have various ways to gain knowledge. Once the knowledge is gained, pharmacists receive various credentials. A *credential* is documented evidence of a pharmacist's qualification. A credential can be in the form of a diploma, a certificate, a statement of continuing education, or certification.

Formal Education

Today, students of pharmacy must study for at least 6 years at the college level to earn the doctor of pharmacy degree (Pharm.D.). The first 2 years (60 semester credits) are considered prepharmacy requirements that can be earned at a college or university before being accepted into a college or school of pharmacy. Most of the prepharmacy requirements are in biology, chemistry, and liberal studies, and some schools also require physics and calculus.

In the fall of 2004, 89 colleges of pharmacy in the United States offered accredited degree programs, and this number keeps growing. To be admitted to most pharmacy schools, the candidates must have above average grades, especially in mathematics, biology, and chemistry. They also must have strong interpersonal skills and enjoy working with and helping people, especially sick people.

High ethical behavior is a must. It also helps if the candidate loves to learn. Other traits of pharmacy school applicants are understanding, drive, flexibility, perseverance, being goal oriented, being decisive, having a good knowledge of pharmacy, and having varied personal interests. Having some or all the skills and virtues common to pharmacists (discussed later in this chapter) also helps.

Accreditation is the process by which a private association, organization, or government agency, after initial and periodic evaluations, grants recognition to an organization that has met certain criteria or standards. The American Council on Pharmaceutical Education (ACPE) is the organization that grants accreditation for colleges of pharmacy in the United States.

The 4 years of pharmacy school following the 2 years of prepharmacy include didactic courses in basic science, pharmacy administration, and clinical science. In addition, there are introductory (during the first 3 years) and advanced (during the first year) clinical rotations. Although some pharmacy schools can be expensive, particularly private schools, educational loans are plentiful, as are jobs as pharmacy technicians or interns.

In at least one state (Tennessee), pharmacists may use the designation "PD" after their names. This is not a designation of an earned educational degree like the doctor of pharmacy degree (Pharm.D.), but may be used by any pharmacist licensed by that state's board of pharmacy.

Internship

Pharmacy interns are pharmacy students licensed by a state board of pharmacy to work with a licensed pharmacist and learn how to practice pharmacy. Their work hours count toward meeting the training requirement of the board (usually 1000 to 2000 hours). Pharmacy students usually acquire internship hours during holidays and vacations. In some states, academic experiential training is accepted as partial fulfillment of internship hours. Pharmacy interns can do most, but not all, of the work pharmacists do as long as they work under the direct (within earshot) supervision of a licensed pharmacist.

Licensure

Once pharmacy students complete the educational requirements of a school of pharmacy, they graduate. Once they graduate and have completed internship requirements in their states, they may sit for the board examination. The *board examination* involves passing the national pharmacy examination (North American Pharmacy Licensure Examination, NAPLEX) or a state examination, a state jurisprudence (law) examination, and sometimes a laboratory examination or an oral examination. Licensure indicates that the pharmacist has met the minimum requirements of the state in which he or she intends to practice.

The NAPLEX is a computer-adaptive, competency-based examination that assesses the candidate's ability to apply knowledge gained in pharmacy school to real-life practice. The NAPLEX was developed by the National Association of Boards of Pharmacy (NABP). The NAPLEX is available for use by state boards of pharmacy to assess competence to practice pharmacy.

The NAPLEX helps the state boards of pharmacy in fulfilling one of their responsibilities — safeguarding the public health and welfare. Most states also require candidates to take a state-specific pharmacy law examination. Most states use the Multistate Pharmacy Jurisprudence Examination (MPJE) from NABP. The NAPLEX and MPJE examinations are administered by daily appointment throughout the year at test centers found in all 50 states.

If candidates pass these examinations, they are granted a license to practice in that state. To practice in another state, pharmacists must either take that state's board of pharmacy examination, or reciprocate their license from one state to the other, and pass the jurisprudence examination for the new state. *Reciprocation* is not transferring a license, but it forms the basis for licensure in another state (not Florida or California). Some pharmacists are licensed in more than one state.

Postgraduate Training

Postgraduate training is available in the form of residencies and fellowships. According to the American College of Clinical Pharmacy (ACCP):

> Residencies exist chiefly to train pharmacists in professional practice and management activities. Residencies provide experience in integrating pharmacy services with the comprehensive needs of individual practice settings and provide in-depth experiences leading to advanced practice skills and knowledge. Residencies foster an ability to conceptualize new and improved pharmacy services. Within a given residency program, there is considerable consistency in content for each resident. In addition, accreditation standards and program guidelines produced by national pharmacy associations provide considerable program content detail and foster consistency among programs.

A residency is typically 1 year (PGY1) or may be 2 years (PGY2) in duration, and the resident's practice experiences are closely directed and evaluated by a qualified practitioner–preceptor. A residency may occur at any career point following an entry-level degree in pharmacy (however, most start their residency on July 1 following graduation from pharmacy school). Individuals planning practice-oriented careers are encouraged to complete all formal academic education before entry into a residency.[3]

Examples of pharmacy residencies include pharmacy practice, infectious disease, ambulatory care, critical care, primary care, community pharmacy, and drug information. A growing number of residencies are in community pharmacy and managed care settings, in part because of a partnership between the American Society of Health-System Pharmacists (ASHP), APHA, and AMCP for the purpose of fostering such residencies. On successful completion of a residency, the resident receives a certificate of residency training. The annual income offered by residency training programs in 2003–2004 ranged from $25,000 to $49,700, with a median of $30,000.[4]

Residency programs receive accreditation from the ASHP. In 2005, the ASHP accredited 399 PGY1 programs and 213 PGY2. Most pharmacy residencies are in university and community hospitals. During this time there were 1148 (PGY1) pharmacy residents and 292 specialty pharmacy (PGY2) residents.[4]

Fellowships

According to the AACP,[5]

> A pharmacy fellowship is a directed, highly individualized, postgraduate program designed to prepare the participant to become an independent researcher.

> Fellowships exist primarily to develop competency in the scientific research process, including conceptualizing, planning, conducting, and reporting research. Under the close direction and instruction of a qualified researcher–preceptor, the participant (the fellow) receives a highly individualized learning experience that utilizes the fellow's research interests and knowledge needs as a focus for his or her education and training. A fellowship graduate should be capable of conducting collaborative research or functioning as a principal investigator. Fellowships are typically offered through colleges of pharmacy, academic health centers, or specialized health care institutions. Fellowships are usually offered for predetermined, finite periods

of time, often exceeding 12 or even 24 months. Individuals planning research-oriented careers should expect to complete formal education in research design and statistics either before or during fellowship. A fellowship candidate is expected to possess basic skills relevant to the knowledge area of the fellowship. Such skills may be obtained through practice experience or through an appropriate residency and should be maintained during the program.[6]

Examples of pharmacy fellowships include cardiology, drug development, infectious disease, oncology, pharmacoeconomics, pharmacoepidemiology, pharmacokinetics, psychiatry, and transplantation. There were 83 fellowships available in 2005–2006. The annual stipend for a first-year fellow in 2004–2005 ranged from $27,500 to $60,000, with a median of $35,000.[5]

Residency candidates need to select the right residency. The search is less daunting when candidates know what kind of residency they would like to do and perform a thorough search and investigation of available programs.[6] The starting point for finding available residencies and fellowships is accessing the ASHP and ACCP Web sites concerning residencies and fellowships (these Web sites are listed at the end of this chapter). Signing up for the residency matching program and attending the ASHP Residency Showcase and Personal Placement Service at ASHP's Mid-Year Clinical (MYC) meeting that takes place in early December are highly recommended.

It is important that candidates for pharmacy residencies understand the criteria residency directors and preceptors use to select residents. In 2003, the number one criteria for selecting pharmacy residents was the personal interview.[7] Other highly ranked criteria, in descending order, were: clinical course grades, letters of recommendation, pharmacy-related work experience, rotation grades, and the candidate's personal statement.[8] The criteria most commonly deemed least important were the reputation of the college of pharmacy attended, publications, prepharmacy or undergraduate grades, and the completion of rotations at the institution to which the applicant is applying.[9]

The first, or screening, face-to-face interview is usually conducted at ASHP's MYC meeting. The residency candidate should thoroughly investigate a residency program prior to going to the MYC meeting. It is recommended that the candidate write for an onsite interview and send a *curriculum vitae* (resumé) to programs of interest *before* the MYC meeting. The residency candidate should dress well and be on-time for the interview. The interview goals for candidates are to discuss what they do not know about the residency program, and if interested, to impress the interviewer so they will eventually invite you to their program for an on-site interview.

Completing an accredited pharmacy residency makes a difference in a career. Many pharmacy practice leaders have completed pharmacy residency programs. Being a leader in pharmacy is the preeminent expectation when you complete a residency program.[10] This means a personal commitment to improve the profession by leading change.

Specialty Certification

Pharmacists who specialize in a field (e.g., pharmacotherapy, psychiatric pharmacy, nuclear pharmacy, nutrition support, or oncology [cancer]) may seek *board certification* by voluntarily sitting for a rigorous examination. The Board of Pharmaceutical Specialties (BPS) oversees the certification process. Pharmacists who pass the examination for the specialty practice may use designations after their names to show this competency. This is how the designation would appear: Thomas R. Jones, Pharm.D., BCPS. The BPS designations are as follows: pharmacotherapy (BCPS), nuclear pharmacy (BCNP), nutrition support pharmacy (BCNSP), psychiatric pharmacy (BCPP), and oncology pharmacy (BCOP).

In December 2005, more than 5000 pharmacists held BPS certification, distributed as follows: pharmacotherapy (3191), nutrition support pharmacy (348), nuclear pharmacy (495), psychiatric pharmacy (463), and oncology pharmacy (557).[11] Pharmacists who want to keep BPS certification must confirm their competency every 7 years through a recertification process. All five examinations are given on a single day, once a year, in roughly 35 sites throughout the United States and in several other countries.

The BPS also recognizes pharmacists who meet rigorous requirements for *added qualifications* in cardiology or infectious disease, but only after the pharmacist has passed the board examination in pharmacotherapy.

The Commission for Certification in Geriatric Pharmacy (CCGP) certifies pharmacists in geriatric practice. Consultant pharmacists practice in extended care facilities (such as independent living facilities and nursing homes) or specialize in helping senior patients. The designation for a board-certified geriatric pharmacist is CGP. As of January 2006, 1300 pharmacists (721 in 2001) had earned the CGP credential. Pharmacists who wish to keep their CGP credential must successfully complete a computer-based examination or complete the professional development program for recertification every 5 years.[12]

Continuing Education

Being a pharmacist means being a lifelong learner. The rate of new drug development has accelerated. Many drugs taught in pharmacy school are replaced by newer agents shortly after graduation. Pharmacists must keep up, and the primary way to do this is through *continuing education* (CE).

Colleges of pharmacy, professional pharmacy organizations, and pharmaceutical manufacturers offer most of the CE programs for pharmacists. Most state boards of pharmacy require pharmacists to complete a certain number of CE units (CEUs) annually before they can renew their licenses. The CEUs must be earned through participation in a CE program whose provider has been approved by the ACPE. CEUs may be earned by attending education seminars, teleconferences, and meetings; reading approved journal articles; or completing home-study courses or computer-assisted instruction. On completion of a CE program, participants are provided documentation that they attended the program.

Another form of CE is *certificate training programs.* Unlike a typical CE program that may be an hour or two of lecture, certificate training programs are structured, systematic education programs. These are smaller in extent and shorter in duration than degree programs. Certificate training programs are designed to instill, expand, or improve practice competencies through the systematic gaining of knowledge, skills, attitudes, and behaviors. The focus of certificate training programs is narrow. For example, there are certificate training programs in asthma, diabetes, immunization therapy, and dyslipidemias.[13]

Certificate training programs are offered by national and state pharmacy organizations and by schools of pharmacy and other educational groups. A certificate is awarded on successful completion of the course, and usually CE credit is awarded if the program is approved by the ACPE.

Certificate training programs for pharmacists in managing disease states such as diabetes are becoming more important. A few insurance programs and pharmacy benefits management companies (PBMs; companies handling pharmacy claims for the insurance companies or employers) are starting to pay pharmacists for *cognitive services*. Pharmacists are starting to be paid for monitoring therapy, adjusting therapy, and educating patients about their chronic disease, but only if the pharmacist has a certificate of training in that disease state.[14] One state (Mississippi) is paying pharmacists who have a certificate of training to help manage Medicaid patients with diabetes, asthma, and hyperlipidemia and those taking anticoagulants.[15]

Postgraduate Education

The pharmacy field also has masters (M.S. or M.A.) and doctor of philosophy (Ph.D.) degrees conferred after attending graduate school and meeting requirements. Common fields of study for master's programs include business administration, clinical pharmacy, public health, and pharmacy administration. Common fields for Ph.D. studies include pharmaceutical chemistry (chemical properties of drugs), pharmaceutics (physical properties of drugs and dosage forms), pharmacology (the action of drugs), and social and administrative sciences. There also are some combined degree programs such as Pharm.D./Ph.D. and Pharm.D./MBA (masters in business administration).

CHARACTERISTICS OF PHARMACISTS

Pharmacists receive formal education and training in the basic, clinical, and social sciences. They must have a certain knowledge base to be competent at what they do. Beyond knowledge, certain characteristics make pharmacists excellent practitioners. These characteristics are divided into three broad areas: skills and traits, virtues and character, and habits.

Skills and Traits

Skills are expertise that comes with training and practice. The skills common among pharmacists usually existed in childhood or young adulthood, were instilled by a parent or a teacher, or existed or improved while attending pharmacy school. Once the candidate is judged to be able to do the academic work, some pharmacy schools use these skills to screen pharmacy school applicants during the interview process.

The following traits are common to pharmacists:

Empathy is the ability to sense what the patient is feeling and experiencing. This is a basic trait pharmacists need to help care for the patient.

Self-confidence is needed to excel as a pharmacist. Patients notice and want this feature in all health care providers, unless it is overstated.

Being organized is needed to lessen confusion and to be efficient.

Assertiveness helps with patients who are undecided about health matters. It also helps in dealing with other health care providers when pharmacists need to protect patients from poor or dangerous drug therapy.

Common sense is often needed to help solve patient problems and sometimes is the only thing to rely on in solving complex situations.

The ability to *analyze situations* and judge them is an asset common among pharmacists, and is frequently called for.

Some pharmacists come by *critical thinking* naturally, whereas others pick it up when taking certain coursework such as physics and calculus. This trait helps when you are confronted with complex patient problems.

The ability to *problem solve* is a skill pharmacy schools work diligently at instilling in pharmacy students. It goes hand and hand with the skills of analysis and critical thinking.

Paying attention is a must for being accurate, doing high-quality work, and practicing safely.

Being a *good communicator* is an asset appreciated by most patients. This is mostly a learned skill, and communication is an important course in the pharmacy curriculum. There are some good sources of information on this important trait.[16,17]

Being a *team player* is critical, as health care and pharmacy are team professions. Little gets done, and gets done efficiently, without teamwork.

Being a *lifelong learner* is critical to maintain competency as a pharmacist, to provide the best care for patients, and to continue to practice.

Character

It takes more than knowledge, skill, and traits to be a good pharmacist. A good pharmacist is distinguished from the technically skillful pharmacist. Other than knowledge, skill, and technical ability, what is the essence of a good pharmacist?

Pharmacists relate to patients in a special way, because they claim to be helpers and therefore assume duties to the people who need them. A covenantal relationship is established between the patient and the pharmacist. The relationship is based on medical need and trust by the patient and help by the pharmacist. Pharmacists promise to help patients make the best use of their medication, and in return patients allow access to confidential information. This relationship and promise by the pharmacist results in a legal duty to the patient.

Based on the duty to help patients, the good pharmacist develops a healing ethos or way of being. A bond, a trust, and a friendship develop between the good pharmacist and the patient. This human partnership is referred to as the *pharmacist–patient relationship*. Based on this relationship, pharmacists are held to higher standards of conduct than the public. The dimensions of the pharmacist–patient relationship, like the physician–patient relationship, are varied.[18]

The *medicinal* dimension concerns the therapeutic needs of the patient. The pharmacist focuses on the patient's pathology and diagnosed and undiagnosed needs and develops strategies to provide quality drug therapy. Quality drug therapy is safe, effective, timely, and cost-effective.

The *spiritual* dimension involves the verbal and nonverbal communication between the patient and pharmacist, some of which may be
confidential. Good pharmacists routinely talk with and counsel their
patients effectively.

The *volitional* dimension concerns important decisions that need to
be made about the patient. Concerns are expressed between the
patient and the pharmacist. The good pharmacist helps patients
explore alternatives to their health problems and concerns and helps
guide them to a decision they (patients) make for themselves.

The *affective dimension* involves the feelings pharmacists and patients
have for each other. It is important for the pharmacist to have a
positive feeling for the patient and vice versa. Good pharmacists
have empathy for patients and try to be tolerant of and ignore the
poor behavior of certain patients, some of whom may be physically
sick and or emotionally upset.

The *social dimension* is about the broader, societal features of medical
problems. There are social causes of disease, and illness can make
the patient socially unacceptable. Good pharmacists never turn their
backs on any patient, no matter how infectious, diseased, or socially
unacceptable the patient may be.

The *religious dimension* is about guidance that often touches on
confidential and emotional matters. In these situations, the good
pharmacist listens well, asks good questions, and offers guidance.
This is what makes it possible for the good pharmacist to be
satisfactory to every patient need.

As eloquently described by Zellmer in his Whitney Award address, it
is critical that the soul (character) of individual pharmacists be nourished
to make sure the pharmacy profession survives as a clinical profession.[19]
Character is formed by virtues.

Virtues

The act of pharmacy, like all the healing professions, is personal. Buerki
and Vottero write that by the end of the nineteenth century, the practice
of pharmacy in the United States emerged as a socially necessary function.[20] Pharmacists of this generation prided themselves on personal service. They displayed a genuine concern for their patients that earned them
respect and the informal title of "Doc." The basic value of pharmacy was
built on personal service. This affirmed pharmacists' belief in themselves
as health care professionals.

To fulfill successfully the dimensions of the pharmacist–patient relationship takes more than courage and practice. To be a good pharmacist, certain virtues must be present and practiced daily.

Beneficence

The good pharmacist is benevolent. This is the essential medical virtue. The good pharmacist displays personal caring and compassion. There is goodness in the sense of treatment of illness and also in how the pharmacist relates to the patient. There is openness to a real relationship despite the patient's problems, and there is a commitment by the pharmacist to carry out medical acts according to the highest ethical standard. This also means the pharmacist believes what the patient says until proven otherwise.

Truthfulness

Effective communication is the lifeblood of a good pharmacist–patient relationship. Talking is the verbal expression of benevolence and a willingness to help. It is how the good pharmacist carries out generosity. The good pharmacist seeks and always speaks the truth. The virtue of truthfulness in the pharmacist disposes real communication to meet the patient's need. Truthfulness is the foundation of character. Therefore, without it, there is lack of character.

Respect

Being cognitive, patients are autonomous beings. Therefore, they have the right to decide for themselves about their health care. Good pharmacists train themselves to reverence free acts by which patients carry out their best interests and to use restraint when disagreeing with the patient's decision. In other words, the pharmacist is not paternalistic. Respect is the essential medical virtue that guards against insensitivity and paternalism.

Friendliness

People who interact must feel something for each other. Love is the deepest foundation of pharmacy. The good pharmacist's love of the profession and pharmacy's healing mission should overcome any negative feelings toward the patient. If the love is great, the fruits drawn from it will be great. Doing this successfully means feeling the patient's vulnerability. Although friendliness can increase healing, it is the most endangered virtue today: "I don't have enough time for me. How can I have time for you?" When older practitioners say pharmacy is not fun anymore, they may mean it is not friendly and humane anymore.

Justice

Justice is about giving patients their due. It is also about fairness that is tempered by intelligence. Fairness does not mean treating everyone equally. Some patients need more help than others. The greatest injustice in the U.S. health care system is not simply that some individuals get more or better medical treatment than others, but that some get the best treatment and others get none at all. The good pharmacist helps lessen this disparity. Unfortunately, special effort is needed for the pharmacist to gain the virtue of justice, as little attention has been paid to justice in pharmacy training. However, this trait can be taught and modeled.

Fidelity

This virtue is about faithfulness. Good pharmacists live by their promises and hold confidentiality well. Patients want assurance that the pharmacist can be trusted and is reliable. They also look for consistent service and performance. They want to be able to say "my pharmacist" rather than "the pharmacist."

All of these virtues are dependent on recognizing the value and dignity of human life. Without this belief, the virtues are hollow and meaningless.

Habits

Zellmer has written about habits that help make pharmacists successful: (a) the habit of empathy, (b) the habit of translating complexity into simplicity, and (c) the habit of recognizing and acting on the obvious.[21]

Empathy

"Successful pharmacists have empathy. Empathy with patients whose lives can be improved by the appropriate use of medicines. Empathy with patients whose health has been compromised by the inappropriate use of medicines."[22] Pharmacy will not reach its potential as a true clinical profession until most of its practitioners are driven by a deep and enduring need to help people make the best use of their medication. You know you are emphathetic when you feel the patient's vulnerabilities.

Translating Complexity into Simplicity

This is about clear thinking and the power of simple words. "People judge the pharmacy profession by how pharmacists act and by what they say. Every time pharmacists speak to nonpharmacists about their work, they can influence what someone else thinks about the value of pharmacists."[21]

All pharmacists have thousands of opportunities through their lifetime to influence those outside the profession. The pictures that can be created and the feelings that can be evoked with words have great power.

Zellmer goes on to say, "Imagine a pharmacist telling a nonpharmacist something like this, after being asked: 'What do you do for a living?'"

> I have one of the best jobs in the world. I devoted more than 6 years of my life to preparing for this career, although the learning has never really stopped. I work closely with doctors, nurses, and patients, and my job is to help them make the best use of medicines. Medicines have tremendous power to do good or to do harm. Achieving the good is my area of expertise. I am a pharmacist.

Recognizing and Acting on the Obvious

It is easy "to accept as *normal* the things that we see in our everyday lives that in fact are *not normal* and that could be improved with concentrated effort. Much of what pharmacists accept as *normal* does not square with pharmacy being a true clinical profession. And, unfortunately, because of the public's stereotype of the pharmacist, strangers passing through the community do not notice the disparity. But, a good pharmacist having this habit, recognizes the obvious difference and tries to lessen the gap between what is and what should be, and improving the image of pharmacy."[21]

Professionalism

Public trust is what sanctions a profession. To hold that trust, pharmacists must act professional at all times. It is difficult to teach professionalism — it is best modeled. The American Pharmaceutical (Pharmacists) Association has a pledge of professionalism for pharmacy students.[22]

------------------------------ ▼▲▼ ------------------------------

As a student, I will:

DEVELOP a sense of loyalty and duty to the profession by contributing to the well-being of others and by enthusiastically accepting responsibility and accountability for membership in the profession.

FOSTER professional competency through life-long learning. I will strive for high ideals, teamwork, and unity within the profession in order to provide optimal patient care.

SUPPORT my colleagues by actively encouraging personal commitment to the "Oath of a Pharmacist" and the "Code of Ethics for Pharmacists" as set forth by the profession.

DEDICATE my life and practice to excellence. This will require an ongoing Reassessment of personal and professional values.

MAINTAIN the highest ideals and professional attributes to ensure and facilitate the covenantal relationship required of the pharmaceutical care giver.

—————————————— ▲▼▲ ——————————————

WHAT PHARMACISTS DO

Pharmacists do various tasks, and not all pharmacists do the same things because of the variety of job titles and job settings available today and the extent of education and training the pharmacist possesses. In general, pharmacists have the following roles:

Quality Controller

This term applied to a pharmacist may surprise anyone outside pharmacy. Most nonpharmacists would probably have guessed the first function mentioned would be supplying the medication — retrieving the medication, typing the label, and counting out the medication. Think about it: Does it take someone with 6 years of college education and an internship to be able to do that? Most anyone who can read, find a bottle of medication that is placed on a shelf alphabetically, and type a label — even with two fingers — can fill (correct word is *dispense*) a prescription.

No, the primary function of pharmacists is to see that the medication is appropriate for the patient. *Appropriate* means the best medication for that patient. The first thing the pharmacist asks is, "Is the medication safe for this patient?" Then, "Will it work for the patient's problem?" Next, "Is there a better medication?" Then, "Is there a cheaper medication that is as safe and as effective?" The pharmacist asks many other questions when receiving a prescription to dispense a medication for a patient. These points will be discussed in more detail in Chapter 7, Pharmaceutical Care.

The pharmacist's role as medication quality controller is broad. In organized health care settings — hospitals, clinics, managed care and extended care facilities — the pharmacist is responsible for something called the *drug-use process*. Laws, rules and regulations, and standards set by various organizations and government agencies have made the director of pharmacy — the *chief pharmacist* — responsible for seeing that the drug-use process is safe and efficient. The drug-use process is broad and complex. It includes drug procurement and storage, prescribing, preparation, dispensing, and administration of drugs and keeping records of all these things. This will be further explained in Chapter 4, The Drug-Use Process.

The function of making sure the drug-use process is safe and efficient is critical to the public's health. Society requires a pharmacist in the health care system to oversee the process of using medication (legitimate drugs). State boards of pharmacy license pharmacists to help protect the public from harmful medication errors — prescribing, dispensing, and administration — in the medication process, not to dispense medication.

Caregiver

Pharmacists are also caregivers. This is obvious from the dimensions of the pharmacist–patient relationship. The patient — not the physician, nurse, or any other health care provider — is the primary focus of the pharmacist. Good pharmacists dispense more than medication. At times they dispense empathy, compassion, advice, and an encouraging word. They also make sure the patient understands what the medication is for, how to take it, and when the patient should contact his or her physician. On each refill of a prescription, the pharmacist should check on side effects and the patient's compliance with taking the medication as prescribed.

Clinician

For pharmacists to fulfill their role as caregiver, they must be clinicians.[23] A clinician in pharmacy is called a *clinical pharmacist*. Being a clinician requires knowledge of disease (anatomy, physiology, and pathology), drug therapy (medicinal chemistry, pharmacology, and therapeutics), and drug literature evaluation (drug information, research design, and biostatistics) and being able effectively to understand and talk with patients (psychology and communication). This knowledge is used to assess patients and advise physicians and other health practitioners on drug selection, proper dosage, interactions, and side effects and how properly to monitor the drug.

In a strict sense, not all pharmacists are clinical pharmacists. However, all pharmacists practice some clinical pharmacy. A clinical pharmacist practices and sees patients on a full-time basis and rarely dispenses medication. Most, but not all, clinical pharmacists practice in organized health care settings. They are often a part of patient care teams in the clinics or inpatient areas of the hospital.[24] This is discussed in more detail in later chapters of this book.

Problem Solver

Pharmacists have a professional responsibility to problem solve the medication-use process and the complex medical system on behalf of their patients. In 1986, Rucker outlined a method by which pharmacists may evoke assistance to help minimize patient risk that is not readily controlled at the treatment level when prescription therapy is authorized.[25] The approach is still applicable today.

Advisor

The pharmacist is well qualified and in a unique position to help patients with their use of medicine and, in general, to advise them on health concerns. The good pharmacist listens carefully to patients' questions and problems and clarifies the situation by asking good questions. After listening and assessing the situation, the pharmacist has three options: (a) refer the patient for medical attention, (b) discuss various over-the-counter (OTC) medications with the patient, or (c) put the patient's mind at ease by letting him or her know the condition is self-limiting.

Unfortunately, the pharmacist's advisory role is underutilized by the public. This may be because most patients are unaware of the pharmacist's qualifications to fulfill this role. Many patients still think the pharmacist has only one role — to supply the medication. This problem is reinforced when the pharmacist looks busy with the dispensing process and is therefore not available to advise patients. This is further aggravated by the increasing volume of prescriptions to be dispensed in a given day.

Teacher

Pharmacy students are taught that when they become pharmacists they will also be teachers. Some will teach on a full-time basis and become faculty members at a college of pharmacy. Others will be teachers at their practice sites. The pupils are patients, pharmacy technicians, pharmacy students, pharmacy interns, pharmacy residents, and nurses. Pharmacists also train the staff working in the pharmacy about pharmacy, business, and the preferred way to provide service to patients. If pharmacists do not teach, then they are not practicing pharmacy as handed down from previous generations of pharmacists and as they have been taught.

An important distinction is needed here. Pharmacists do more than just teach pharmacy interns and residents. What they do is provide mentoring. This is different from teaching. *Mentoring* is a close and continuous relationship between a master and an apprentice that involves teaching, training, discussion, continuous monitoring by the master, and generous feedback to the apprentice.[26]

Manager, Supervisor, and Leader

Pharmacy students receive coursework and training in management. These students learn proven methods in managing resources (human, physical, and fiscal). This prepares them for possible promotion into management positions in large pharmacies, hospitals, managed care organizations, and the pharmaceutical industry. Excellent supervisors are often promoted to managers, and the best managers often become leaders or chief executive officers of companies. However, to rise to management positions, pharmacists may need additional education by taking business courses and earning a degree in business administration (M.B.A.).

Owner

Some pharmacists like working for themselves and seek the opportunity to be an entrepreneur. The joys and challenges of owning a pharmacy are well known. Owning a pharmacy used to be the dream of most new pharmacy graduates. Ownership today is more challenging because of third-party reimbursement, differential pricing of drugs by some drug manufacturers, and increasing competition by chain drugstores. However, this can be counterbalanced by providing new services and providing friendly, patient-focused care to patients.

Researcher

Some pharmacists with advanced education and training perform basic scientific and clinical research on drugs. Most basic scientists (pharmacologists, pharmaceutical chemists, those working in pharmaceutics) have earned a Ph.D. degree. They hold positions in academia, the pharmaceutical industry, or in private research companies. Most of the work is in the laboratory (*in vitro* experiments) and in animal models (*in vivo* experiments).

There are also pharmacist researchers in the social, management, and administrative pharmacy areas. These researchers usually work in academia, hold an M.A., Ph.D., or Pharm.D., and have administrative and management training experience. Most of this work is performed by administering scientifically designed surveys that are statistically evaluated. Pharmacists working in clinical research usually have a Pharm.D. and advanced training to include a 1-year residency and a 2-year clinical fellowship in a defined area such as infectious disease, cardiology, psychopharmacy, or clinical pharmacokinetics, to name a few.

Sales Representative

Some pharmacists elect to work for a pharmaceutical company as a sales representative. Their job is to convince physicians to use their company's drug. This can be difficult, as pharmacists are trained to treat a disease and to be aware of the advantages and disadvantages of all drugs available to treat a disease. At times, the company's drug may not be the best drug to treat the patient. This results in an ethical dilemma for the pharmacist, who must choose between being loyal to the company and keeping his or her ethical commitment to the profession. Fortunately, these difficulties do not occur often.

Today, many companies are hiring pharmacists with Pharm.D. degrees and residency training. These pharmacists hold the title of *clinical liaison* rather than sales representative. These pharmacists practice differently than pharmaceutical sales assistants, who may not be pharmacists but are people with management or business training. Clinical liaisons call on targeted physicians (usually *opinion leaders* — those who influence other physicians) or physicians needing the latest clinical data on the company's drugs.

Quality Reviewer

As previously mentioned, directors of pharmacy in organized health care settings are responsible for the drug-use process within their institutions. To see how the drug-use process is doing, it must be monitored. In the treatment phase of the drug use process, this monitoring is called *drug-use review* and *drug-use evaluation,* and they involve peer review. Drug-use review is a potent tool for measuring the use and cost of drug therapy. Drug-use evaluation measures the process and outcome of drug therapy and compares these results to national or local standards developed by an expert group of practitioners.

TITLES AND CAREER PATHS

In Chapters 8 through 19, the various settings pharmacists work in are discussed in detail. There are other aspects of working as a pharmacist that need to be mentioned here: job titles and careers paths for pharmacists.

Job Titles

Job titles are important, as they describe and differentiate the job being done. Pharmacists also receive varying compensation depending on the job title held. Job titles in pharmacy include pharmacist (also called staff pharmacist) and clinical pharmacist. Sometimes there are levels of these two kinds of pharmacists, often designated by the roman numerals I, II, or III after the title (e.g., clinical pharmacist II). Other titles for pharmacists include supervisor, assistant or associate director, and manager or assistant manager. These titles are for management positions in pharmacy.

Career Paths

If the pharmacist's title has a Roman numeral after it, such as Staff Pharmacist II or Clinical Pharmacist III, it probably means there is a *career development ladder* in place. Career development ladders are common in hospitals. Each succeeding level requires more experience, exceptional annual performance reviews, and sometimes more training.[27] Career development ladders are helpful, as they encourage learning and growth. As pharmacists move up the ladder, they receive more pay. Sometimes there is a bridge between the staff pharmacist ladder and the clinical pharmacy ladder. The Department of Veterans Affairs has a career ladder program with clinical privileges for pharmacists.[28]

EXPECTATIONS OF PHARMACISTS

Doctors, nurses, and patients have differing expectations of pharmacists. In 2002, Smith et al. surveyed 2600 practicing physicians in California. The authors concluded that, overall, doctors do not know what to expect of pharmacists.[29] Using a Likert scale of 1 to 5 (5 = strongly agree), scores above 4 included: "I expect pharmacists to be knowledgeable drug therapy experts"; "I expect community pharmacists to educate my patients about the safe and appropriate use of their medications"; and "I expect pharmacists to assist my patients in selecting appropriate nonprescription medications." Only one score was above 4 for physicians' current experience with pharmacists: "In my experience, pharmacists are a reliable source of general drug information (i.e., specific facts about drugs which can be found in standard references)."

More work needs to be done in determining the expectations nurses have of pharmacists. A study matching the expectations patients and community pharmacists have of each other is discussed in Chapter 8, Ambulatory (Community) Pharmacy.

SUPPLY AND DEMAND FOR PHARMACISTS

In 2004, there were about 230,000 pharmacists and about 72,000 pharmacies.[1] About three of five pharmacists worked in community pharmacies either independently owned or part of a drugstore chain, grocery store, department store, or mass merchandiser. Most community pharmacists are salaried employees; the balance are pharmacy owners.

About one-fourth of salaried pharmacists work in hospitals, whereas others work in clinics, mail-order pharmacies, pharmaceutical wholesalers, long-term care, home health care agencies, academia, or the federal government. About one in five practicing pharmacists work part-time exclusively.[30]

American pharmacy can be proud that women were included in the profession almost from its beginning. However, until 1970, most pharmacy students were men. This has changed a great deal. Today, almost two-thirds of pharmacy school enrollments are women, and 13% are under-represented minority students.

Pharmacy has been fortunate. Unlike other professions, there has rarely, if ever, been a time when there have been too many pharmacists. However, there have been a few times when there have not been enough. One such time is right now, during the first part of the twenty-first century. According to a report from the U.S. Department of Health and Human Services (HHR), entitled "The Pharmacist Workforce: A Study of the Supply and Demand for Pharmacists," "there is an emergence of a shortage of pharmacists."[31] A similar shortage occurred during the 1980s.

A 2005 report indicates that the nation's 37,000 chain store pharmacies had almost 6,000 open pharmacist jobs.[32] Pharmacy schools that numbered 72 in 1985 and 92 in 2005 graduated 8158 students in 2005 versus 7500 students 3 years earlier, but this increase is still not meeting demand.

The pharmacy manpower project seeks to collect, analyze, and disseminate data on the supply of licensed pharmacists in the United States, the demand for pharmacy services and related pharmacy student and workforce issues for educational, scientific, or charitable purposes. Data is routinely reported by a panel of persons who participate in the hiring of pharmacists on a direct and regular basis. It is intended that the panel represent the major geographic and practice sectors of pharmacy practice in the United States.[33] The pharmacy manpower project routinely assesses the supply and demand for pharmacists by using an aggregate demand index (ADI):

5 = High demand: difficult to fill open positions
4 = Moderate demand: some difficulty filling open positions
3 = Demand in balance with supply
2 = Demand less than the pharmacist supply available
1 = Demand much less than the pharmacist supply available

In March of 2006, the ADI was 4.21 versus 3.88 a year earlier. The ADI for community pharmacies was 3.83, and for institutional pharmacies, 4.16.

The HHR report outlines a few of the reasons for the emerging shortage of pharmacists: a sharp increase in the demand for pharmacy services, declines in pharmacy school applications (but not enrollments), expanded health care coverage for prescriptions, and a resultant increase in administrative paperwork. The report also cited movement to the 6-year Pharm.D degree from the 5-year B.S. degree and expanding pharmacy practice into nontraditional areas such as managed care, mail-order pharmacy services, and internet-based pharmacy services.

The HHR report goes on to say the factors causing the shortage are not likely to lessen without fundamental changes in pharmacy practice and education. Results of the shortage include less time for pharmacists to counsel patients, job stress, poor working conditions with reduced professional satisfaction, longer working hours, less schedule flexibility, greater potential for fatigue-related pharmacist errors, and fewer pharmacy school faculty.

Some proposals to combat the emerging shortage of pharmacists include using more pharmacy technicians to perform repetitive, nonjudgmental tasks and freeing up pharmacists to focus on tasks they alone are authorized to do. Another proposal is greater use of pharmacy automation to increase efficiency and safety and to reduce pharmacists' workloads.

The rising numbers of prescriptions is a major issue in all of this. As shown in Table 2.2, the number of prescriptions dispensed between 1992 and 2000 rose by 50%.[34] The number of prescriptions dispensed between 2000 and 2005 rose 33%. Three key factors are driving this increase: (a) the number of prescriptions dispensed (42%), (b) newer, higher-priced drugs replacing older, less expensive drugs (34%), and (b) manufacturer price increases (25%).[35] Colleges of pharmacy do not have the resources, nor can they gear up fast enough to graduate enough qualified pharmacists to meet this demand. Thus, being more organized and using more pharmacy technicians and automation is a must.

Table 2.2 Estimated and Projected Prescription Volume in the United States, 1992–2005

Year	Prescriptions (Billions)
1992	2.0
1994	2.2
1997	2.6
2000	3.0
2005	4.0

Source: Data taken from Knapp, KK. *J Manag Care Pharm.* 1999;5:324–328.

THE REWARDS OF BEING A PHARMACIST

According to accepted theory, the rewards for work are based on intrinsic and extrinsic factors.[36] The theory goes on to explain that an employee will be motivated if the task allows for: (a) achievement, (b) recognition for achievement, (c) increased responsibility, (d) opportunity for growth (professional), and (e) chance for advancement.

Intrinsic Factors

Intrinsic factors — or motivators — include achievement, recognition, the work itself, responsibility, and advancement. Most pharmacists pride themselves on the work and the quality of their work. Most also feel good about helping patients. Positive feedback from patients is a reminder of why pharmacists are doing what they are doing. Pharmacists, like most people, like accomplishing things and having their good work noticed and appreciated. Some also like receiving more responsibility.

Pharmacists also like to be promoted, but this is a problem if the pharmacist prefers patient care and is not interested in management. In well-developed clinical pharmacy services in hospitals, there is someone who coordinates clinical pharmacy services called the *clinical coordinator*. The clinical coordinator provides clinical leadership and supervises other clinical pharmacists. However, beyond this position, there is little promotion opportunity for clinical pharmacy specialists other than management.

Extrinsic Factors

Extrinsic factors — also called hygienes — include company policy and administration, supervision, salary, interpersonal relations with coworkers, and working conditions. These nonsalary factors are important to pharmacists. It is nice to work for a company or individual who can be trusted and is ethical, fair, and consistent in making decisions. It is equally important to report to someone who is trustworthy and fair. Most pharmacies and pharmacy staffs are small; therefore, it is important that everyone work together as a team.

Pharmacists usually work in clean, well-lit, and well-ventilated areas. However, most pharmacists spend all day on their feet. In hospitals, pharmacists may prepare sterile medication and must wear protective garments. In these settings, pharmacists can be exposed to potentially harmful substances such as oncology drugs, infectious diseases of patients, and contaminated blood. Of course, most pharmacists accept this, and all are trained in handling these situations.

Many community and hospital pharmacies are open 24 hours a day; thus, some pharmacists must work the evening (usually 3 p.m. to 11 p.m.)

and the night (often 11 p.m. to 7 a.m.) shifts. There is usually a shift differential in salary (usually 5 to 10%) to work these off shifts. In addition, pharmacists often work weekends, holidays, and overtime. Most full-time pharmacists work about 40 hours per week.[31] Some — including most self-employed pharmacists — work more than 50 hours per week.

In 2005, the median salary for a staff pharmacist in the United States was $95,627 (25th percentile was $90,647 and the 75th percentile $100,179).[37] The salary may vary by the amount of experience, location, and type of pharmacy.[38] Salaries for pharmacists are highest on the West Coast. Some pharmacists, especially those working for for-profit companies receive bonuses, overtime, and profit sharing.

Because of the shortage of pharmacists, salaries are increasing based on supply and demand. Sometimes (based on location, hours, and competition), pharmacists make more than $100,000 a year, and those bold enough to step outside the bounds of traditional practice, such as consulting or starting an entrepreneurial venture, can reap $150,000 a year or more, but they must be willing to take a risk.[39]

Salaries for pharmacists working in hospitals generally lag behind community pharmacy salaries, but eventually improve owing to shortages and to retain staff. However, pharmacists in hospitals usually advance in their salaries and careers at a faster rate.

Pharmacists working for the federal government fall into several categories. First is the uniformed service commissioned officer pharmacists who work for the Department of Defense (DoD); these officers are active duty military working throughout the extensive network of DoD military installations and related organizations worldwide.

Next is the uniformed service Commissioned Corps pharmacists who work for the U.S. Public Health Service (USPHS) and serve on active duty with the Department of Health and Human Services and other federal agencies (e.g., Centers for Disease Control, National Institutes of Health (NIH), Federal Drug Administration, Environmental Protection Agency, Bureau of Prisons, Indian Health Service, etc.). USPHS Commissioned Corps Officers, like DoD pharmacy officers, wear a uniform comparative to the U.S. Navy and hold rank like Naval Officers. However, USPHS pharmacy officers are not considered part of the "military" contingency and may be activated to "military" service at the discretion of the President only in times of national or worldwide wars or disasters.

Last, there are civil service pharmacists—nonmilitary federal employees who hold pay grades within the General Schedule (GS) system of the federal government. These pharmacists may serve wherever there is need for a federal GS pharmacist both within the United States (i.e., Veterans Administration, NIH, DoD hospitals, etc.) and, in federal facilities located overseas. These pharmacists have no relation to the military, and their jobs do not usually require relocation to meet the national or international needs of the military.

Most USPHS Commissioned Corps pharmacist officers enter active duty at a grade level of 0-3, which is equivalent to a captain in the U.S. Army or a lieutenant commander in the USPHS. In 2006, these officers received roughly $53,448 to $78,444 per year in base salary, depending on the extent of housing allowance. The housing allowance and other subsistence account for 12 to 15% of this salary, and these are nontaxable benefits. Grade level 0-4 officers with over 10 years of service can earn a base salary of $90,648 to $118,212, and grade level officers 0-6 with over 20 years of service can earn a base salary of $117,252 to $147,384. There is no cost to USPHS Commissioned Corps pharmacists for health care benefits, dental coverage, or use of commissaries, post exchanges and other facilities located on military installations. In addition, USPHS Commissioned ffficers (as with other uniformed services) may fly at no cost anywhere in the world on DoD aircraft when seating is available.[40]

Finally, USPHS Commissioned Corps pharmacists have the benefit of a 20 to 30 year noncontributory retirement (retirement after 20 years is voluntary and is prorated upward yearly until the officer reaches 30 years, when retirement is mandatory).

Considering benefits, the salary for commissioned pharmacy officers could easily equate to $70,000 a year. The USPHS has in recent years been successful in passage of a Congressional bill that allows a $30,000 initial sign-on bonus for first time pharmacy officers.

The second category of federal government pharmacists work for the Department of Veterans Affairs or the NIH. Pharmacists grades are GS-9 (graduate pharmacist or staff pharmacist with B.S. degree), GS-11 (staff pharmacist with a Pharm.D.), GS-12 (clinical pharmacists I and II), GS-13 (clinical pharmacist with board certification), GS-14 (clinical pharmacist with board certification plus experience), and GS-13-15 (management positions). Salaries depend on the job description, education, and experience and are adjusted according to location (cost of living). At the time of this writing (2006), pharmacists with a Pharm.D. degree and completion of a residency were usually starting in the high $90,000s to the low $100,000s.

Salaries for full-time faculty at schools of pharmacy appointed for a calendar year vary by rank, years in rank, discipline, and school (private or public). Salaries for the 2005 to 2006 school year were: dean ($179,619 to $185,931), associate dean ($112,000 to $140,285), assistant dean ($95,505 to $101,676), full professor ($111,843 to $136,803), associate professor ($87,322 to $93,560), assistant professor ($76,923 to $85,791), and instructor ($68,327 to 72,658).[41]

Job Satisfaction

Nine of ten pharmacists are satisfied with their choice of pharmacy as a career.[42] The highest degree of satisfaction is for those working in hospitals, women, and those who thought the future of pharmacy was bright. This survey revealed that the major reasons for satisfaction were personal contact and counseling patients.

According to a survey on institutional and ambulatory pharmacists, pharmacists with training beyond a B.S. degree in pharmacy were more satisfied with their jobs than those whose highest degree was a B.S. degree in pharmacy.[43] Job satisfaction was influenced by perceived utilization of skills, staffing, and education. The practice setting, job title, and age were significantly related to perceived utilization of skills.

Things that detract the most from pharmacist satisfaction in community pharmacy are excessive record-keeping chores and handling insurance forms and third-party claims. Others problems include not having enough time to counsel patients, spending too much time trying to reach physicians, and poor working conditions, stress, and lack of time to complete tasks.

In another survey of job turnover of pharmacists licensed in four states, the average turnover was 11% yearly.[44] The average median tenure of pharmacists who left their jobs was 32 months. The percentage of pharmacists citing stress as a reason for leaving increased, and the percentage of pharmacists citing salary decreased.

Job Stress

The main source of stress in pharmacy is workload. In a national study of independent and chain store pharmacists commissioned by *Drug Topics*, 52% classified their work as *heavy*, 30% as *moderate*, 17% as *extremely heavy*, and only 2% as *light*.[45]

Pharmacists taking part in this survey said they worked an average of 10 hours per day. Overall, these retail pharmacies dispensed an average of 182 prescriptions per day, with chain pharmacies dispensing more (236) than independently owned pharmacies (151). Individually, the pharmacist respondents reported dispensing an average of 120 prescriptions per day. Pharmacists working for chain pharmacies dispensed more (154 each) than pharmacists working in independently owned pharmacies (101).

North Carolina's board of pharmacy pioneered a regulation holding employers equally liable (with the employee pharmacist) for medication errors when a pharmacy's daily load exceeds 150 prescriptions. A recent proposal by this board would prohibit pharmacy owners from requiring their pharmacists to work more than 12 continuous hours per workday.[46] Other state boards of pharmacy are struggling with how to protect pharmacists from stress and work overload and yet not severely infringe on the rights of pharmacy owners.

LIFELONG LEARNING AND CAREER PLANNING

Graduation from pharmacy school is a beginning rather than an ending. Who teaches the pharmacist after the commencement exercise is over? No one. The pharmacist must learn independently about the latest drugs, diseases, and drug therapy to remain competent.

Each new pharmacist needs to develop a strategy to keep up-to-date. Some of this will involve the consistent reading of clinical journals such as *Pharmacotherapy, JAMA,* and the *Annals of Internal Medicine* or a specialty journal in the pharmacist's practice area. In addition, the pharmacist will want to keep up on the latest drugs and subscribe to a publication such as *The Medical Letter* or *The Pharmacist Letter.* It is recommended that pharmacists belong to some professional pharmacy organizations — local, state, and national — to keep abreast of what is happening in pharmacy. Most organizations have a journal and professional meetings throughout the year where pharmacists can take part in CE programs.

Lifelong learning and career development do not end until retirement (and sometimes not even then).[47] The challenge is to continually think about and plan for a career that will change several times before retirement. For example, a survey of 337 clinical pharmacists who began practicing clinical pharmacy during the years 1965 to 1974 and were about 40 years old at the time of the survey, were found to have changed jobs 2.1 times.[48] The percentage of the job functions of hospital pharmacist and pharmacy faculty declined over time, whereas those in hospital pharmacy administration, academic administration, and the pharmaceutical industry increased. Thus, many pharmacy clinicians became managers, and clinical activity declined for these pharmacists.

It is also wise to consider differentiating. *Differentiation* develops competencies that collectively create a quality distinction.[49] Why is this important? It positions the pharmacist to compete more successfully for the most rewarding career opportunities. Two strategies may help make this happen. The first is to specialize in a narrowly defined area and become an expert. The second strategy is combining pharmacy and another discipline, such as business, information management, physician assistant training, law, publishing, sales, or education.

Career planning is also about coming to grips with balancing a career and a family. It can mean trying to deal with job issues when you wish or feel you should be home with your family.[50] This creates stress and guilt. Pharmacists working under these circumstances should develop coping mechanisms and have an adequate support system to be successful at both their jobs and their personal lives.

Another career planning issue involves two-pharmacist marriages. This situation can involve lifestyle issues, potential conflicts, and stress beyond what the average married couple experiences.[51] Time and home management need to be carefully worked out. What happens when both pharmacists have good careers and one wants to make a career change or move to a new city? Stress! Pharmacists thinking about marriage to another pharmacist should know what lies ahead and talk with pharmacists married to other pharmacists before getting married to one. More information on career planning is provided in Chapter 20.

JOB OUTLOOK

The job outlook for pharmacists during the next 10 to 20 years looks promising. The U.S. population is growing and aging. The first wave of baby boomers reached 60 in 2006. This large population segment and the Medicare prescription benefit that started January 1, 2006, will result in more prescriptions to dispense and patients to counsel. Cost-conscious insurers and quality-of-care managers will want to stress the role of pharmacists in primary and preventive services. In addition, advances in drug therapy, including genomics, will make drugs more complex to prepare and use. The pharmacist will be involved in all of this and will continue to help patients make the best use of their medication.

SUMMARY

Pharmacists are health care practitioners who help patients make the best use of their medication. They work in a variety of settings, and the patient is their number one concern. Pharmacists receive rigorous education and training and are licensed to protect the patient from harm. Pharmacists are vigilant about providing quality drug therapy, are caregivers, clinicians, listeners, advisors, teachers, and lifelong learners. Good pharmacists dispense more than medication — they are empathetic and concerned about the patient. Pharmacists are proud members of a trusted profession.

CHALLENGES

1. One estimate is that there will be shortage of 157,000 pharmacists (out of 417,000 needed) in the United States in the year 2020. For extra credit and with the approval of your professor, prepare a concise report concerning the possible options for meeting the

prescription and medication needs of patients in 2020, state conclusions, and state what you think is the best option for solving
this problem.

2. Based on increased education and training and perceived needs,
    pharmacists are expanding their scope of practice into new respon-
    sibilities and are providing cognitive services. However, routine
    payment for these services has been slow. For extra credit, and
    with the permission of your professor, prepare a concise report
    providing convincing arguments on why payers should pay phar-
    macists for their cognitive services.

DISCUSSION QUESTIONS AND EXERCISES

1. The mission of pharmacy is for pharmacists to help patients make
    the best use of their medication. How can pharmacists best do this?
2. Some pharmacists go on to do a pharmacy residency. What do you
    see as the advantages of doing this? What do you see as the
    disadvantages of doing this?
3. Do the advantages of doing a residency outweigh the disadvantages
    of not doing a residency?
4. Some pharmacists achieve board certification in a specialty area of
    practice. Is this something that interests you? Why? Why not?
5. As a pharmacist, what characteristic do you feel will be prominent
    in your dealing with patients?
6. When you receive a Pharm.D. degree, you will be entitled to be
    called "doctor." How do you feel about this?
7. Currently there is a shortage of pharmacists. Is this good or bad
    for pharmacy?
8. Being a pharmacist means being a lifelong learner. What does the
    term *lifelong learner* mean to you?
9. What will be your strategy for being a lifelong learner?
10. Part of being a pharmacist is teaching others one-on-one. How do
    you feel about this?

WEB SITES OF INTEREST

U.S. Bureau of Labor Statistics: http://www.bls.gov/oco/ocos079.htm
NAPLEX®/MPJE®: http:/www.nabp.net
Residencies/Fellowships:
 http://www.ashp.org/rtp/index.cfm?cfid=14127718&CFToken=
 26670281

Residency Standards (PGY1): http://www.ashp.org/rtp/PDF/PGY1_std_vs_prevstd.pdf

Residency Standards (PGY2): http://www.ashp.org/rtp/PDF/PGY2_vs_oldspecstd.pdf

Residency Matching Program: http://www.natmatch.com/ashprmp/

Fellowship Guidelines: http://www.accp.com/resandfel/?page=guidelines

Board Certified Specialties: http://www.bpsweb.org/

Certification in Geriatrics: http://www.ccgp.org/index.htm

Pharmacy Manpower Project: http://www.pharmacymanpower.com/about.html

USPHS Pharmacy: http://www.hhs.gov/pharmacy/recruit.html.

REFERENCES

1. Bureau of Labor Statistics, U.S. Department of Labor, *Occupational Outlook Handbook*, 2006–07 Edition, Pharmacists. Available at http://www.bls.gov/oco/ocos079.htm. Accessed April 12, 2006.
2. U.S. National Center for Health Statistics, Advance Data. No. 343. May 27, 2004. Available at http://www.cdc.gov/nchs/data/ad/ad343.pdf. Accessed April 11 2006.
3. American College of Clinical Pharmacy. Residencies and Fellowships. Available at http://www.accp.com/resandfel/?page=definition. Accessed April 11, 2006.
4. American Society of Health-System Pharmacists. ASHP Resident Match Program. Available at http://www.natmatch.com/ashprmp/. Accessed April 11, 2006.
5. American College of Clinical Pharmacy. Fellowships for 2007. Available at http://www.accp.com/resandfel/directorynon.php. Accessed April 11, 2006.
6. American College of Clinical Pharmacy. Program Characteristics. Available at http://www.accp.com/resandfel/?page=use. Accessed April 11, 2006.
7. American Society of Health System Pharmacists. Selecting the right residency. *Am J Health-Syst Pharm.* 2005;62:1138, 1140.
8. Mancuso CE, and Paloucek FP. Interview selection processes and interview selection criteria for pharmacy practice residents. ASHP Midyear Clinical Meeting, December 2003, Vol 38, pp. P–17(E).
9. Khorana KS, and Paloucek F. Survey of selection criteria for pharmacy practice residents. ASHP Midyear Clinical Meeting, Dec 2002, Vol. 37, pp. P–340E.
10. Zellmer WA. Doing what needs to be done in pharmacy practice leadership: a message for residents. *Am J Health-Syst Pharm.* 2003;60:1903–1907.
11. Board of Pharmaceutical Specialities. Available at http://www.bpsweb.org/. Acessed April 11, 2006.
12. Commission for Certification in Geriatric Pharmacy. Available at http://www.ccgp.org/index.htm. Accessed April 11, 2006.
13. *Credentialing in Pharmacy.* The Council on Credentialing in Pharmacy. Washington, DC, 2000.
14. Wickman, JM, Jackson, RA, and Marquess, JG. Making cents out of caring for patients. *J Am Pharm Assoc.* 1999;39:116–119.

15. Meinhardt, RA. Pharmacists manage to get paid in Mississippi (it could happen in your state, too). *Drug Ben Trends*. 1999;11:32, 55.

16. Tindall, WN, Beardsley, RS, and Kimberlin, CL. *Communication Skills in Pharmacy Practice*. Lea & Febiger, Philadelphia, 1994.

17. Rantucci, M. *Pharmacists Talking with Patients: A Guide to Patient Counseling*. Williams & Wilkins, Baltimore, MD, 1997.

18. Drane, JF. *Becoming a Good Doctor: The Place of Virtue and Character in Medical Ethics*. Sheed and Ward, The Catholic Health Association. Kansas City, MO, 1988.

19. Zellmer, WA. Searching for the soul of pharmacy. *Am J Health-Syst Pharm*. 1996;53:1911–1916.

20. Buerki, RA, and Vottero, LD. *Ethical Responsibility in Pharmacy Practice*. American Institute of the History of Pharmacy, Madison, WI, 1994.

21. Zellmer, WA. The habits of successful pharmacists. *Am J Health-Syst Pharm*. 2000;57:1794–1796.

22. Traynor, AP, and Ferguson, HR. Professionalism is a lifelong commitment. Available at http://www.aphanet.org/STUDENTS/leadership/psm/professionalism%20is%20lifelong%20committment.pdf. Accessed April 11, 2006.

23. Gonzalez, LS. What are pharmacists, and what do they do? *Am J Health-Syst Pharm*. 2005;62:2039.

24. Chandler, C, Barriuso, P, Rozenberg-Ben-Dror, K., and Schmitt, B. Pharmacists on a primary care team at a Veterans Affairs medical center. *Am J Health-Syst Pharm*. 1997;54:1280–1287.

25. Rucker, TD. Problem solving: the professional responsibility of pharmacists. *Drug Intell Clin Pharm*. 1986;20:556–560.

26. Pierpaoli, PG. Mentoring. *Am J Health-Syst Pharm*. 1992;49:2175–2178.

27. Meyer, JD, Chrymko, MM, and Kelly, WN. Clinical career ladders: Hamot Medical Center. *Am J Health-Syst Pharm*. 1989;46:2268–2271.

28. Swanson, KM, Hunter, WB, and Trask, SJ. Pharmacist career ladder with clinical privilege categories. *Am J Health-Syst Pharm*. 1991;48:1956–1961.

29. Smith WE, Ray MD, and Shannon, DM. Physicians' expectations of pharmacists. *Am J Health-Syst Pharm*. 2002;59:50–57.

30. Thompson CA. *ASHP News*. One in five pharmacists work part-time exclusively. Available at http://www.ashp.org/news/ShowArticle.cfm?id=14636. Accessed April 1, 2006.

31. Report to Congress: *The Pharmacist Workforce: A Study of the Supply and Demand for Pharmacists*. Health Resources and Services Administration, Bureau of Health Professions, Washington, DC, 2000.

32. Schmit J. Helped wanted at the drugstore. *USA Today*. Page B3, August 17, 2005.

33. The Pharmacy Manpower Project. The aggregate demand index. Available at http://www.pharmacymanpower.com/about.html. Accessed April 12, 2006.

34. Knapp, KK. Charting the demand for pharmacists in the managed care era. *J Managed Care Pharm*. 1999;5:324–328.

35. Kaiser Family Foundation. Prescription drug trends. October, 2004. Available at http://www.kff.org/rxdrugs/upload/Prescription-Drug-Trends-October-2004-UPDATE.pdf. Accessed April 12, 2006.

36. Herzberg, F. *Work and the Nature of Work*. World Publishing, Cleveland, OH, 1966.

37. Salary.com. Salary Wizard. Available at http://swz.com/salarywizard/layoutht-mls/swzl_compresult_national_HC07000011.html. Accessed April 12, 2006.

38. Allied Physicians. Pharmacist Salaries. Available at http://allied-physicians.com/salary-surveys/pharmacy/. Accessed April 12, 2006.

39. Gebhart, F. Superpharmacists finding cash rewards in nontraditional practice. *Drug Top.* 1999;143(Dec 6):111.

40. Pharmacy's Best Kept Secret. U.S. Department of Health and Human Services. 2006. Available at http://www.hhs.gov/pharmacy/recruit.html. Accessed April 14, 2006.

41. *2005-2006 Profile of Pharmacy Faculty.* The American Association of Colleges of Pharmacy, Alexandria, VA, 2001.

42. Gosselin, RA, and Robbins, J. *Inside Pharmacy: The Anatomy of a Profession.* Technomic, Lancaster, PA, 1999.

43. Cox, ER, and Fitzpatrick, V. Pharmacists' job satisfaction and perceived utilization of skills. *Am J Health-Syst Pharm.* 1999;56:1733–1737.

44. Mott, DA. Pharmacist job turnover, length of service, and reasons for leaving, 1983–1997. *Am J Health-Syst Pharm.* 2000;57:975–83.

45. Fleming, H, and Gannon, K. No rest for the weary. *Drug Top.* 1999;143:50–52, 55–56.

46. Ukens, C. Pharmacy boards revisit R.Ph. workload and dispensing errors. *Drug Top.* 1998;142:40.

47. Rucker, TD. The importance of career planning. *Am J Hosp Pharm.* 1984;41:879.

48. Angaran, DM, Hepler, CD, Bjornson, DC, and Hadsall, RS. Career patterns of pioneer clinical pharmacists. *Am J Hosp Pharm.* 1988;45:101–108.

49. O'Connor, TW. For pharmacists, two distinct career paths. *Pharm Times.* 1995;45:42.

50. Shane, R. Women in pharmacy: balancing career and family. *Top Hosp Pharm Manage.* 1986;6:56–61.

51. Wackowiak, JI, and Wackowiak, LR. Two career couple: dual pharmacists' perspective. *Top Hosp Pharm Manage.* 1986;6:46–55.

3

PHARMACISTS AND THE HEALTH CARE SYSTEM

Pharmacists do not practice in isolation, but are a part of a health care team functioning within the health care system. The health care system in the United States is complex — so complex that no one can adequately describe it in all of its detail.

This chapter is about the pharmacist and the parts of the health care system where there is an interface between the two. The chapter will present an overview of disease, the health care system, its expenditures and financing, the delivery of care, the health professions, and the place of drugs. It will end with discussion of how pharmacists play an important part in the health care system

LEARNING OBJECTIVES

After reading this chapter, you should be able to:

- State the five leading disease causes of death in the United States
- State the five major causes of death in the United States
- Provide a concise overview of the health care system in the United States
- Briefly explain how the health system in the United States is financed
- List the five major factors driving up the cost of health care in the United States
- Provide a brief explanation of how health care is delivered in the United States
- Provide a brief explanation of Medicaid

- Provide a brief explanation of Medicare
- Explain the place of drugs in the health care system
- Explain the primary and emerging roles of the pharmacist in the health care system
- Explain Medicare's Part D Prescription Benefit
- Define and explain the term *medication therapy management program*
- Discuss HIPAA and what it means for pharmacists

DISEASE BURDEN

Disease burden is the effect on society of both disease-related mortality and disease-related morbidity.[1] For example, the major causes of death and disease burden in the world during 2005 were communicable diseases, maternal/perinatal conditions, and nutritional deficiencies (39%), chronic diseases (32%), injuries (13%), cardiovascular diseases (10%), and cancer (5%).[2]

Figure 3.1 shows the leading causes of death by disease in the United States in 2003. Heart disease, cancer, and stroke represent almost 70% of all deaths. The contrast of disease burden between the United States and the rest of the world is striking.

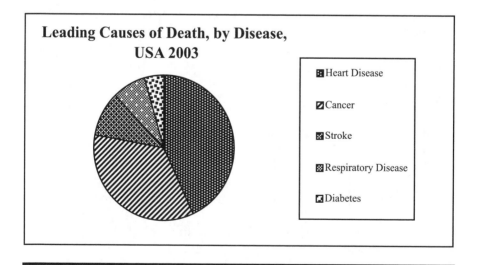

Figure 3.1   Leading causes of death, by disease, in the United States in 2003. (Source: Centers for Disease Control and Prevention. *The Burden of Chronic Disease and the Future of Public Health.* **2003.)[4]**

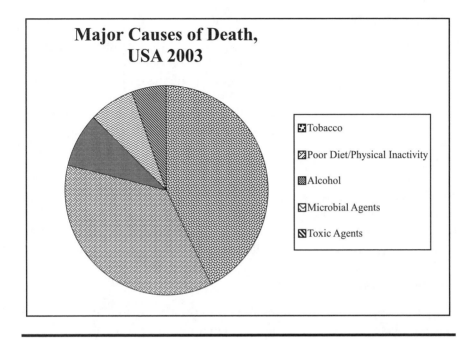

Figure 3.2   Major causes of death in the United States in 2003. (Source: Centers for Disease Control and Prevention. *The Burden of Chronic Disease and the Future of Public Health 2003, and the Actual Causes of Death in the United States, 2000.*)[4,5]

Despite great improvements in the overall health of the nation, compelling evidence indicates that Americans who are members of racial and ethnic minority groups and those who are poor are more likely than whites to have poor health and die prematurely.[3]

Figure 3.2 shows the major attributable causes of death by risk factor during 2003. The major risk factors were the use of tobacco, poor diet, and physical inactivity.

OVERVIEW OF THE HEALTH CARE SYSTEM IN THE UNITED STATES

The health care system in the United States is complex — so much so that no one can adequately describe it in all of its details. Furthermore, it seems to be getting even more complex with the advent of Medicare's Part D prescription benefit.

Health care systems can be compared using five basic parameters: access, quality, cost, financing, and how providers are paid.

Access to Care

The United States is probably best in the world for its quantity and quality of health practitioners and medical facilities and our access to them, but it probably is the worst for the proportion of the population that has limited access to care because of having no health insurance or being uninsured. The United States is the only country in the developed world, except for South Africa, that does not provide health care for all of its citizens.

The Medicare Part D prescription benefit implemented on January 1, 2006, will do more to reduce the cost of medication than provide better access to care. One major impediment to insuring more people is small businesses that cannot afford to provide insurance coverage for their employees. Only Congress can solve this problem, and their interest and priority for doing so remain on the back burner.

Quality of Care

Many U.S. citizens probably think the United States has the highest quality of health care in the world, but this not true. It depends on how you measure quality. In a World Health Organization (WHO) report, the United States ranked 37th out of 191 countries ranked.[6] France was ranked number one and Italy number two. That does not mean the French are the healthiest people — Japan won that distinction.

The WHO compares a population's health with how effectively its government spends its money on health, how well the public health system prevents illness instead of just treating it, and how fairly the poor, minorities, and other special populations are treated.

In another comparison, the United States ranked an average of 12th (second from the bottom) for 16 available health indicators.[7] The best countries were Japan, Sweden, Canada, France, and Australia. The worst ratings for the United States were low birth weight percentages (13th [last], neonatal mortality and infant mortality overall (13th), and years of potential life lost (excluding external causes) (also 13th). Note: the U.S. health care system is the best in responsiveness — the extent to which caregivers are responsive to patient expectations with regard to nonhealth areas such as being treated with dignity and respect.

Although the use of tobacco and alcohol use in excess are clearly harmful, their use does not explain the relatively poor position of the United States on health indicators. One author has suggested that the United States' poor health ratings may be the result of three factors: (a) a relatively poor primary care infrastructure; (b) a high numbers of deaths from unnecessary surgery, medication errors, other medical errors, nosocomial infections, and adverse drug reactions; and (c) a high degree of income inequality.

Cost

Despite the low ranking for health care in the United States, the country spends the most per person on health care.[6] In 1999, the United States spent a stunning $3724 per person on health care each year. Japan (ranked 10th) spent the equivalent of $1759 per person on health and France (ranked 1st) spent $2125. Note: In 2003, the United States spent $5671 per person on healthcare. While the United States is good at expensive heroic care, it is woefully inadequate at the low-cost preventative care that keeps Europeans healthy.[6]

The United States is spending more and more of its gross domestic product (GDP) on healthcare and spends the highest of all countries, at 15%.[8] In comparison, many countries that have better quality care spend far less of their GDP on health care and have longer life expectancies.

There are many reasons why health care in the United States is so expensive. Some undisputed reasons include the rising costs of medical technology and prescription medication, the latter of which is subsidizing the cost of medication in many other countries. The pharmaceutical companies have no shame about this and charge what the market bears. Perhaps the biggest reason for expensive healthcare in the United States is the administrative costs associated with operating a multipayer system, which are estimated at 19.3 and 24.1% of the total dollars spent on health care in the United States.[9]

The higher proportion of uninsured and underinsured in the United States also contributes to expensive health care because conditions that could be treated inexpensively at the early stages of illness can later develop into health crises that are much more expensive.

Another factor is that Americans who are covered by health insurance have little incentive to limit their consumption or to look at less expensive treatment options.[10] Also, American consumers remain relatively uninformed about health care, are heavily dependent on their health providers to direct their health care purchases, and usually are not provided options concerning their care.

Financing

The United States' spending for health care is enormous — $1.7 trillion in 2003.[11] Table 3.1 shows the money spent on health care in the United States from 1960 to 2003.

Table 3.1 Health Care Expenditures in the United States, 1960–2003

	1960	1970	1980	1990	2000	2003
Amount in Billions ($)						
National Health Expenditures	26.7	73.1	245.8	696.0	1309.9	1678.9
Private	20.1	45.4	140.9	413.5	717.5	913.2
Public	6.6	27.6	104.8	282.5	592.4	765.7
Amount Per Capita ($)						
National Health Expenditures	143	348	1067	2738	4560	5671
Private	108	216	612	1627	2498	3084
Public	35	131	455	1111	2062	2586
As Percent of Gross National Product						
National Health Expenditures	5.1	7.0	8.8	12.0	13.3	15.3

Source: Centers for Disease Control and Prevention, Center for Health Statistics. Health, United States, 2005.

Health care in the United States has undergone three distinct evolutions. It is currently in the fourth, moving from the era of rugged individualism to more control by the federal government.[12] For example, the proportion of health care spending using public funds in 1960 was 24.7%. In 2003, this proportion was 45.6%. With the advent of Medicare's Part D prescription benefit, started January 1, 2006, even more health care will be financed with public funds, and this may be a tipping point for financing health care in the United States and put pressure on Congress to finally address the question, Is health care a right or a privilege?

Private Sector Funding

Most employees of large employers in the United States receive or have access to health care insurance. Most of these companies use an insurance company to provide health care benefits for their employees, and some are self-insured.

In the beginning, all insurance premiums were paid by employers, but today more and more of the cost of premiums is being shifted to employees. Some employees struggle to pay their share of the premium and the co-payments and deductibles associated with their health insurance. A *deductible* is the amount the individual pays per year before the insurance payment goes in to effect. A *copayment* is a percentage of the charge paid by the individual. For example, the individual may have to pay the first $300 of health care costs in a given year before any costs are paid by the insurance company. After the deductible is paid, the individual may have to pay a percentage (for example 10% in network; 30% out of network) of the charge.

The employee may be able to choose the type of health plan (e.g., managed care, preferred provider organization, or a point-of-service plan) (see Chapter 10, Managed Care Pharmacy).

Public Sector Funding

Public sector funding for health care comes from the federal and state governments.

Medicare

Medicare, Title 18 of the Social Security Act, was enacted in 1965. Medicare is a social insurance program. Eligibility is strictly determined by age (62 and over) and is independent of means tests. Benefits are earned. The scope of benefits is narrow but getting broader, and financing is through special taxes paid by employees and employers. Programs are administered centrally with uniform rules by the Centers for Medicare and Medicaid.

There are several parts to Medicare. The Part A benefit is mandatory and covers hospital services, nursing home services, home health services, and hospice services. The Part B benefit is optional and covers medical and surgical services and entails an annual deductible and coinsurance. Unlike Part A, where payment is in full, a charge by a physician may not be fully paid by Medicare.

Congress created Medicare's Part C benefit under the Balanced Budget Act of 1997 to incorporate the cost-saving measures of managed care into the Medicare program. It covers everything that Part A and Part B cover but offers this coverage in a new manner that may take the form of a health maintenance organization, preferred provider organization, medical savings account, or other new type of health plan.

The Part D benefit comes as a result of the Medicare Modernization Act of 2003. This legislation provides seniors and people with disabilities with the first comprehensive prescription drug benefit ever offered under the Medicare program, and the most significant improvement to senior health care in nearly 40 years.

Since January 1, 2006, everyone with Medicare, regardless of income, health status, or prescription drug usage, has had access to prescription drug coverage. Medicare prescription drug coverage is insurance that covers both brand name and generic prescription drugs at participating pharmacies.

Medicare prescription drug coverage provides protection for people who have very high drug costs. There are two ways to get Medicare prescription drug coverage: (a) through a stand-alone Medicare prescription drug plan or (b) through a Medicare Advantage Plan or other Medicare Health Plans that offer medical and drug coverage. Like other insurance, beneficiaries pay a monthly premium, which varies by plan, and a yearly deductible. They also pay part of the cost of their prescriptions, including a copayment or coinsurance. There is additional help for those with limited incomes and resources — some may not have to pay a premium or deductible.

Individuals have the option of having the premium taken from their Social Security check, paying the premium directly, or having the premium taken directly from a bank account. Those with the Part D benefit must pay the first $250 each year, and then Medicare will pay 75% of the next $2000 worth of drugs on the plan's formulary. After that, they have a gap in coverage called the "doughnut hole." During this gap period, the beneficiary pays all the costs of drugs until he or she has paid another $2850 out-of-pocket. At that point, Medicare will begin paying about 95% of the cost of covered drugs until the end of the calendar year. This is known as catastrophic coverage. The total out of pocket cost for drugs on the plan's list of drugs was $3600 for 2006.

Medicaid

Medicaid, or Title 19 of the Social Security Act, is a federal and state program for insuring the indigent or poor and is a welfare program. Eligibility for Medicaid is based on a means test, financing is through general revenues, and the administration is at the state level. Each state administers its own program within federal guidelines. Some services are mandated. These include inpatient and outpatient services, physician services, lab and x-ray services, skilled nursing facility services, family planning, home care services, and several others. Some services are optional, and a state may or not cover them, for example, prescription drugs, intermediate care facilities, and dental services. In general, Medicaid services cover more than Medicare services.

When the Medicare Part D prescription benefit was started on January 1, 2006, many *dual eligibles* (people who qualify for both Medicare and Medicaid) were shifted from Medicaid to Medicare.

Paying Providers

The two basic methods of payment to providers (hospitals and health practitioners) are (a) cost charged-based methods, the most common of which is fee-for-service, and (b) prospective reimbursement.

In the *fee-for-service* model, providers are at no risk and are responsible for providing all needed care. There is no incentive to contain costs —the more service you provide, the more you are paid. Hence, this model has largely been abandoned by payers.

In the *prospective reimbursement* model, providers are paid ahead of time, based on formulas. The provider is at risk — using more services than necessary may cause the provider to loose money. Prospective payment using *diagnosis-related groups* (DRG) and *capitation* is the way hospitals are paid for government patients — a set amount per diagnosis or the way health management organizations (HMOs) are paid per member per time period. Prospective reimbursement provides incentives to produce care efficiently; if the hospitals' and HMOs' costs are less than the diagnosis-related group or capitation rates, they get to keep the difference.

Physicians and other health professionals are paid in one of two ways on a fee-for service basis: fee schedules or usual and customary charges. In the first instance, a *relative value scale* compares procedures with respect to their length and complexity. Usual and customary charges are based on the typical amount charged by all physicians in the local area.

Few patients pay for prescription themselves (private pay). Most prescriptions are paid for by a third party. Third-party programs involve two administrative entities: the insurance company (which pays on behalf of the employer) and the pharmacy benefits manager, who administers the benefit (working with pharmacies, enrollees, and prescribers; sometimes handles the drug formulary; adjudicating claims; monitoring utilization and cost and undertaking cost containment measures). The most common way of paying pharmacies is to reimburse them on the acquisition cost of the drug plus a dispensing fee.

THE DELIVERY OF CARE

Meeting patient needs means meeting patients at their point of need and where they are in the health care continuum. The *health care continuum* starts with self-care and flows through ambulatory care (Chapter 8), acute care (Chapter 9), critical care, home care (Chapter 11), long-term care (Chapter 12), and hospice care. Problems can occur when patients move from one part of care to another.

The process of care in the United States in fairly standardized in the patient–doctor relationship and when care is provided in a hospital. It is also standardized for routine dispensing of medication, but less so for the delivery of pharmaceutical care, something that needs attention. Patients generally know what to expect and how to act when dealing with physicians, less so with hospital personnel, and not at all with the pharmacists trying to be more patient-centered.

Patient-Centered Care

The patient-provider interface in the United States has generally been paternalistic, and leaders in the health professions are advocating a more patient-centered approach to care, which has not yet reached a tipping point. Table 3.2 lists the tenets of patient-centered care.[13] Every patient secretly hopes for these promises, but observation reveals a disappointing compliance with these promises in most health care settings.

The Health Care Team

The health care team is composed of many individuals — doctors, nurses, pharmacists, and other health care professionals all available to help the patient. In general, the health professions are empowered by society through a covenant that says, "If you will use all of your abilities and talents to help me and will protect my privacy, I will allow access to my body and provide information that may be confidential."

In general, the health professions in the United States have done a good job of holding up their end of the covenant, but they have not always done it in a patient-friendly way. Patients do die of what we do or do not do, they have pain that is undertreated, they often feel helpless and wait a lot, and there is a great deal of waste. The problem is that not a lot has changed in the delivery of care from the patient's point of view, and they feel helpless to change the system. Only the health professions can do that.

However, the health professions seem more concerned with manpower issues that need addressing. The medical profession is dominated by specialty practice because of the payment system that favors this group. There are shortages of nurses and pharmacists, and the perfect storm — a growing older population — is nearing the shore.

Table 3.2   The Attributes of Patient-Centered Care

No needless death	Don't kill me
No needless pain	Don't hurt me
No helplessness	Don't make me feel helpless
No unwanted waiting	Don't make me wait
No waste	Don't waste money

Source: Berwick, DM. Request for Proposals: Replacing Don's Right Knee. Institute for Health Care Improvement. December 4, 2003. Used with permission.

Prescribing Authority

Those allowed by regulation to prescribe prescription drugs are controlled by state law. In general, in the United States, those who may prescribe drugs include doctors (MDs and DOs) and dentists, veterinarians, some physician assistants, and some nurse practitioners within their scopes of practice. The irony is that most of these prescribers have less education in pharmacology and therapeutics than pharmacists with the Pharm.D. degree. The educational weakness of pharmacists to prescribe medication is in the area of diagnosis. That is why the best therapeutics may result from the collaborative practice of doctors (expert at diagnosis) and pharmacists (expert at drugs). This is the model used in the clinics of the Veterans Administration and in some innovative health care organizations.

Patient Confidentiality

Protecting the confidentiality of patient information is an ethical standard found in all health professions. The Health Insurance Portability and Accountability Act (HIPAA) was passed by Congress in 1996.[14] The regulations under the act apply what are called "covered entities": healthcare providers, health plans, and healthcare clearinghouses who transmit any health information in electronic form in connection with a transaction covered under HIPAA. The regulations are made up of three distinct parts:

Transaction Standards: The transaction standards call for use of common electronic claims standards, common code sets, and unique identifiers for all health care payers and providers.

Privacy Regulations: The privacy rules govern the release of individually identifiable health information, specifying how health providers must provide notice of privacy policies and procedures to patients, obtain consent and authorization for use of information, and tell how information is generally shared and how patients can access, inspect, copy, and amend their own medical records.

Security Regulations: The security regulations dictate the kind of administrative procedures and physical safeguards covered entities must have in place to ensure the confidentiality and integrity of protected health information.

Needless to say, all pharmacists need to be very careful and only share patient information with those who have the need to know and have the authorization of the patient to know.

THE PLACE OF DRUGS IN THE HEALTH CARE SYSTEM

Prescription drugs serve as complements to medical procedures, substitutes for surgery and other medical procedures (e.g., lipid-lowering drugs that lessen need for bypass surgery), and provide new treatments where there previously were none. Some of the major advances in public health — the near eradication of polio and measles and the decline in infectious diseases — are largely the result of vaccines and antibiotics. As the understanding of genetics increases, the possibility for pharmaceutical and biotechnology interventions will increase.

The elderly and people with disabilities are particularly reliant on prescription drugs. Not only do they experience greater health problems, but these problems tend to include conditions that respond to drug therapy.

Prescription drugs are the number one modality used to improve patients' health and to get them out of the hospital sooner, rather than later. They frequently prevent or control ailments and diseases, but rarely cure.

Over-the-counter medications are used by most of the public to help with self-limiting health problems, and these agents serve a useful role in self-care. The roles of alternative therapies (herbs, folk medicine, megavitamins, and homeopathic remedies), although widely used, in most cases are yet to be validated scientifically.

THE ROLE OF PHARMACISTS IN THE U.S. HEALTH CARE SYSTEM

Pharmacists have always been a part of the health care system (see Figure 3.3) in the United States, but that role has changed and continues to change with time.[15] Society sanctions each health profession from the standpoint of need. If there were no need for pharmacy, the profession would not exist.[16]

Pharmacy's Societal Purpose

To discover what pharmacy is and what it is to become, one must start with its societal purpose. In 1985, the pharmacy profession took a hard look at itself and critically evaluated its societal purpose at an invited conference of 150 thought leaders in pharmacy. This consensus conference concluded that "pharmacy is *the* healthcare profession most concerned with drugs and their clinical application"[17] and that the fundamental purpose of the profession is to serve as a force in society for safe and appropriate use of drugs.

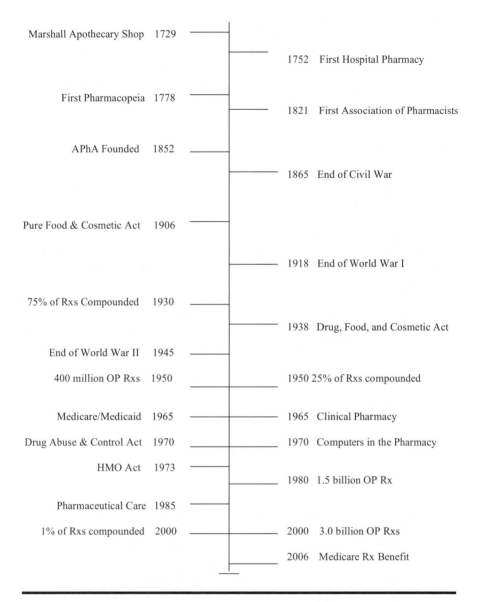

Marshall Apothecary Shop 1729	
	1752 First Hospital Pharmacy
First Pharmacopeia 1778	
	1821 First Association of Pharmacists
APhA Founded 1852	
	1865 End of Civil War
Pure Food & Cosmetic Act 1906	
	1918 End of World War I
75% of Rxs Compounded 1930	
	1938 Drug, Food, and Cosmetic Act
End of World War II 1945	
400 million OP Rxs 1950	1950 25% of Rxs compounded
Medicare/Medicaid 1965	1965 Clinical Pharmacy
Drug Abuse & Control Act 1970	1970 Computers in the Pharmacy
HMO Act 1973	
	1980 1.5 billion OP Rx
Pharmaceutical Care 1985	
1% of Rxs compounded 2000	2000 3.0 billion OP Rxs
	2006 Medicare Rx Benefit

Figure 3.3 Timeline of the history of pharmacy in the United States.

The reader should take note that the purpose of the profession is not to dispense drugs. In the broadest sense, pharmacy should promote health by promoting the optimal use of drugs. The profession seeks to advocate rational drug therapy rather than merely react to treatment decisions made by others. A broader role for pharmacists as public health advisors is yet to be explored.

Pharmacy's Destiny

Where the profession evolves is highly dependent on how pharmacists see themselves. If most pharmacists see themselves as dispensers of medication, this is largely how others (the public, the media, and other health professionals) will view them. If most pharmacists see themselves as clinical practitioners, the profession is most likely to reach a tipping point and go in that direction, especially if there is a thoughtful plan in place to achieve this goal. When the country truly gets serious about health care reform, pharmacists need to be at the forefront with evidence of what they can and will do for patients and the health care system.

However, forces are at play that may prevent pharmacy from meeting its desired destiny. One of those is the unexpected growth in medication use that is outpacing the supply of pharmacists.[18] In 2005, one dean was overheard to say, "If we double the enrollments of pharmacy students at all schools of pharmacy, we still will not have enough pharmacists in 2030." Increasing workload (see Table 3.3) has deterred many pharmacists from being more patient-centered and from practicing pharmaceutical care. The answers to meeting prescription workload demand and achieving the goals of pharmaceutical care are the use of more supportive personnel, loosening restrictive barriers on the use of supportive personnel, and using much more pharmacy technology and automation.

Opportunity

Pharmacy has a golden opportunity to move more toward its goal of being viewed (by the public, other health professions, and the media) as a clinical profession. Under Medicare's Part D prescription benefit, every

Table 3.3 Retail Prescription Volumes, Prescriptions per Pharmacist, and Retail Prescription Sales, United States, 1992–2000

	1992	1994	1996	1998	2000
Retail prescriptions dispensed (millions)	1,947	2,016	2,221	2,481	2,843
Prescriptions dispensed per pharmacist	16,500	16,900	18,200	19,000	22,200
Retail Prescription Sales (billions)	$46.6	$54.6	$67.2	$87.2	$121.8

Source: Adapted from Cooksey, JA, Knapp, KK, Walton, SM, and Cultice, JM. *Health Affairs.* 2002;21(5):182–188. With permission.

health plan offering this benefit must have a *medication therapy management program* (MTMP), and plans can use and pay pharmacists to perform the MTMP role for their enrollees. Additionally, billing codes have been developed to bill for a pharmacists' cognitive services.

The keys to this opportunity for pharmacists are: (a) having a strong desire and the time to do it, (b) having the skills to do it, (c) getting a health plan to allow them to do it, (d) having a process in place to document interventions and outcomes, and (e) having a billing mechanism in place. Many pharmacy organizations have MTMP tools available for pharmacists.[19–22]

SUMMARY

The health care system in the United States is complex, responsive, and wasteful. Forty million people in the United States do not have health insurance, and minorities and the poor receive disparate care. The quality of care in the United States is not as good as 36 other countries, yet its care is by far the most expensive. Critics feel the health care system in the United States is broken and needs reform.

Pharmacists are a part of a health care team, functioning within the health care system. Pharmacy's societal roles are to serve as a force for safe and appropriate use of drugs and to help patients make the best use of their medication.

The new Medicare Part D prescription benefit, started on January 1, 2006, may be a major step in health care reform that is proceeding slowly. Medicare's requirement for MTM is an opportunity for pharmacy to display a value-added service that will help achieve pharmacy's long-term goals of being viewed as a clinical profession.

DISCUSSION QUESTIONS AND EXERCISES

1. Contrast and compare the disease burden of the United States with that of the rest of the world. Explain differences.
2. Of the five leading disease causes of death in the United States, in which disease are we making the most progress? The least progress?
3. Make a convincing argument on what the United States should do to improve the quality of its health care.
4. What primary method should pharmacists use to help improve the quality of health care in the United States?
5. Make a convincing argument on what the United States should do to decrease the cost of care without decreasing quality.

6. What primary method should pharmacists use to help decrease the cost of care in the United States?
7. What has been the impact of Medicare's Part D prescription benefit on Medicaid?
8. Under HIPAA, can a pharmacist discuss a patient's drug therapy with the patient's spouse without the patient's written permission?
9. Does medication therapy management differ from disease management? If yes, how?
10. Do you think there is an expanded role for pharmacists in public health? If so, how would this work?

CHALLENGES

1. Pharmacy is trying to be viewed as a clinical profession. For extra credit, and with the permission of your professor, prepare a concise report listing and explaining the steps the profession should go through to achieve this goal.
2. Under Medicare's Part D prescription regulations, each health plan providing the Part D benefit must have an MTMP. Investigate and visit a pharmacy performing MTM for a health plan and prepare a concise report on what you saw and discovered about MTP being performed by pharmacists.

WEB SITES OF INTEREST

Center for Medicare and Medicaid: http://www.cms.hhs.gov/default.asp
HIPPA: http://www.hhs.gov/ocr/hipaa/
Medication Therapy Management: http://www.hhs.gov/ocr/hipaa/
Health Care Reform: http://www4.nationalacademies.org/onpi/webextra.nsf/web/chasm?OpenDocument

REFERENCES

1. U.S. Environmental Protection Agency. Draft Report on the Environment 2003. Available at http://www.epa.gov/indicators/. Accessed May 19, 2006.
2. World Health Organization. World Health Statistics 2006. Available at http://www.who.int/whosis/whostat2006/en/index.html. Accessed May 19, 2006.
3. Centers for Disease Control and Prevention. Disease Burden and Risk Factors. Available at http://www.cdc.gov/omh/AMH/dbrf.htm. Accessed May 19, 2006.

4. Centers for Disease Control and Prevention, National Centers for Health Statistics. Health: The United States, 2005. Available at http://www.cdc.gov/nchs/data/hus/hus05.pdf. Accessed May 19, 2005.

5. Centers for Disease Control and Prevention. Actual Causes of Death in the United States, 2000. Available at http://www.cdc.gov/nccdphp/publications/ActualCauses/pdf/methods.pdf. Accessed May 19, 2006.

6. Nerrgaard, L. Shame, shame: U.S. ranked 36 for health care. June 21, 2000. Available at http://www.dir.salon.com/story/health/wire/2000/06/21rankings/index.xml. Accessed May 2, 2006.

7. Starfield, B. Is US health really the best in the world? *JAMA*. 2005; 284(4):483–485.

8. OECD Observer. Life values. April, 2006. Available at http://www.oecdobserver.org/news/printpage.php/aid/1831/Life_values.html. Accessed May 20, 2006.

9. Bureau of Labor Education, University of Maine. The U.S. Health Care System: Best in the World, or Just the Most Expensive? Summer, 2001. Available at http://dll.umaine.edu/ble/U.S.%20HCweb.pdf. Accessed May 20, 2006.

10. Anonymous. The U.S. health care system in transition. *CPA J Online*. Available at http://www.nysscpa.org/cpajournal/old15410211.htm. Accessed May 20, 2006.

11. Centers for Disease Control and Prevention, Center for Health Statistics. Health, United States, 2005. Available at http://www.cdc.gov/nchs/data/hus/hus05.pdf#119. Accessed May 21, 2006.

12. Scott, DM. Overview of health care in the United States. In *Pharmacy and the U.S. Health Care System*, 2nd ed. Fincham, JE and Wetheimer, AI, eds. Pharmaceutical Products Press, Binghamton, NY, 1998, chap 2.

13. Berwick, DM. Request for Proposals: Replacing Don's Right Knee. Institute for Health Care Improvement. December 4, 2003. Available at http://www.ihi.org/IHI/Topics/Improvement/ImprovementMethods/Literature/RequestforProposalsReplacingDonsRightKnee.htm. Accessed May 21, 2006.

14. Walden, DC, and Craig, RP. The health insurance portability and accountability act of 1996 (HIPAA) and the pharmacy benefit: implications for health plans, PBMs, and providers. *J Managed Care Pharm*. 2003;9(1):66–71.

15. Desselle, SP. The pharmacist and the pharmacy profession. In *Introduction to Health Care Delivery*. McCarthy, RL, and Schafermeyer, KW, eds.. Jones and Barlett Publishers. Boston, MA. 2004, chap. 3.

16. Hepler, CD. Pharmacy as a clinical profession. *Am J Hosp Pharm*. 1985; 42:1298–1306.

17. Zellmer, WA. Achieving pharmacy's full potential. *Am J Hosp Pharm*. 1985;42:1285.

18. Cooksey, JA, Knapp, KK, Walton, SM, and Cultice, JM. Challenges to the pharmacist profession from escalating pharmaceutical demand. *Health Affairs*. 2002;21(5):182–188.

19. National Association of Chain Drugstores. Medication therapy management: training and techniques for MTM services in community pharmacy. Available at http://www.nacdsfoundation.org/wmspage.cfm?parm1=1044. Accessed April 28, 2006.

20. Academy of Managed Care Pharmacy. Medication therapy programs described. April 6, 2006. Available at http://www.amcp.org/amcp.ark?c=news&type=pr&id=454. Accessed April 28, 2006.

21. American Pharmaceutical Association. Medication therapy management in community pharmacy. Available at http://www.aphanet.org/AM/Template.cfm?Section=Pharmacy_Practice_Resources&Template=/CM/ContentDisplay.cfm&ContentID=3303. Accessed May 21, 2006.

22. American Society of Health System Pharmacists. MTM Quality Measures. Available at http://www.ashp.org/medicare/mtm.cfm#6. Accessed May 21, 2006.

4

THE DRUG-USE PROCESS

Once a drug is approved for use in the United States, there is a process of how the drugs are distributed and used. This process is organized, complex, and controlled and is called the *drug-use process*. Pharmacists are intimately involved in the drug-use process. They are accountable for controlling parts of the process so the drugs are used safely and effectively and not diverted into the wrong hands.

This chapter will focus on how drugs make their way to the patient after being made by the manufacturer. The chapter will begin with discussion of drug distribution, the self-use of medication, and the prescribing and dispensing of *prescription-only medication.*

Drug pricing, quality drug therapy, and patient outcomes from taking medication will also be discussed. The chapter will end with information on the control of the drug-use process and some current issues concerning this process.

LEARNING OBJECTIVES

After reading this chapter, you should be able to:

- Discuss how drugs are distributed, prescribed, and administered
- Discuss how drugs are priced
- List five general categories of drugs
- Explain the how the use of drugs is increasing and why
- Discuss how pharmacists help control the drug use process
- Discuss the concept of self care as it relates to the use of medication
- Define quality drug therapy
- Explain the term *patient outcomes*

WHAT IS THE DRUG-USE PROCESS?

The drug-use process is complex. A whole book could be written about it. As a minimum, it involves the process of manufacturing, storing, distributing, prescribing, pricing, dispensing, administering, using, controlling, and monitoring drugs and their effects and outcomes.

DRUG DISTRIBUTION

The United States has the most complex, yet the most efficient, drug distribution system in the world. Automation such as bar coding, computerized inventories, robots, and automated information systems keep the products flowing. As drugs flow through the distribution system, they increase in value.[1]

Drug manufacturers, wholesalers, and retailers are the major firms responsible for the supply and distribution of medication in the United States. *Drug manufacturers* develop and produce the pharmaceutical products. *Drug wholesalers* distribute medication, medical devices and appliances, health and beauty aids, and other products to pharmacies, and all of these, except prescription drugs, to other retailers. *Retailers* (like pharmacies) distribute these products to the patient.

The Drugs

Table 4.1 shows the national supply of pharmaceuticals. There are no less than 29,000 drug products (Rx and over the counter [OTC]) in the United States. In general, there are five types of medication: (a) prescription

Table 4.1　The National Supply of Pharmaceuticals

Number[a]	Type
1,200	Chemical entities
2,000	Pharmaceutical products (single entity plus combination products)
8,000	Pharmaceuticals from supplies (branded and generic products)
10,000	Pharmaceutical products with unique product strength
14,000	Pharmaceuticals with dosage form with unique product strength
15,000	OTC and herbal products

[a] Since new drug products come into the market place frequently, and some products are withdrawn from the market as well, these estimates should be regarded as close approximations. However, true figures are larger since there has been no way to estimate compounded prescriptions.

drugs, (b) controlled substances, (c) OTCs, (d) investigational drugs, and (e) alternative medicines that may be prescription or OTC.

Prescription medication is only available when the pharmacist receives a legal prescription or drug order from a licensed prescriber. Prescription medication used to be called *legend medication,* as it was labeled with the U.S. Food and Drug Administration's (FDA) required legend — "Caution: Federal law prohibits using this medication without a prescription." The FDA now requires the phrase "Rx only." This has freed space on the label for other important information that may help decrease errors in use by the patient.

Controlled substances, which are also prescription-only products, are drugs classified by the U.S. Drug Enforcement Agency (DEA) as being addicting or misused. These drugs have varying levels of control on their distribution and use based on the drug's addiction liability and potential for abuse. The Comprehensive Drug Abuse Prevention and Control Act of 1970 placed controlled substances into five schedules:

Schedule I: The drug or substance has a high potential for abuse and no currently accepted medical use in treatment in the United States. There is a lack of safety for use of the drug or other substance under medical supervision. Examples of drugs in schedule I are marijuana, heroin, and lysergic acid (LSD).

Schedule II: The drug or other substance has a high potential for abuse, is currently accepted for medical use in treatment in the United States, or has a currently accepted medical use with severe restrictions. Abuse of the drug or other substance may lead to severe psychological or physical dependence. Examples of drugs in schedule II are morphine, cocaine, and methadone.

Schedule III: The drug or other substance has a potential for abuse less than the drugs or other substances in schedules I and II and has a currently accepted medical use in treatment in the United States. Abuse of the drug or other substance may lead to moderate to low physical dependence. Examples of drugs in schedule III are barbiturates, amphetamines, and codeine.

Schedule IV: The drug or other substance has a low potential for abuse relative to the drugs and other substances in schedule III and has a currently accepted medical use in treatment in the United States. Abuse of the drug or other substance may lead to limited physical dependence relative to the drugs or other substances in schedule III. Examples of drugs in schedule IV are stimulants other than amphetamine and tranquilizers such as chlordiazepoxide (Librium) and diazepam (Valium).

Schedule V: The drug or other substance has a low potential for abuse relative to the drugs and other substances in schedule IV and has a currently accepted medical use in treatment in the United States. Abuse of the drug or other substance may lead to limited physical or psychological dependence relative to the drugs and other substances in schedule IV. Examples of drugs in schedule V include codeine when mixed with other ingredients to make a cough syrup and small amounts of opium when mixed with other medicinal ingredients.

OTC drugs may be sold without a prescription. Some of these drugs may have started out as a prescription drug and have been converted to OTC status after being found to be safe. Patients seeking an OTC medication for a health problem present a good opportunity for pharmacists to guide and help patients. Most vitamins, minerals, and nutrients are OTC.

Investigational drugs are drugs that are being investigated and are not yet approved by the FDA for marketing. They are also defined as drugs labeled with the legend "Caution: New drug, limited by Federal Law to investigational use."

All drugs must make their way safely and efficiently from the manufacturer to the physician (all drugs), the doctor (all drugs), nonpharmacy retailer (OTCs), or the investigator (prescription and investigational drugs).

Alternative medications are prescribed or OTC medications that are out of the main stream of treatment options. They are considered unproven and not accepted by most medical practitioners as generally safe and effective or as safe and effective as FDA-approved medication.

Distribution of Drugs from Pharmaceutical Manufacturers

Most of the pharmaceutical products made by manufacturers go directly to drug wholesalers and to other major distribution centers. This can be tricky — production needs to meet demand. If production of a drug is high and demand is low, too much is available. This represents a cost and a storage problem for the manufacturer. If demand is high and production is low, there will be a shortage of the drug.

Unlike in the past, community pharmacies rarely are able to order drugs directly from the manufacturer, and if they can, the required minimum dollar amount to be ordered is quite high.

Pharmaceutical companies also distribute their products to distribution centers set up by chain pharmacies (such as CVS, Rite Aid, and Walgreens), mass merchandisers (such as Kmart, Target, and Wal-Mart), and grocery store chains that have pharmacies (such as Krogers and Publix).

Although some hospitals can buy directly from the manufacturer, most buy their medication through an arrangement called *group purchasing*. Most hospitals are part of a group of hospitals (such as the University Hospital Consortium and the Voluntary Hospitals of America), and pharmaceutical companies will ship large quantities of drugs to the buying group warehouses of these hospital groups or to wholesalers. The distribution can be similar for most managed care organizations (such as Aetna, Cigna, Kaiser Permanente, and Prudential), also called MCOs.

Distribution from Drug Wholesalers

The basic function of the *drug wholesaler* is to ensure the smooth, safe, and efficient distribution of products to retailers, such as community pharmacies (independent, chain, and grocery stores), mass merchandisers, and mail-order pharmacies. At the wholesaler, large pallets of drugs delivered from the manufacturer are broken down into smaller units for distribution to pharmacies, other distribution centers, and drug repackagers.

Drug wholesalers (such as Amerisource, Bergen Brunswig, Cardinal, and McKesson) store manufactured goods in strategic geographical locations so they can quickly send the products to hospitals, managed care facilities, clinics, and community pharmacies. The Healthcare Distribution Management Association estimates that there are about 60 wholesale corporations that run about 225 distribution centers throughout the United States.[2]

Drug wholesalers are licensed in the state in which they are located and in the states in which they do business. As most handle controlled substances, they must also have a DEA license. They are required to adhere to strict storage and handling requirements. Drug wholesalers also must ensure the integrity of the medications they distribute. Thus, temperature and humidity must be controlled. They must also protect against medications into the wrong hands.

In addition to filling orders for customers, drug wholesalers provide other services such as supplying important order and inventory information for their customers, help with claims processing, and provide computer support. Some drug wholesalers will help clients in counting their inventory once a year.

Distribution from Distribution Centers and Repackagers

The distribution centers of chain drugstores, mass merchandisers, food store pharmacy chains, hospital groups, and groups of independent pharmacies break down the products shipped to them from the manufacturer and ship needed supplies to their pharmacies.

There are also service centers called *repackagers*. After receiving the drugs from the pharmaceutical company or drug wholesaler, the repackager packages the drug exactly the way the customer (the pharmacy) wants it. For example, the product may be put into individual, single-dose packages with labeling and bar coding so the hospital or nursing home pharmacy does not need to do this. Another example of repackaging is *prepackaging* the drug in a container for a 30-day supply so the pharmacy does not have to do this. However, the label information on the repackaged medication must be identical to the label information on the original container, as approved by the FDA.

Most repackaging is done by pharmacy chains for their pharmacies. However, now that automation is available, some repackaging and the addition of bar coding to the products is being done in the hospital. The repackager needs to have a pharmacy license and must follow laws carefully so as not to misbrand (mislabel) or adulterate (change the nature of) the product.

COUNTERFEIT DRUGS

The problem of stolen and counterfeit drugs surfaced in 2004 when it was reported that the United States ranked first in worldwide incidents.[3] As the largest market for pharmaceuticals, the United States will continue to be a target for the distribution of contraband. The Internet has made it easier for consumers to obtain — sometimes without a prescription or a doctor's approval — prescription medication illegally. The World Health Organization (WHO) estimated in 2003 that $200 million in prescriptions were counterfeit or tainted and that counterfeit drugs are a $32-million-a-year business.[4]

SELF-CARE AND THE ROLE OF OTC MEDICATION

It is important for pharmacists and pharmacy technicians to understand illness and the patient's reaction to it. Seldom do people go to a physician when they first become ill — at least not right away. Most people see how they are feeling and how the illness progresses. Some will deny they are ill. Some will seek the advice of family or friends. Still others will take control and seek out as much information as they can about their problems.

Self-Care

People taking a more active role in their health care form a new generation of patients. The partnership between these types of patients and health care providers is termed *lifestyle medicine*.[5] Documentation of increased interest in self-care is witnessed by the many self-help books, TV programs, newspaper articles, and talk shows covering the topic.

It is difficult to discover what spawned this self-care revolution. However, one thing is obvious — consumers are increasingly self-medicating with nonprescription drugs. The Nonprescription Drug Manufacturers Association has surveyed many consumers to learn about their attitudes about this practice:[6]

- Almost 7 of 10 consumers prefer to fight symptoms without taking medication, if possible.
- Among consumers, 85% believe it is important to have access to nonprescription medication.
- About 9 of 10 consumers realize they should take medication only when necessary.
- Of consumers who ended the use of their nonprescription medication, 90% did so because their medical problem or symptoms resolved.
- Even though a medication may be available without a prescription, almost 95% of consumers agreed that care should be taken when using it.
- Nearly 93% of consumers report that they read instructions before taking a nonprescription medication for the first time.

OTC Medication

Some ill patients and those who experience a health problem will find their way to a pharmacy to browse the OTC aisle for a cure. Many will try reading the labels of various OTC medications to see if the medication will cure what ails them.

Three-fifths (59%) of Americans have taken an OTC in the past 6 months.[7] This is slightly higher than taking a prescription drug in the past 6 months (54%). Three-quarters (78%) of Americans taking an OTC in the past 6 months have done so to relieve pain. Other use includes cough, cold, flu or sore throat (52%); allergy or sinus relief (45%); heartburn, indigestion, or other stomach problems (37%); constipation, diarrhea, or gas (21%); infections such as athletes foot or yeast infection (12%); skin problems (10%); and other (3%).

Unfortunately, self-medicating is incomplete and imperfect. How do people seeking OTC remedies know their true diagnoses? How do they know if the problem is self-limiting, or if they need to see a physician, or even if they need to go directly to an emergency room? How do they discover if the product they are about to buy will work for the problem they are experiencing or if there is something better?

The system of self-medication works better if the patient seeks the advice of a pharmacist in the search for relief of the problem. It is even better if the pharmacist is aware of a patient walking the OTC aisles of the store looking for a product. Pharmacists can do the following for these patients:

■ Try to identify the real problem.
■ Determine the seriousness of the problem.
■ If serious, refer the patient to his or her physician, to an emergency room, or call 911.
■ If the condition is self-limiting, recommend the best OTC product or other treatment.
■ Recommend how the product should be used to have the best results.
■ Offer to be available for follow-up.

Unfortunately, too many pharmacists are too busy filling prescriptions to be available for OTC counseling. Thus, they lose a wonderful opportunity to make a difference for these patients in need of help. In addition, OTCs are sold in places other than pharmacies. For these purchases, the consumer has no place to turn to for proper counsel.

It is fortunate that there is a system of self-medication in the United States and that OTC medication can be found everywhere — drugstores, convenience stores, supermarkets, and mass merchandisers. If this were not so, we would need many more physicians and health care facilities. A survey on patient satisfaction with pharmacy services found that patients' highest awareness of OTCs was for cold remedies, vitamins, and dental products, and that satisfaction was high with these products.[8]

Complementary and Alternative Medications

It is estimated that 30 to 50% of Americans use complementary and alternative medications (CAM) such as herbs, acupuncture, or chiropractic care.[9] Some of the reasons people use CAM include: belief that the combination with conventional medicine would help (54.9%), belief that it would be interesting to try (50.1%), at the suggestion of a medical professional (25.8%), and because conventional medicine was too expensive (13.2%).

A 2003 survey asked pharmacists about their beliefs and attitudes about CAM.[10] The percentages of pharmacists completely agreeing or somewhat agreeing with the following statements were: alternative medicines are safe (33%), alternative medications are effective (48%), I consider myself knowledgeable about alternative medicines (47%), and I am comfortable providing information about alternative medicines (47%). Pharmacy schools should take note of these results.

Dietary Supplements

The use of dietary products continues to grow despite knowledge of problems surrounding their use — safety, effectiveness, interactions with drugs and foods, and high cost.[11] Motivation for using these products may be: (a) that they are safe because many of the products are derived from "natural sources," (b) easy access, (c) lack of motivation to use exercise and diet, and (d) hopes for a quick fix to a weight problem. Counseling opportunities in this area abound for the patient-oriented pharmacist.

Tips for Consumers

Consumers who would like to use medication wisely are offered the following tips:

- Talk to your doctor and pharmacist about your medication.
- Know what you are taking, why, and how much and how often you should take it.
- Know for how long you should take your medicine.
- Know which side effects of the medication you are taking need attention.
- Avoid alcohol when taking drugs affecting the central nervous system.
- Read prescription labels.
- Keep medicines in their original containers.
- Know the names of drugs you are allergic to and tell your doctor and pharmacist, even if they do not ask.
- Know if you need to be routinely monitored for the drugs you are taking.
- Know if your drug interacts with other drugs or foods.
- Use the same pharmacy for all of your medication.

Should There Be a Third Class of Drugs?

The danger with OTC use is that patients may try to self-medicate with the wrong medication or need to seek medical attention rather than self-medicate. As stated before, many OTCs are sold in places other than retail pharmacies. Therefore, there may be a health care risk. How big a risk is unknown and needs study. If the risk is larger than expected, one solution may be a third class of drugs.

The two categories of drugs — prescription only (Rx drugs) and OTCs — leaves no room for error. Although the FDA works at discovering whether a prescription drug can be switched to OTC status, these decisions are difficult. Is the drug safe enough to put on a retail store shelf that allows patients to make their own decisions? When the drug was prescription only, it was only used after a physician examined and diagnosed the patient, and the drug was double-checked by a pharmacist. When a drug goes from prescription only to OTC, these controls disappear.

Many countries have a third category of drugs — drugs available on the advice of a pharmacist but without a prescription (RPh-only drugs). There probably are some OTC drugs that should be in this category and some Rx drugs that could be switched to this category. It would also be safer for the FDA to move Rx drugs to RPh-only drugs for a period of time before giving them OTC status.

PRESCRIBING DRUGS

An important part of the drug-use process is how drugs are prescribed. This involves a process that is more complex than most people realize. It starts with a patient need and the prescriber's — usually a physician or dentist — willingness to help. In some states, the prescriber might be a physician's assistant or nurse practitioner; however, these categories of health care workers have limited prescribing privileges. Veterinarians may also prescribe, but only for animals, and certain drugs can be prescribed only by veterinarians and dispensed on the order of a veterinarian.

Once the physician establishes the *doctor–patient relationship*, the physician asks about the patient's *chief complaint* — the main reason the patient is seeking the physician's advice. Next are questions about history of the present illness, followed by questions about the patient's past medical history. Once this is done, the physician performs a physical examination of the patient (historically called the *laying on of hands*).

While working through this process, the physician is trying to rule out what the problem is not. The physician then may order laboratory tests to help confirm the patient's diagnosis. When all of the information is complete, the patient will be told the physician's opinion of the health problem. Sometimes it may be necessary to discuss severity and prognosis (prediction of probable outcome). Treatment alternatives are discussed next. Nonmedical treatment such as exercise or rest or medication, radiation, or surgery may be advised. In any case, the role of the pharmacist assumes drug therapy is the therapy of choice.

The Prescription

If the condition warrants a prescribed medication, the drug is ordered using a prescription. A *prescription* — the slang term is *script* — is an order by a prescriber requesting the pharmacist to *dispense* — prepare, package, and label — specific medication for a patient at a particular time.[12] Before the 1960s, most prescriptions were written using Latin phrases and symbols. Thus, physicians and pharmacists needed to know Latin. Although some Latin terms are still used today, most prescriptions are written in English.

The prescription may be written on a prescription blank — a piece of paper, usually 4 by 6 inches, preprinted with terms, lines, and space to write information. However, there is no legal requirement that the information be on such a form. It may be on any piece of paper, even a restaurant napkin. There is no requirement that the prescription be in writing. Most prescriptions can be provided to the pharmacist orally. It should be documented in the prescriber's records that the medication was ordered for the patient. The pharmacist, on receiving an oral prescription from a prescriber, must, under legal requirement, immediately record the prescription in writing or in electronic format.

Parts of a Prescription

A model prescription is shown in Figure 4.1. The legal requirements for a prescription vary from state to state. However, every prescription has eight essential features.[6]

Date: The prescription should be dated the same day it is written or ordered by the physician. It should be presented to the pharmacist within a reasonable time of seeing the physician.

Name and address of patient: It is important to identify the patient correctly. Names instead of initials should be used to keep from confusing a patient with someone else. All names should be correctly spelled. An address and telephone number are important in case it becomes necessary to contact the patient at a later time. Age and gender are other important information that can be gathered in the pharmacy.

Superscription: The "Rx" symbol is the superscription that heads the introduction to the prescribed medication. Rx in Latin meant "recipe."

Inscription: This part of the prescription contains the name, strength, and quantity of medication to be prepared.

Subscription: This section may include any special instructions or directions to the pharmacist about the method of preparation and dispensing.

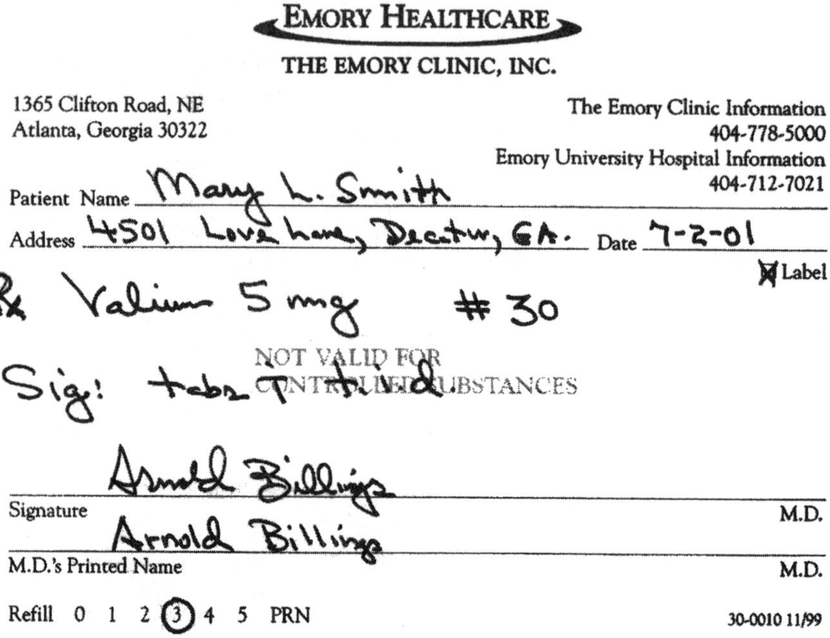

EMORY HEALTHCARE

THE EMORY CLINIC, INC.

1365 Clifton Road, NE
Atlanta, Georgia 30322

The Emory Clinic Information
404-778-5000
Emory University Hospital Information
404-712-7021

Patient Name Mary L. Smith

Address 4501 Love Lane, Decatur, GA. Date 7-2-01

X Label

Rx Valium 5 mg #30

NOT VALID FOR CONTROLLED SUBSTANCES

Sig: tabs ī t.i.d.

Arnold Billings
Signature M.D.

Arnold Billings
M.D.'s Printed Name M.D.

Refill 0 1 2 (3) 4 5 PRN

30-0010 11/99

Figure 4.1 An example of a prescription.

***Signatura*:** This section of the prescription is usually shortened "sig." In Latin, *signatura* means "take." The sig. is the directions to be typed on the label of the prescription container. If safe, the pharmacist must put the amount of medication to be taken at one time and the number of times a day on the prescription label, as prescribed by the prescriber. However, the pharmacist may add directions to the label that help in taking the medication correctly. Other information added to the label may be the medication's lot number and expiration date.

Refill information: It is important for patients to know if their medication can be refilled without returning to the prescriber. If there is no refill, it is better to put this on the label than to put nothing.

Signature, address, and registry number of the prescriber: The prescription must be signed by the prescriber. The signature and address of the prescriber authenticate the prescription. If the prescription is a narcotic or controlled substance, the physician's DEA registry number needs to be added.

Other requirements for narcotic and other controlled substance prescriptions are beyond the scope of this book.

Types of Prescriptions

There are all types of prescriptions — new ones, refills, trade name, generic, narcotics, controlled substances, and compounded (ones made from scratch).

Writing the Prescription

The writing of the inscription, subscription, and *signatura* is filled with specific terminology and often uses Latin terms and abbreviations and apothecary, avoirdupois, or the more standard metric units of measurement. This is why most patients cannot read or understand them — or maybe it is because of poor handwriting, which pharmacists become masters at reading. However, when in doubt, the pharmacist must always call the doctor for clarification.

Drug Orders

It is important to recognize that physicians write *drug orders* for patients in organized health care settings — such as hospitals, MCOs, and nursing homes — rather than prescriptions. The differences between a drug order and a prescription are in definition, legal status, and how they are written.

A drug order is a medication order written to a pharmacist by a legal prescriber for an inpatient — a patient confined to a bed — of an institution. A drug order has legal requirements that exempt it from having all the information needed on a prescription, but it needs to have information beyond a prescription, such as the patient's location (room number). An example of a drug order is shown in Figure 4.2.

When prescribing drugs in an organized health care setting, the physician normally must prescribe only those drugs found in the organization's *formulary*. A formulary is a listing of *drugs of choice* — as determined by relative drug product safety, efficacy, and effectiveness — along with information about each drug approved by the medical staff of that organization for use within the organization. More information on drug formularies is provided in Chapter 9, Hospital Pharmacy.

Drug Samples

Sometimes a patient may receive a sample of the medication or a sample of the medication and a prescription for it. These drug samples are small quantities of the drugs supplied to the physician, usually by sales representatives of drug companies. The idea behind samples is for the patient to try the medication to see if it works and is tolerated before having their prescription *filled* (slang for dispensed) at a pharmacy.

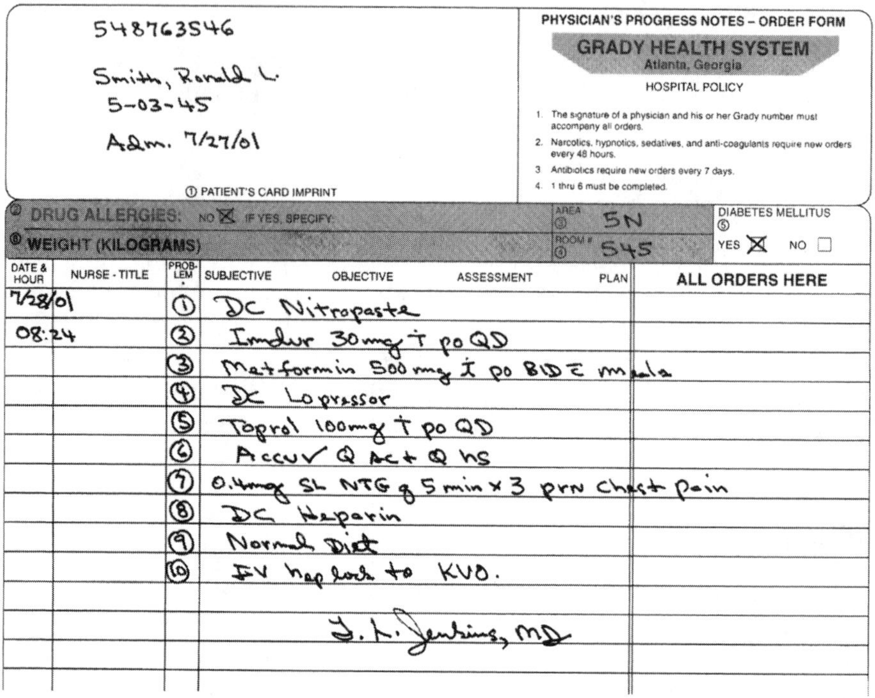

548763546
Smith, Ronald L.
5-03-45
Adm. 7/27/01
① PATIENT'S CARD IMPRINT

PHYSICIAN'S PROGRESS NOTES – ORDER FORM
GRADY HEALTH SYSTEM
Atlanta, Georgia
HOSPITAL POLICY
1. The signature of a physician and his or her Grady number must accompany all orders.
2. Narcotics, hypnotics, sedatives, and anti-coagulants require new orders every 48 hours.
3. Antibiotics require new orders every 7 days.
4. 1 thru 6 must be completed.

② DRUG ALLERGIES: NO ☒ IF YES, SPECIFY:
⑥ WEIGHT (KILOGRAMS)
AREA ③ 5N
ROOM # ④ 545
DIABETES MELLITUS ⑤ YES ☒ NO ☐

DATE & HOUR	NURSE - TITLE	PROB-LEM •	SUBJECTIVE OBJECTIVE ASSESSMENT PLAN	ALL ORDERS HERE
7/28/01		①	DC Nitropaste	
08:24		②	Imdur 30 mg ī po QD	
		③	Metformin 500 mg ī po BID c̄ meals	
		④	DC Lopressor	
		⑤	Toprol 100 mg ī po QD	
		⑥	Accu✓ Q Act Q hs	
		⑦	0.4 mg SL NTG q 5 min × 3 prn chest pain	
		⑧	DC Heparin	
		⑨	Normal Diet	
		⑩	IV hep lock to KVO.	
			J. L. Jenkins, MD	

Figure 4.2 An example of a drug order.

Pharmacists, and some regulators, such as state boards of pharmacy, health departments, and the Joint Commission on Accreditation of Healthcare Organizations (JCAHO), frown on sample giveaways because of lack of control over samples, and even though they are dated, they sometimes go out-of-date before they are given to patients. In addition, some physicians feel they may become biased toward a certain drug or cause them to start prescribing the most expensive drugs if they are provided samples. Therefore, some physicians refuse to accept them.[13]

DISPENSING

Once the patient receives a prescription, he or she will decide whether or not to take the prescription to a pharmacist to be filled. Surprisingly, some patients do not do this.[14,15] If a patient decides he or she would like the prescription filled, the next step is selecting a pharmacy. There are various considerations in making this decision, which are discussed in Chapter 8, Ambulatory (Community) Pharmacy.

Types of Retail Pharmacies

Patients have a variety of choices for filling their prescriptions.

Independent Community Pharmacies

These pharmacies are owned and operated by a pharmacist (a sole proprietorship) or a pharmacist with other pharmacists or nonpharmacists (a partnership). Independent community pharmacies were the first pharmacies in the United States, and for many years they were the only pharmacies.

Chain Store Pharmacies

These pharmacies are usually owned and operated by large companies. However, there are a few, small, usually family-owned local chains. Chain pharmacies are run according to corporate policy, and most of the people in upper management who oversee the pharmacies in the company are not pharmacists. Examples of chain store pharmacies are CVS, Rite-Aid, and Walgreens.

Mass Merchandiser Pharmacies

These pharmacies are also owned by large corporations and run according to the procedures of the corporations. Like chain pharmacies, most of the people in upper management who oversee the pharmacies in the corporation are not pharmacists. Examples of mass merchandiser pharmacies are Kmart, Target, and Wal-Mart.

Food Store Pharmacies

These pharmacies are located within grocery store chains. They try to fit into the "one-stop and shop" concept. Like chain and mass merchandise pharmacies, these pharmacies are owned by large corporations. The people within the corporation who have control over the pharmacies at the corporate level may not be pharmacists. Examples of food store pharmacies are Krogers and Publix.

Mail-Order Pharmacies

These pharmacies can be divided into two categories: (a) those affiliated with large *pharmacy benefits management* (PBM) companies and (b) smaller, independent operations. PBMs are employed by employers, or the insurers of employers, to manage and handle pharmacy claims.

Mail-order pharmacies accept new prescriptions from patients through the mail, fill the prescriptions, and send them back through the mail to the patients. Refills for medication are requested by telephone, electronic mail, or postcard.

About 7% of patients obtain their medication from mail-order pharmacies.[14] Eighty-seven percent of mail-order users were "very satisfied" or "extremely satisfied" with the service. About 75% believed the prices they paid were lower than a community pharmacy would charge. Ninety percent of the prescriptions were for refills, versus 46% of prescription refills brought into a community pharmacy. Nearly half (46%) of mail-order customers were 55 years of age or older, compared with 29% of all age categories.

Sometimes the mail-order pharmacy is located in a state other than the state where the patient lives. The lack of one-on-one contact with a pharmacist and the delay in receiving medication are the main reasons people do not use mail-order pharmacies. Examples of mail-order pharmacies are those associated with the American Association of Retired Persons (AARP), Express Scripts, Medco, Advance PCS, and Pharmacare Direct.

Outpatient Pharmacies in Hospitals

Some larger hospitals have outpatient pharmacies within the hospital, usually close to the entrance, the clinics, or the emergency room. These pharmacies dispense medication to *ambulatory patients* — those who are not hospitalized (outpatients). These pharmacies fill prescriptions written by physicians on the hospital staff. They also dispense the first filling of a new prescription for a patient being discharged from the hospital and prescriptions for employees of the hospital.

Internet Pharmacies

Recently, some *cyberpharmacies* have emerged. The first question about these is usually "Are they legal?" They are if they are licensed in the state in which they are located and in the states where they are doing business. These pharmacies run much like mail-order pharmacies, but with a few new wrinkles. Some Internet pharmacies establish personal contact between pharmacists and patients via e-mail, using patient profiles, offering OTC sales, and providing a wide choice of delivery options, including mail, express delivery, or pick up at an affiliated retail pharmacy. Examples of Internet pharmacy services are Drugstore.com, Planet-Rx, and Soma.com.

The Dispensing Process

The dispensing of medication, a prescription, is much more than meets the eye. Most patients have never been behind a prescription counter to see what takes place. It is much more than "count and pour" (the medication) and "lick and stick" (the label). Here are the recommended steps in dispensing a prescription:

- Accepting the prescription and establishing the pharmacist–patient relationship
- Reviewing the prescription and patient information
- Reviewing the patient's medication profile
- Checking for drug interactions and proper dosage
- Reviewing the insurance coverage
- Retrieving the drug or ingredients from storage
- Preparing or compounding (making) the medication
- Labeling the container
- Checking and dispensing the medication and preparing the label
- Counseling the patients about their medication

Each of these steps is discussed in more detail in Chapter 8, Ambulatory (Community) Pharmacy.

DRUG DISTRIBUTION IN ORGANIZED HEALTH CARE SETTINGS

Although some organized health care settings, such as hospitals, have outpatient pharmacies that dispense medication on the order of a prescription for its ambulatory patients, most of the medication dispensed is for *inpatients* — patients confined to beds.

Inpatients receive their medication by refined, organized drug distribution systems such as unit dose and centralized IV admixture services. Thus, pharmacy in organized health settings is practiced much differently than the way pharmacy is practiced in the community. Besides medication distribution, which is becoming more automated, the clinical services provided by pharmacists in organized health care settings are more extensive and more specialized.

Further information on how medications are prepared and distributed within organized health care settings is presented in Chapter 9.

Table 4.2   Growth of Prescription Expenditures (in Billions) in the United States, 1999–2004

Year	Total	Increase	Total Private	Total Public	
1999	$104.7	—	$81.6	$23.1	(22.1%)
2000	$120.8	13.3%	$93.2	$27.6	(22.8%)
2001	$138.6	12.8%	$105.5	$33.0	(23.8%)
2002	$157.9	12.1%	$118.7	$39.2	(24.8%)
2003	$174.1	16.2%	$128.0	$46.1	(26.5%)
2004	$188.5	7.6%	$136.6	$51.9	(27.5%)

Source: From The United States Centers for Medicare and Medicaid Services. National Health Expenditure Estimates, 2005.

DRUG SALES

Drugs Are Big Business

Today, drugs are big business — big business for the drug manufacturers, their investors, drug wholesalers, and corporate drugstore chains. How big is big drug business? As shown in Table 4.2, prescription medication is approaching a $200 billion dollar industry in the United States[16] and it is getting bigger. In 2005, the wholesale prices for brand name drugs rose 6%, faster than inflation.[17]

In 2004, the percentage of private funding for prescriptions was about 72.5%.[16] The balance was paid with public funds. As shown in Table 4.2, the percentage of private funding for prescriptions is dropping, while the percentage of public funding is increasing. With the Medicare starting to pay for prescriptions on January 1, 2006, these numbers will shift dramatically. The actual dollar expenditures, by payer, are shown in Table 4.3.

Of concern is that spending on prescription drugs has increased much more rapidly than spending on other health care services. As shown in Table 4.4, beginning in 1995, the spending for prescription drugs grew twice as fast as other health care spending, and at double-digit rates.[16]

Why Costs for Drug Prescriptions Are Rising

There are many reasons for this prescription growth:[18,19]

Spending growth in a few heavily advertised drug categories: Most of the increases in total drug spending have been among a few therapeutic categories that are heavily advertised by the drug companies. Four drug categories are increasing dramatically: oral

Table 4.3 Prescription Drug Expenditures (in Billions) in the United States, Distribution by Source of Funds, 1997–2004

Year	Out of Pocket	Total Private	Total Public	Federal	State and Local
1997	$25.7	$35.6	$16.4	$9.0	$7.4
1998	$27.5	$42.1	$19.0	$10.7	$8.3
1999	$30.4	$51.2	$23.1	$13.2	$9.9
2000	$33.4	$59.7	$27.6	$15.8	$11.8
2001	$36.2	$69.3	$33.0	$19.2	$13.8
2002	$40.0	$78.7	$39.2	$23.1	$16.2
2003	$43.7	$84.2	$46.1	$28.1	$18.1
2004	$46.9	$89.7	$51.9	$31.9	$20.0

Source: From The United States Centers for Medicare and Medicaid Services. National Health Expenditure Estimates, 2005.

Table 4.4 National Health Expenditures: Annual Growth (Billions) by Type of Expenditure, 1960–2004

Service	1960	1980	1990	2000	2004
Hospital Care	$9.2	$101	$251.6	$417.0	$570.8
Physician Services	$5.4	$47.1	$157.5	$288.6	$399.9
Home Health Care	$0.1	$2.4	$12.6	$30.6	$43.2
Nursing Home care	$0.8	$19.0	$52.6	$95.3	$115.2
Prescription Drugs	$2.7	$12.0	$40.3	$120.8	$188.5

Source: From The United States Centers for Medicare and Medicaid Services. National Health Expenditure Estimates, 2005.

antihistamines, antidepressants, cholesterol reducers, and the anti-ulcerants.

Generic drugs have a small market share despite lower prices: Although the proportion of generic drug use has been rising, the proportion of total drug sales for generic drugs has been dropping — from 11% in 1993 to 8% in 1998.

Spending is up because of higher prices and increased use: The proportionate increase for drugs because of rising prices is 64%, whereas the percentage because of increased use is 36%.[18] A reason for the higher prices is the introduction and widespread use of costlier new drugs. Two reasons for increased use are (a) new drugs for diseases previously unable to be treated and (b) the aging population.

Employers and health plans have increased the coverage for prescription drugs: Coverage for prescription medication has increased. Also, patients having all or a portion of their prescription drugs covered by an employer insurance plan use more medication. This is because they are insulated from knowing the true cost of their medication.

An increase of elderly individuals with treatable chronic conditions: The population in the United States is aging. With aging comes chronic health care conditions, many of which can be treated or controlled with prescription medication.

Direct marketing by pharmaceutical companies to consumers: The FDA allows drug companies to advertise directly to the consumer on television and through popular magazines. Advocates claim this increases awareness and sends more patients to their physicians for treatment. Critics argue that direct to consumer advertising results in patients pressuring physicians for the latest, most expensive drugs even when older, less costly, and equally or more effective drugs can be used.

Economic and foreign trade relations: These often allow countries outside the United States to buy drugs at lower prices than consumers pay in the United States.

Increased cost of conducting clinical trials: The cost of clinical trials has been rising rapidly, which means only companies with the hopes of producing a "blockbuster" drug will eventually be able to afford to do clinical research. This may lessen competition and increase prices further.

Some Possible Solutions

The current pattern of rising costs suggests that the current controls for drug costs are not enough. New ways to ensure the proper use of drugs are needed — ones that focus on effectiveness, safety, and cost. The American Medical Association (AMA) has suggested some ideas:[19]

Increase patient choice and responsibility: Most employees have little or no choice in drug coverage. They receive what is offered through their employer's health care plan. Patients need choices. Tiered fees will do this and probably save the employer money.[20] Those who want the most comprehensive drug coverage with the fewest limits and lowest out-of-pocket expense should be allowed to get it at a higher premium cost. Those wanting less coverage with more limits should be allowed to get it, but at a higher out-of-pocket expense.

Stronger and more consistent formularies: Formularies are lists of drugs of choice approved for use by the medical staff of a hospital, by a government agency, or a payer. The benefits of a formulary are achieved by channeling prescribing to more cost-effective medications and by negotiating better prices through volume buying.

More support for clinical effectiveness studies: Formularies can be made stronger by making formulary decisions based on unbiased clinical effectiveness studies of drugs in the same therapeutic class. The key issue should not be the cost of a drug but the overall cost of treating a disease or condition.

Messages to consumers about medications: The public mistrusts MCOs, the general feeling being that MCOs are interested in saving money at the expense of quality care. National medical and pharmaceutical organizations need to speak out more on the issue of inappropriate drug therapy. The extent of profiteering by MCOs also confuses the picture.

Greater information coordination for patients with multiple medical problems: Patients who see multiple physicians represent an opportunity for improvement. In these cases, one physician may not know what the other one has prescribed for the patient. Thus, there may be overlapping therapy, too many drugs (*polypharmacy*), or drug interactions. The same can be said for patients going to more than one pharmacy. When this happens, the pharmacist will have less of an opportunity to catch these problems. Patients receiving all of their medical care from one organization, such as an MCO or a health care system, with good integrated databases are more likely to discover these problems.

Higher health care premiums: No one likes to think or hear about this, but new and innovative drug therapy comes with a cost. Taking a drug from the laboratory to the shelf may cost over $500 million today, which is up from $125 million just 10 years ago.[21] Patients need to understand that if they want these new drugs, they must expect to share in the increased cost.

Responses to Rising Drug Costs

Payers of drugs are responding in different ways to the problem of rising drug costs.

Employers

Reining in rising drug expenses is now a primary goal of many managed care organizations, pharmacy benefits managers (PBMs), and employers. In

1999, some companies increased their medical costs 4% to 6%, whereas the increase in pharmacy costs may rise as much as 18%.[21] Employers are demanding cost controls by the government and meanwhile are asking their health benefit managers to raise employee premiums for their health care.

Some health benefit managers are taking a new, innovative approach to the problem of rising medication costs. For example, instead of focusing solely on drug costs, Active Health Management, Inc. is focusing on clinical outcomes and patient satisfaction.[22] Active Health Management is using patient data to manage quality of care instead of managing costs.

State Government

State governments buy large quantities of drugs for Medicaid patients and state employees. One state has taken a bold approach to rising drug costs.[23] Maine recently passed a law that will have the state negotiate with drug manufacturers to gain large discounts and pass these savings on to consumers. If negotiations fail to reduce prices significantly, price controls will be put in place. This new law is being challenged by the Pharmaceutical Research and Manufacturers of America (PhRMA), which represents about 100 brand name drug companies. A federal appeals court denied a petition by the PhRMA to review the court's ruling to lift an injunction on Maine's discount drug and price control program. Thus, Maine is free to negotiate lower prices with pharmaceutical companies for its 325,000 uninsured and underinsured residents.[24]

Federal Government

Various members of Congress are being pressured by various groups, including patients, to develop prescription drug pricing bills.[25] These bills would require the pharmaceutical industry to remove its practice of charging different prices for different buyers and making medicines more affordable for seniors.

Patients

Many patients have to purchase drugs out of pocket. These are the patients hurt the most by rising drug costs. Some seniors on limited budgets have to choose between buying all of their drugs or buying other essential items such as food, heat, and electricity.

Patients are pressuring consumer support groups and their elected officials to do something. Some patients are using other alternatives for getting their drugs; for example, mail-order and Internet pharmacies, which often have lower prices, and buying drugs outside the country. As we will see later, pitfalls may exist with some of these choices.

MEDICATION USE

How often is medication used? How is it administered? Do people always take it as prescribed? How should medication be monitored?

Medication Use in the United States

According to a national survey, over half (51%) of American adults take two or more medications each day.[26] In addition, almost half of Americans (46%) take at least one prescription medication each day, whereas more than a quarter (28%) take multiple prescription medications daily.

The rates of prescription medication use are highest among older Americans. Of those age 65 years old or older, 79% reported taking one prescription medication each day compared with respondents aged 55 to 64 (63%), aged 45 to 54 (52%), and aged 44 years or younger (28%). Americans aged 65 years or over who take prescription medications take an average of four each day.

Among respondents who reported the use of a prescription medication within the past week, the majority (61%) indicated that the medication was for a long-term health condition. Twenty-four percent said they were treating a recurring health problem, whereas 10% indicated that they were treating a short-term, acute health condition.

Besides increased OTC sales in the United States, the use of alternative medicine (e.g., herbal supplements, megavitamins, and other nontraditional remedies) is increasing dramatically. Overall, 4 of 10 Americans are trying alternative health treatments. In the American Society of Hospital Pharmacists survey, more than one-third (39%) of respondents reported taking an average of four herbal supplements and vitamins in the past week.[26] Forty percent reported taking an average of two herbal supplements or vitamins each day.

As well as more medication being taken, there has been a shift in where patients are buying their medication. Although every community pharmacy is filling more prescriptions, the two fastest growing are mail-order and food store pharmacies, and the slowest growing are independent community pharmacies.[27] There is some concern that the independent, corner drugstore may not be able to survive much longer.

DRUG PRICING

In the early days of pharmacy, pharmacists merely set a price for the medicine they prepared. The basis for the charge was the cost of the ingredients used — mostly plant materials and some vehicles (oils, tinctures, ointments), the pharmacist's time, and a little extra for living expenses.

Manufacturers

No one knows for sure how drug companies price their drugs. Every drug company does it differently, although they all probably consider some of the same issues. Because drug companies producing new drugs spend so much money in development, they are allowed to trademark their product and drug name and receive patent protection for 20 years from the time of filing. This allows the company to sell its brand name product without competition for 20 years to help recoup the research and development costs for the drug and for drugs that did not make it.

Interestingly, making the drug product is usually not expensive. Therefore, this is not usually a reason for setting the drug's price. Besides recouping development costs for new drugs, manufacturers also need money for development and for advertising, which is a major expense. Pharmaceutical manufacturers spent 27% of their total revenues on marketing, advertising, and administration promoting their products in the United States.[18] Of this, a large portion is spent for direct-to-consumer advertising and the balance for promoting products to health care professionals. Some groups critical of drug companies say that advertising costs dwarf the research costs of drugs (about 11% of total revenues). Pharmaceutical companies should be allowed to make a reasonable profit. However, there is controversy about 18% being reasonable.

Multitier Pricing

Historically, pharmaceutical manufacturers have set up different drug prices for different buyers, and this has been allowed. Drug companies charged low prices to hospitals, other large buyers like chain drugs stores, and the government, the largest buyer of drugs. Independent community pharmacies and others were charged the most. Today, drug manufacturers are granting large discounts to institutional buyers, such as HMOs, nursing homes, and hospitals.[26] The drug manufacturers are even ignoring large drugstore chains despite volume buys. Independent pharmacies, even the ones in large buying groups, are also being ignored. The National Community Pharmacy Association (NCPA) contends that community pharmacies are paying three to five times more than institutional buyers for the same brand name drug.[27]

The drug manufacturers contend that community pharmacies do not do what institutional buyers do — move market share, use formularies, and educate physicians, which have value to the manufacturers. They say community pharmacies simply fill prescriptions as written by physicians.

Meanwhile, independent community pharmacists are just asking for a level playing field. Seven years ago, thousands of pharmacies and drugstore chains launched a class action price-fixing suit against the drug manufacturers and wholesalers for discriminating pricing. In 1996 and shortly thereafter, 15 drug companies settled the lawsuit for $693 million. Although these companies do not admit to any wrongdoing, they are prevented from further use of two-tier pricing.

Prices for U.S. Made Drugs in Other Countries

One controversy, and one that upsets many patients, is that some U.S. drug manufacturers are selling their drugs outside the United States for substantially lower prices than they charge within the United States. For example, a recent government report found that prices on average are 72% higher in Maine than in Canada, and 102% higher than in Mexico.[28] Some countries have government price controls on drug products.

BUYERS AND SELLERS OF PRESCRIPTION DRUGS

Although drug manufacturers are the only pure sellers of prescription drugs, many others both buy and sell prescription drugs, for example, drug wholesalers, community pharmacists, hospitals, MCOs, and the government. Although specific percentages have been questioned, it has been acknowledged that U.S.-produced drugs are being sold for less in Canada and Mexico.[29] This issue has recently resulted in the U.S. Congress considering bills that allow the reimportation of U.S.-made drugs into the country. The question is, Are the drugs coming back into the United States safe and effective?

Drug Wholesalers

Drug wholesalers, such as AmerisourceBergen, Cardinal, and McKesson, purchase their drugs directly from the drug manufacturers at a price called the wholesale average cost (WAC). Distribution through drug wholesalers has increased from 47% in 1970 to about 80% in 2006.[30] Drug wholesalers do not make much money on the sale of an individual item (about 1 to 2%).[29] Although profit margins have been dropping, drug wholesalers run efficient operations and make money by selling large amounts of many items. In 2004, Cardinal Health ranked number one in customer satisfaction.

Community Pharmacy

Community pharmacy includes all retail pharmacies in the community — independent, chain drugstores, food stores, and mass merchandisers.

Buying

All drug pricing is based on a figure called AWP. This is the cost assigned to the product by the manufacturer and listed in a regularly published source such as the *Drug Topics Red Book* or *American Druggist Blue Book*.[31] The AWP is typically *not* the average price at which the drug is sold by wholesalers. A common joke among pharmacists is that AWP stands for "ain't what's paid." Despite its inaccuracy, the AWP is what *third-party payers* — insurance companies and PBMs — historically have based their reimbursement for a prescription's ingredient cost.

Based on discussion with community pharmacists, the actual acquisition cost of a product is typically 10 to 15% less than the AWP. The *actual acquisition cost* is dependent on two things — volume and loyalty. The more drugs the pharmacy buys, and the more they buy from one source — a drug wholesaler or buying group — the less the drugs will cost.

In trying to develop a more accurate figure for what pharmacists pay for drugs, third-party payers have developed the *estimated acquisition cost*. This is usually defined as AWP less some percentage discount (e.g., AWP less 10%). A recent innovation is for drug wholesalers to sell their products to the buyer at WAC plus 2 or 3%. WAC is generally about AWP minus 16.66%.

Selling

The only flexibility pharmacists have in pricing medication is for *private-pay patients* — those who pay for their medication out of their own pocket. Historically, community pharmacists have used three methods for pricing medication: (a) a percentage mark-up on the cost of the drug (cost plus 25% of cost), (b) cost of the drug plus a professional fee (cost plus $3.00), or (c) a sliding scale (cost of the drug plus a sliding fee based on the cost of the drug).

Each method has pros and cons; however, today most community pharmacists use the sliding scale method of pricing prescriptions for private-pay patients. For generic prescriptions, many community pharmacies price these at 60% of the charge for the comparable trade name product.

Third-Party Contracts

As shown in Table 4.3, about 73% of the prescriptions in the United States are paid by someone other than the patient. Insurance companies and PBMs (such as Express Scripts, Merck Medco, and PCS), who handle prescription claims processing for the health plans of various employers, set up prices they will pay pharmacies for prescriptions dispensed to their clients. Community pharmacies are paid much less for dispensing third-party prescriptions than they are for dispensing prescriptions to private-pay patients. For example, a repayment for dispensing third-party prescriptions is AWP minus 12% plus $3.00. Community pharmacy owners decide on a plan based on whether it is worthwhile to take part.

Medicaid Patients

Prescriptions of patients paid by the government under the Medicaid program are reimbursed differently. Each state sets reimbursement.[32] For example, in 2000, the Medicaid reimbursement to pharmacies in one state was AWP minus 10% plus $4.63, and the patient paid a $0.50 copay for each prescription. In New York, the reimbursement rate was AWP minus 10% plus $3.50 for a brand name drug and AWP minus 10% plus $4.50 for a generic drug. Patient copays were $0.50 for a generic drug and $2.00 for a brand name drug. In California, the reimbursement rate was AWP minus 5% plus $4.05. The copay was $1.00 for each prescription.

Medicare Patients

Patients receive Medicare after they retire, so they are usually 65 years of age or older. This age group uses more medication than any other age group, and retirees are usually on fixed incomes.[33] The Medicare Modernization Act, authorizing payment for outpatient prescriptions for Medicare beneficiaries, is covered in Chapter 3, Pharmacists and the Health Care System.

Gross Margin, Reimbursement, and Making a Profit

It is increasingly difficult for community pharmacies to stay in business. Over the past several years, many community pharmacies in the United States have closed.[34] The profitability of community pharmacies has declined, because third-party reimbursement programs have increased and these programs pay less than cash-paying customers. Because of this, a subsidy is being paid by the private-pay patient to compensate the pharmacy for costs involved in serving third-party customers.[19]

To stay in business, pharmacies need to make a profit. Therefore, the price paid for a prescription needs to cover three elements: (a) the price the pharmacy pays for the product, (b) the cost of dispensing the prescription, and (c) net profit.

A study was conducted to estimate the reimbursement necessary to provide community pharmacies in Georgia with a reasonable profit on third-party prescription programs.[35] It was discovered that pharmacies in

Georgia bought single-source prescription drugs — brand name drugs with no competing product — for AWP minus 17.2% and multisource drugs — drugs produced by more than one company — for AWP minus 45.1%.

The difference between the purchase price and the selling price of a drug is its *gross margin*. To compute profit, the cost of dispensing must be subtracted from the gross margin. The cost of dispensing includes salaries, supplies, and overhead — costs such as electricity, heat, and taxes. It was discovered that the median cost of dispensing a prescription was $6.41. The range was $5.18 (for mass merchandisers) to $7.19 (for traditional chain drugstores). A reasonable profit was set at 12%. This translated into making $0.54 per prescription.

The study concluded that for pharmacies in Virginia to earn a reasonable profit on third-party prescriptions, the repayment needed to be AWP minus 15% plus $6.95 for single-source drugs and minimum acquisition cost (MAC) plus $6.95 for multisource drugs. This is much higher than the reimbursements currently provided in most third-party programs.

As this shows, there is much more opportunity for pharmacies to make up some of the pricing disparity on multisource drugs, most of which are generics. Most community pharmacies price prescriptions for generic drugs at 60% of the price of the brand name equivalent. This provides patients with cost savings and at the same time increases the pharmacy's gross margin.

Hospitals

There are over 5000 hospitals in the United States, and they all buy, dispense, and charge for many drugs.

Buying

As previously mentioned, hospitals often receive discounts when buying large quantities of drugs. Today, almost all hospitals have joined large buying groups to gain the lowest prices on drugs. Hospitals receive large discounts when buying drugs, because they have favored status with the drug companies, which annoys many community pharmacists. A drug bought by private and nonprofit hospitals through group buying may cost only a fraction of what a community pharmacist pays for a drug, and a city or county government hospital will even pay less.

The federal government is the largest single buyer of drugs. It buys drugs for Veterans Affairs hospitals, the Department of Defense (DoD), and the U.S. Public Health Service. The government buys drugs using the Federal Supply Schedule. The Federal Supply Schedule catalog prices are interpreted as prices to "most-favored customers" such as large insurance companies and HMOs.[29] These prices are considered to be the lowest. The patients in Veterans Administration hospitals do not pay for their medication.

Formularies

Hospital formularies promote rational prescribing, but they also reduce the cost of drugs by lowering therapeutic overlap. For example, rather than having every benzodiazepine (e.g., Valium), there is only one. This raises the amount of the one drug ordered, lowers inventory cost, and decreases the cost of the medication. This is because of the price reduction manufacturers are willing to give if their product is the only one on the formulary within a particularly therapeutic class. If every hospital in the buying group commits to using the same drug in a drug class, and only that drug, the price goes even lower.

Projecting Drug Costs

Projecting drug costs for the next year's budget in hospitals has become a major problem.[36] Drug costs are going up in hospitals at unprecedented rates. This is because (a) many new drugs are much more expensive than the drugs they are replacing, (b) new drugs have been developed for conditions previously untreated (e.g., HIV), (c) increasing drug use because of an increasing intensity of illness and an older patient population, and (d) drug pricing inflation.

Selling

Hospitals establish drug charges based on what they expect private-pay patients to pay. This charge is sometimes referred to as the *usual and customary charge*. Each hospital has its own basis for setting the charge, and the pricing strategy usually varies by category of drug — oral solids, injections, intravenous solutions. Many of the drugs used in a hospital are not found in community pharmacies (many are injectable), but for the ones that are, the hospital charge is many times higher than is charged in the community. This, so say hospitals, is to offset the necessary parts of the hospital, such as the personnel department, hospital administration, and the maintenance department, that do not directly charge for their services.

Reimbursement

Less than 10% of hospital patients are private pay. The balance of hospital patients have their bills paid by private insurance, Medicaid, or Medicare.

Private insurance (such as Blue Cross–Blue Shield) negotiates prices for its patients. Medicaid sets the prices it pays for inpatient medication, just like it does for patients receiving prescriptions from a community pharmacy. The big difference is for Medicare patients.

Medicare pays for the drugs Medicare patients receive while they are in the hospital, but does so indirectly through a hospital reimbursement program called *prospective reimbursement.*[37] This is how it works: A single national reimbursement rate has been set for 467 *diagnosis-related groups* (DRGs). Each DRG is weighted for the extent of care needed. For each weight there is a reimbursement figure that is reset each year. Hospitals bear the financial risk of exceeding the cost of care for each DRG. If the cost exceeds the DRG rate, they loose money. However, if they provide care at a lower cost than the DRG rate, they are rewarded with the difference. The cost of drugs is part of the overall cost of care. Thus, Medicare does not pay for each drug provided to the patient. It pays one rate for treating a patient with a specific diagnosis regardless of how many drugs or how expensive the drugs are that are used for that case.

Since the implementation of prospective reimbursement by Medicare in 1983, the DRG system of reimbursement has been adopted by other payers, including some insurance companies and many state governments. The reimbursements by third parties, such as insurance companies and state and federal governments, have been making many hospitals struggle for survival. Because of low third-party reimbursement, there is a cost shift to private-pay patients, who pay more for the care they receive.

Managed Care

The 1990s saw explosive growth in managed care. Opponents of managed care call it "managed cost," stating that MCOs care more about cost than care. Rising drug costs are a major concern of MCOs. Although drugs comprise less than 12% of total health care costs, they are rising at a much faster rate than medical expenses.

Buying

MCOs buy their drugs for use for inpatients at preferential rates based on volume and the ability to control how drugs are used within their organization. MCOs also pay for the prescriptions their members receive as outpatients through either their own pharmacies, mail-order pharmacies, or community pharmacies. MCOs are able to arrange prescription discounts with community pharmacies based upon the number of clients they have who may have their prescriptions filled. The pharmacy receives payment on a *fee-for-service basis,* which pays for the ingredient cost plus a professional fee, or on a *capitation basis*, which pays a set amount per patient every month plus a patient copay for each prescription dispensed.[38] The latter method is risky for pharmacists, and most do not elect to do it.

Because the administration of managed care pharmacy programs is complex and requires a large prescription volume to be conducted efficiently, MCOs usually have prescription claims managed by PBMs. Reimbursement by PBMs is usually substantially lower than private-pay prescription prices. The average HMO reimbursement to network pharmacies in 1997 was AWP minus 14.2% plus $2.38.22

Selling

Technically, MCOs do not make money selling drugs. MCOs put themselves at risk by contracting with employer groups to provide medical care for employees of various companies for an annual, negotiated employee fee called *capitation*. The employees become members of the MCO. At the end of the year, it is hoped — and carefully calculated — that the MCO will spend less for the health care of its members than it collected in capitation fees from employers. The MCOs sell these plans to employers by touting their ability to manage costs. Thus, it is usually in the best interest of the MCOs and their investors not to spend money. Thus, they are always looking for ways to spend less for drugs.

A recent development is the possibility of having the members of MCOs buy their drugs through Internet pharmacies such as Rx.com rather than through traditional community pharmacies.[38] These pharmacies promise prices between those charged by retail pharmacies and mail-order pharmacies and more service. However, the safety and legality of these types of pharmacies are being scrutinized.[39]

PATIENTS

Patients often have many choices of where to go to have their prescriptions filled. The cost of the prescription is only one factor to consider. Most patients have to have their prescriptions filled at a pharmacy that will accept their insurance program. However, most community pharmacies accept most insurance programs. Thus, the decision should be based on something other than price or insurance. For many, it will be convenience. Beyond this, it comes down to where the patient feels the most comfortable. Patients feel comfortable when they feel welcomed and when they know the pharmacist is competent and cares.

ECONOMIC VALUE OF PHARMACEUTICALS

Despite the high and rising cost of pharmaceuticals, drugs may represent the best way to erase or control disease. They also may be the most cost effective. Researchers discovered that the total cost of treating depression in the United States fell by 25% from the early to the mid-1990s. In addition, outcomes improved because of advances in medical treatment and antidepressant drugs.[40] A leading selective serotonin reuptake inhibitor (SSRI) is safer and more tolerable than older drugs. Despite its higher cost, the total treatment cost for the SSRI was equal to or lower than the treatment cost of using the older agents.[41]

In another study, patients suffering from migraines benefited from taking a pain medication. Taking this medication resulted in fewer migraine-related disabilities and fewer severe migraines and fewer hospital stays, emergency room visits, physician office visits, and disability days associated with migraine headaches. Despite the medication cost of $44 a month, overall treatment costs dropped $391 per employee per month.[42]

MEDICATION ADMINISTRATION

Patients usually receive medication one of three ways: (a) self-administration, (b) administration from a friend or relative, or (c) administration from a nurse.

Self-administration is the way most medication is taken. It also may be the most dangerous. Unless the doctor, nurse, or pharmacist counsels the patient on taking the medication, the chances of the patient taking it correctly diminish. The patient should understand the name of the medication, what it is for, and what to expect from it. Most importantly, the patient needs to understand how to take the medication correctly. Does taking one tablet three times a day mean three times during the waking hours or spread out every 8 hours? Does it need to be taken with water or can it be taken with fruit juice or milk? Can patients stop taking the medication when they feel better or do they need to take it until it is all gone? If they miss a dose, should they take twice as much next time? How should the medication be stored? What about side effects?

Medication administered by a friend or relative is needed when the patient is sick and at home. This method of medication administration may be safer than self-administration. Most people are more careful when responsible for others. They also tend to ask more questions and are afraid to do anything wrong. Friends and relatives also are better at giving the medication on a schedule or reminding the patient when the medication is due to be taken.

Nurse-administered medication is the most accurate method of administering medications. Nurses know medication and how to give it, and if they do not, they have been trained to find out. Nurses pride themselves on this important function. They also have developed ways to get the most ornery patient or youngest child to ingest the medication.

No matter who administers the medication, it is easy to make an error such as forgetting to give it, giving the wrong drug, giving too much or too little, or giving it at the wrong time. This is unfortunate, as so much effort went into going to and seeing the physician, getting a diagnosis and a prescription, and getting the prescription filled. Not taking the medication properly can result in an extended illness, going back to the physician, having an adverse reaction, or possibly having to go to the emergency room or hospital. All of this results in more time and expense.

Compliance with Taking the Medication as Prescribed

The Problem

Some people never have their prescription filled, or if it is called into the pharmacist, never pick it up. How big of a problem is this? One study looking at this problem in community pharmacies found that about 2% of people never picked up their prescriptions.[15] This translates into 40 million prescriptions not being picked up and $1 billion in lost sales. Reasons cited by patients for this problem were: recovery (39%), having a similar drug at home (35%), not feeling they needed it (34%), and not liking to take medication.

The problem of unclaimed prescriptions is also a problem for outpatient pharmacies in hospitals. A 1995 study showed that 1.6% of patients did not pick up their medication.[43] One proposed solution to this problem is to call the patients to remind them their medication is ready for pick up.

Even if a person has a prescription filled, it does not mean he or she will take it as prescribed. Forgetting or purposely not taking medication as prescribed is called *noncompliance*. Noncompliance is a big problem. There are various means of discovery rates of medication compliance, such as urine tests, serum tests, pill counts, patient interviews, and record reviews.[44,45] As reported in the literature, rates of noncompliance with prescribed therapy vary between 15 and 93%. The variance is explained by different patient populations, the category of drugs, how often the medication is prescribed per day, and by differences in study design. Table 4.5 provides medication compliance rates for several disease states.[46-55]

The underlying problems associated with medication noncompliance are patient actions (decisions and behaviors).[56,57] Patients decide whether

Table 4.5 Rates and Possible Consequences of Noncompliance with Medication Requirements for Important Conditions

Condition	Rate of Noncompliance (%)	Possible Consequence	Reference
Epilepsy	30–50	Relapse	47
Arthritis	55–71	Condition worsens	48
Hypertension	40	Hospitalization	49
Diabetes	40–50	Loss of control	50
Contraception (pill)	8	Unwanted pregnancy	51
Asthma	20	Attacks, hospitalization	52
Alcoholism	48–56	Relapse, hospitalization	53
Organ transplant	18	Rejection, death	54
Anticoagulants	30	Bleeding, hospitalization	55
Estrogen deficiency	57	Symptoms, osteoporosis	56

Source: From *Noncompliance with Medications.* The Task Force for Compliance, Baltimore, MD, 1994. With permission.

to take a medication and how often. Reasons for patients not taking their medication or not taking it as prescribed include cost, feeling better, side effects, not realizing the importance, and forgetting.

Cost

The cost of medication noncompliance is high in lives lost, time lost, and added care needed. It has been estimated that 125,000 Americans die each year simply because they fail to take their medication as prescribed.[58] Equally disturbing are the unnecessary hundreds of thousands of extra hospital admissions resulting from medication noncompliance. In one study, 36 of 89 medication-related admissions were related to medication noncompliance.[59] Of these, 54% were because of intentional noncompliance.

Another study examined the records of seven patients not taking their medication as prescribed.[60] More than $14,000 was spent on outpatient visits, hospital days, and emergency room visits over 1 year as a direct result of medication noncompliance.

There is also the cost of time, such as having to stay home or leave work or school to seek medical attention. The estimated cost is a loss of 20 million workdays a year, or about 1.5 billion dollars in lost earnings.[58] The annual economic cost of medication noncompliance in the United States is estimated to be more than $100 billion dollars.[61]

Solutions

Many groups of people, such as physicians, nurses, pharmacists, the AARP, the Task Force for Compliance, and the National Council on Patient Information and Education (NCPIE) have been working on the problem of medication noncompliance. A lot has been learned, and more still needs to be done. Each patient not taking his or her medication as prescribed has a different reason, or set of reasons, for not being in compliance. Thus, the solution for getting the patient to be compliant will differ from one patient to the next.

Once it has been determined that there is a noncompliance problem, the pharmacist should try to find out why. The most common issues are (a) cost, (b) need, (c) fear of the medication not working or causing adverse effects, and (d) forgetfulness:

Cost: The pharmacist can sometimes help with this by arranging for a generic equivalent drug or arranging with the doctor to prescribe a drug as good as the more expensive drug but at less cost.

Need: If the patient does not feel he or she needs the drug, the pharmacist's understanding of the diagnosis and severity of illness should be able to help convince the patient to take the drug. If not, the patient should be referred to the physician.

Fear of the medication not working or causing adverse effects: Again, the pharmacist understands the drug well — its benefits and its potential side and adverse effects — and therefore should be able to help reassure the patient.

Forgetfulness: The pharmacist can also help with this problem. Pharmacy computer systems can now be programmed to calculate when a refill is needed and to print a list of patients due for a prescription refill. Postcards, telephone calls, or e-mail reminders can be sent to patients. In addition, compliance charts can be printed for patients to put on their refrigerators or bathroom mirrors. There is also reminder packaging available to show if a medication has been taken.

One of the most effective methods of improving medication compliance is for the pharmacist to shift from treating patients as passive pill takers to treating patients as an active participants in making decisions about their health. Patients should be asked if they know why they are taking their medication and what may happen to them if they do not take it or do not take it as prescribed.

The most effective way to improve medication compliance is by understanding why the patient is not taking the medication as prescribed and then using a combination of methods specifically designed to address the patient's reasons for not being compliant. This is not only in the patient's best interest, but also in the pharmacist's best interest both clinically and economically. Unfilled prescriptions and prescriptions not refilled produce an estimated 100 million lost prescriptions valued at $1.2 billion yearly.[58]

QUALITY DRUG THERAPY

There is much more to being a pharmacist than making sure patients receive the drugs prescribed and doing what you can do to make sure they take the drugs as prescribed. Today, pharmacists are trained to help each patient receive *quality drug therapy*, which is safe, effective, timely, and cost-effective drug therapy delivered with care.

Pharmacists used to fill prescriptions written by physicians and were not allowed to question whether the drug prescribed was the best drug for the patient. This has changed for various reasons. First, the drugs are becoming more complex and more potent and there are more of them. Second, physicians cannot know everything about every drug. Third, the clinical education of the pharmacist has expanded, and fourth, the scope of practice and legal duty of the pharmacist to help and protect the patient has expanded.

Physicians prescribe drugs based on what they know and feel is best. Pharmacists see the patient from a different viewpoint, may know things the physician does not know about the drug, or know about other drugs that may benefit the patient. Thus, if the pharmacist thinks the patient may benefit from changing the prescribed drug — its dose, route of administration, or dosage form or changing to another drug — there is obligation to call the physician and discuss it. After all, health care is a team effort. How problems are discussed with the physician is often as important as what is discussed to effect a successful change.

This new pharmacy practice started in the early 1960s and was first called *clinical pharmacy*. Clinical pharmacy has evolved into an even higher level of practice called *pharmaceutical care*. See Chapter 7, Pharmaceutical Care.

HOW DRUG THERAPY IS MONITORED AND REVIEWED

A major emphasis in health care is providing quality care. Part of this care is the drug therapy the patient receives. The quality of drug therapy can be measured. Accreditation bodies, such as the Joint Commission on Accreditation of Healthcare Organizations (JCAHO), require the medical staff of health care organizations to routinely review the quality of their drug therapy and take measures to improve it. The accreditation policies usually say the director of pharmacy will help the medical staff perform these quality reviews.

The method of reviewing the quality of drug therapy is called *drug-usage evaluation* (DUE). DUE programs are formal, structured, ongoing comparisons of drug therapy versus locally developed criteria representing best drug therapy and making recommendations for improvement. DUE programs have evolved over the years and continue to undergo changes. Currently, most DUE programs are measures of the structure and process of prescribing drugs. More sophisticated programs also measure patient outcomes.

The original intent of DUE programs was to review the use of drugs for appropriate use within an organization such as a hospital. Drug classes were selected for review — usually quarterly — based on the opinion of the medical staff that there could be an opportunity for improvement. The director of pharmacy, working with staff pharmacists, would draft criteria for the appropriate use of the drug class under review and submit it to the pharmacy and therapeutics committee (P&T committee) of the Medical Staff for its review, editing, and approval. The director of pharmacy is usually the secretary of this important committee.

DUE criteria can be as simple or as complex as the medical staff wants. The criteria can be positive (how the drug should be used) or negative (how the drug should not be used). Criteria can include when the drug should be used, for what types of patients (such as age and gender), appropriate dosage, length of therapy, and proper monitoring procedures. Some of the items for review may have some exceptions.

Once the DUE criteria are approved, the pharmacy service is usually appointed by the P&T committee to perform the DUE. The P&T committee will select the review, either prospective or retrospective. In *prospective* DUEs, a random sample of patients is followed forward in time as a cohort. Prospective reviews are usually more accurate but take time and manpower. *Retrospective* DUEs go backward in time and take less time and effort. This DUE is performed by selecting a random sample of medical records of patients known to have received the drug under review.

Once data are collected on how the drug was used in the sample of patients being reviewed, the pharmacy service compares the use of the drug versus the preferred way of using the drug, *vis-à-vis* the approved criteria. These results would then be presented to the P&T committee for its review, input, and recommendations.

The JCAHO, during its accreditation visits, is interested in these recommendations. They want to know if the recommendations were ever carried out and if follow-up audits were ever completed to see if the recommendations improved therapy.

The JCAHO is interested in targeted reviews for specific problem areas, data collected prospectively, and the analysis of data with the potential to intervene more immediately in drug prescribing and to continue the process for extended periods of time. It is also pushing for including the measurement of patient outcomes in the DUE criteria. There are some excellent references for further study of the DUE process.[62–64]

PATIENT OUTCOMES

The major drawback of traditional DUE programs has been the focus on the process of drug therapy rather than the outcome of drug therapy. Focusing on the outcomes of drug therapy provides insight into the value of the drug-use process. In general, there are four categories of health outcomes:

Clinical outcomes: Clinical outcomes are the traditional outcomes measured in patients. Examples are less pain, or no pain, better amount and quality of sleep, reduced anxiety, and fewer seizures.

Behavior, functional, and humanistic outcomes: These outcomes have to do with feeling and relating to others better and the ability to do more. Examples are improved school or job attendance, better range of motion, walking further, and perceived therapeutic benefit, health status, and quality of life.

Economic outcomes: These outcomes measure the cost of the various aspects of care, and some measures try to determine the cost of improvement or benefit.

Satisfaction with care: Another improvement measure is the patient's satisfaction with the care received. To measure satisfaction with care (and for quality of life), well-built and validated questionnaires need to be used.

How pharmacists are trying to achieve better patient outcomes is covered in Chapter 7, Pharmaceutical Care.

MEDICATION SAFETY

Although medication can cure an illness or help a patient feel better, it also has the potential for harm.[65,66]

Side Effects

All drugs have *side effects* that may occur in all patients. These are known, usually minor, annoying effects of the drug experienced by most people taking the drug. An example is the drowsiness associated with some antihistamine drugs used for treating hay fever symptoms.

Adverse Drug Reactions

Some drugs can cause more dangerous conditions called *adverse drug reactions*. These are unwanted, more serious, adverse effects of the drug that are not experienced by every patient taking the drug.

Allergic Drug Reactions

Patients allergic to a drug or an ingredient in the medication, even a color dye, can experience drug reactions that can vary from a minor annoyance to a threat to life. It is critical that every pharmacy, patient profile, and computer system contain information on each patient's allergies.

Drug–Drug Interactions

Some drugs interact with other drugs or interact with food or drink the patient is taking. One drug can make another drug inactive or overactive. The outcome of a drug interaction can range from a minor inconvenience to death. Pharmacists must be vigilant about detecting and stopping these interactions from occurring.

Medication Errors

Medication errors rarely occur, when considering the millions of prescriptions and doses of medication patients receive yearly. The incidence is a fraction of a percentage. However, this is meaningless if the error occurs to you or someone you love. Therefore, the public has zero tolerance for medication errors. That means pharmacists and pharmacy technicians have to be perfect all the time and there is no room for errors.

Pharmacists have built good check and balance systems — a safety net — for detecting medication errors before they harm patients. However, medication errors occasionally occur within the drug-use process. These errors usually are the result of a medication system failure rather than the failure of one person.

Adverse drug reactions, allergic drug reactions, drug–drug interactions, and medication errors, as a group are called *drug misadventures* or *adverse drug events.* These are discussed in further detail in Chapter 7, Pharmaceutical Care.

CONTROL OF THE DRUG-USE PROCESS

The drug-use process is extensive and complex. It is also designed with many checks and balances to keep patients from experiencing a preventable drug misadventure.[67] At the center of this control is the pharmacist. Laws, rules and regulations, accreditation policies, and pharmacy tradition have given the pharmacist this important responsibility. Although pharmacists have accepted this responsibility, and they are up to the task, they cannot do it alone. They need the help of pharmacy technicians, other health professionals, automation, and patients who will take responsibility for their own health. They also need infrastructure support.[68]

CURRENT ISSUES IN THE DRUG-USE PROCESS

Some current issues in the drug use process deserve discussion.

Nutriceuticals and Herbal Medicines

Nutriceuticals (nutrient, vitamin, and mineral products), which are often sold in health food stores, represent a challenge to the FDA, United States Pharmacopeia (USP), and health professionals. Although some of these products may be helpful to patients, many are not standardized, and none are regulated. Thus, unsubstantiated claims can, and are, being made for these products without doing any controlled, scientific studies to back up the claims. In addition, several of these products have caused adverse events. Will standards be set for these products (by the USP) and will they be regulated (by the FDA)? How should physicians and pharmacists advise patients about these products?

Direct to Consumer Advertising of Prescription-Only Drugs

The FDA has recently allowed drug companies to advertise directly to patients via television commercials and magazine and newspaper advertisements. This has not been viewed by some health care professionals as wise. Based on seeing one of these ads, some patients come into physicians' offices demanding a certain drug. This puts added pressure on physicians. Even if the drug requested may not be helpful, physicians may succumb to patient pressure and prescribe a drug they know may not help and might even cause some problems in the patient. Even if the physician talks the patient out of using the drug, there may be lingering mistrust of the physician by the patient. Should the FDA continue to allow direct to consumer advertising of prescription-only products?

Importing of Drugs from Other Countries

The recent escalation of drug prices for patients in the United States and cheaper prices for the same drugs in other countries has caused patients, and some Internet-based businesses of questionable legal status, to obtain drugs from foreign sources.

Currently, this is an illegal practice. However, the U.S. Congress is thinking about changing laws to allow the reentry of drugs approved for use in the United States. The basis for this is that some drugs made and approved for use in the United States are shipped for use to Mexico, Canada, and other countries. The prices for these drugs are much lower than patients pay for the same drug in the United States.

Rising Number of Prescriptions and Not Enough Pharmacists

The number of prescriptions filled each year is rising at an unprecedented rate. This rise is the result of increased demand and better drugs. The large baby boom generation will soon be reaching 65 years of age, and individuals often need more medication as they get older. At the same time, the pharmacy profession is being stretched. A shortage of pharmacists is becoming clear because of expanded roles for pharmacists and an increased use of medication.

The profession's response has been to start up more schools of pharmacy. However, from all indications, this may not be enough. To meet the demand, and to preserve or expand the pharmacist's clinical role, pharmacy will need to use pharmacy technicians better, reorganize pharmacies to be more efficient, and increase the use of pharmacy automation and information technology.

SUMMARY

The drug-use process is a complex, structured process involving the manufacture, distribution, prescribing, preparation, storing, dispensing, administrating, monitoring, and review of drugs and their use. The process is controlled, and at the center of this control are various checks and balances, regulations, and the pharmacist. Even with control, the system is not perfect, and thus needs constant attention and improvement.[66,67]

DISCUSSION QUESTIONS AND EXERCISES

1. If you live near a drug company, make an appointment to visit and observe how drugs are manufactured and distributed to drug wholesalers.

2. If you live near a drug wholesale company, make an appointment to visit and observe how drugs are distributed to pharmacies.
3. Make an appointment to visit a hospital pharmacy. Watch how drugs are prepared and distributed to nurses and patients.
4. Make an appointment to talk with the risk manager in a hospital about medication errors. Review at least one medication incident report.
5. A patient hands you (the pharmacist) a prescription. You note that it is a 10-fold overdose and potentially lethal.
   a. How would you handle this?
   b. If you talk to the physician, how would you handle this?
   c. If you talk to the patient, how would you handle this?
6. Go to the FDA's Web site (http://www.fda.gov) and go to the FDA's MedWatch program to learn how serious adverse drug reactions are reported.
7. How do serious adverse reactions to vaccines get reported? Who can report?
8. If pharmacists are responsible for the drug-use process in organized health care settings, and the administration of medication is a part of this process, how can pharmacists assist nurses to administer drugs safely?
9. You are the owner of a small, independent pharmacy and are the only pharmacist. A 55-year-old female patient presents you with a prescription medication used to treat multiple sclerosis. The medication is for 1 month and costs the patient $135. The patient says she can only afford $100. What would you do?
10. Same question (question 9), but this time you are a part-time pharmacist filling in while the owner is off for the day.

CHALLENGES

1. Patients not taking their medication as prescribed is a major public health problem. For extra credit, and with the permission of your professor, investigate and prepare a concise report about the problem and develop three new strategies to help combat this problem.
2. The problem of polypharmacy is real. For extra credit, and with the permission of your professor, and the help of a pharmacist, identify a patient in whom polypharmacy is likely. Write a concise report about this patient's medications (not naming the patient or pharmacy) and recommend how you would reduce the polypharmacy.

WEB SITES OF INTEREST

National Council on Patient Information & Education: http://www.talk-aboutrx.org/index.jsp

REFERENCES

1. Anonymous. *Pharmaceutical Benefits Under State Medical Assistance Programs.* National Pharmaceutical Council, Reston, VA, 1996.
2. Healthcare Distribution Management Association. Healthcare product distribution: a primer. Available at http://www.healthcaredistribution.org. Accessed August 5, 2001.
3. Appleby, J. Stolen: counterfeit drug problems rise. *USA Today.* May 11, 2005, p. 3B.
4. Oldenburg, D. As more shop for drugs online, fakes pose greater health threat. *The Atlanta Journal Constitution.* April 16, 2005, p. EE7.
5. *Handbook of Non-prescription Drugs.* American Pharmaceutical Association, Washington, DC, 2000.
6. National Council on Patient Information and Education. *Attitudes and Beliefs about the Use of Over-the-Counter Medicines: A Dose of Reality.* Bethesda, MD, 2002.
7. *Self-medication in the '90's: Practices and Perceptions.* Nonprescription Drug Manufacturers Association, Washington, DC, 1992.
8. 1999 Retail Pharmacy Digest: Measuring Customer Satisfaction. Ortho Biotech, Raritan, NJ, 1999.
9. Johnson, RF, and Gonzalez, A. Seeking other health solutions. USA Today. July 1, 2004, p. 1D.
10. Dolder, C, Lacro, J, Dolder, N, and Gregory, P. Pharmacists' use of and attitudes and beliefs about alternative medications. *Am J Health-Syst Pharm.* 2003;60: 1352-1357.
11. McQueen, CE, Shields, KM, and Generali, JA. Motivations for dietary supplement use. *Am J Health Syst Pharm.* 2003;60:655.
12. Martin, EW. The prescription. In *Dispensing of Medication,* 7th ed. Mack, Easton, PA, 1971, chap. 1.
13. Japsen, B. Saying yes to free drug samples raises concern. *Atlanta Journal.* January 26, 2001.
14. Hamilton, WR, and Hopkins, UK. Survey of unclaimed prescriptions in a community pharmacy. *J Am Pharm Assoc.* 1997;NS37:341–345.
15. Anonymous. No-show customers cost community pharmacies $1 billion annually. *Am J Health-Syst Pharm.* 1996;53:1236, 1239–1240.
16. The United States Centers for Medicare and Medicaid Services. National Health Expenditure Estimates, 2005. Available at http://www.cms.hhs.gov/National-HealthExpendData/02_NationalHealthAccountsHistorical.asp#TopOfPage.
17. Appleby, J. AARP: brand-name drug prices shot past inflation in 2005. *USA Today.* April 10, 2006, p. 1B.
18. Avorn, J. *Powerful Medicines: The Benefits, Risks, and Costs of Prescription Drugs.* Alfred A. Knopf, New York, 2004.

19. Conway, WA, and Kurtz, S. Pharmaceutical costs: a crisis for provider groups and U.S. health care. American Medical Association, Chicago, IL, 2000. Available at http://www.ama.org. Accessed April 25, 2001.

20. Benko, LB. Patients get choices in drug pricing. *Modern Healthcare*. 2000;30(10):72–74.

21. Knight, W. Too much or too little? The role of pharmaceuticals in the health care system. *J Managed Care Pharm*. 1999;5:296–302.

22. Gebhart, F. Big companies find ways to fight rising drug costs. *Drug Top*. 2000;144:84, 86.

23. Page, L. Maine poised to set nation's first price controls on drugs. *Am Med News*. May 8, 2000.

24. Young, D. Court rules that Maine Rx can move forward. ASHP. Available at http://www.ashp.org/public/news/breaking/ShowArticle.cfm?id=2367. Accessed June 20, 2001.

25. Anonymous. Bill mulled for uniform prescription drug pricing. *Chem Market Reporter*. 1999;255(21):17.

26. Schweitzer, SO. *Pharmaceutical Economics and Policy*. Oxford University Press, New York, 1997.

27. Edlin, M. Drug deals aren't illegal, but some think they're unfair. *Managed Healthcare*. 1998;8(Nov):28–29.

28. *Prescription drug pricing in the United States: drug companies profit at the expense of older Americans*. Minority Staff Report, Committee on Government Reform and Oversight, U.S. House of Representatives, September 25, 1998.

29. Danzon, PM. *Price Comparisons for Pharmaceuticals: A Review of U.S. and Cross-National Studies*. AEI Press, Washington, DC, 1999.

30. Fincham, JE, and Wertheimer, AI. *Pharmacy and the U.S. Health Care System*, 2nd ed. Haworth Press, Binghamton, NY, 1998.

31. Carroll, NV. *Financial Management for Pharmacists: A Decision-Making Approach*, 2nd ed. Williams & Wilkins. Baltimore, MD, 1998.

32. Anonymous. An update on Medicaid reimbursement by state. *Drug Top*. 2001;145(3):79.

33. Press Release. Congressman Pete Stark. Stark calls for affordable Medicare prescription drug coverage for all of America's seniors. Available at http://www.house.gov/stark/documents/perdrugbillann.html. Accessed Marcy 7, 2001.

34. Carroll, NV. Estimating a reasonable reimbursement for community pharmacies in third-party programs. *Managed Care Interface*. 1999;12:73–76, 79–80.

35. McMillan, JA, Carroll, NV, and Kotzan, JA. *Third-Party Associated Cost-Shift Pricing in Georgia Pharmacies*. Studies in Pharmaceutical Economics. Pharmaceutical Products Press, New York, 1996.

36. Mehl, B, and Santell, JP. Projecting future drug expenditures-2000. *Am J Health-Syst Pharm*. 2000;57:129–138.

37. Campbell, CR, Schmitz, HH, and Waller, LC. *Financial Management in a Managed Care Environment*. Delmar, Albany, NY, 1998.

38. Schafermeyer, KW. The impact of managed care on pharmacy practice. *Pharm. Pract. Managed Q*. 2000;19:99–116.

39. Anonymous. Buying drugs over the internet could cost you — in more ways than one. *Tufts Univ Health Nutrition Newsl*. 1999;17:8.

40. Triplett, JE. *Measuring the Prices of Medical Treatment*. Brookings Institution Press, Washington, DC, 1999.

41. Wilde, M, and Benfield, P. Fluoxetine: a pharmacoeconomic review of its use in depression. *PharmacoEcon.* 1998;13:543–561.

42. Legg, R, Sclar, D, and Nemec, N. Cost benefit of sumatriptan to an employer. *J Occup Environ Med.*1997;39(7):652–657.

43. Kirking, MH, Zaleon, CR, and Kirking, D. Unclaimed prescriptions at a university hospital's ambulatory care pharmacy. *Am J Health-Syst Pharm.* 1995;52:490–495.

44. *Prescription Medicine Compliance: A Review of the Baseline of Knowledge.* National Council on Patient Information and Education (NCPIE), Washington, DC, 1995.

45. Salek, MS, and Sclar, DA. *Medication Compliance: The Pharmacist's Pivotal Role.* Upjohn, Kalamazoo, MI, 1992.

46. Leppik, IE. How to get patients with epilepsy to take their medication. The problem of noncompliance. *Postgrad Med.* 1990;88:253–256.

47. Bloom, BS. The medical, social, and economic implications of disease. In van Eimeren, W. and Horisberger, B, *Socioeconomic Evaluation of Drug Therapy.* Springer-Verlag, New York, 1988, pp. 60–71.

48. Clark, LT. Improving compliance and increasing control of hypertension: needs of special hypertensive populations. *Am Heart J.* 1991;121:664–669.

49. Nagasawa, M, Smith, MC, and Barnes, JH. Meta-analysis of correlates of diabetes patients' compliance with prescribed medications. *Diabetes Ed.* 1990;16:192–200.

50. Jones, EF, and Forrest, JD. Contraceptive failure rates based on the 1988 NSFG. *Fam Plan Perspect.* 1992;24:12–19.

51. Bauman, AE, Craig, AR, Dunsmore, J, et al. Removing barriers to effective self-management of asthma. *Patient Ed Counsel.* 1989;14:217–226.

52. Powell, BJ, Penick, EC, Liskow, BI, et al. Lithium compliance in alcoholic males: a six month follow up study. *Addict Behav.* 1986;11:135–140.

53. Rovelli, M, Palmeri, D, Vossler, E, et al. Noncompliance in organ transplant recipients. *Transplant Proc.* 1989;21:833–834.

54. Joglekar, M, Mohanaruban, K, Bayer, AJ, and Pathy, MSJ. Can old people on oral anticoagulants be safely managed as out-patients? *Postgrad Med J.* 1988;64:775–777.

55. Hemminki, E, Brambilla, DJ, McKinlay, SM, and Posner, JG. Use of estrogens among middle-aged Massachusetts women. *DICP.* 1991;25:418–423.

56. The Task Force for Compliance. *Noncompliance with Medications.* Baltimore, MD, 1994.

57. Bentley, JP, Wilkin, NE, and McCaffrey, DJ. Examining compliance from the patient's perspective. *Drug Top.* 1999;143(14):58–67.

58. Robbins, J. Forgetful patient: high cost of improper medication compliance. *US Pharm.* 1987;12:40–44.

59. Col, N, Fanale, JE, and Kronholm, P. The role of medication noncompliance and adverse drug reactions in hospitalizations of the elderly. *Arch Intern Med.* 1990;150:841–845.

60. Smith, M. The cost of noncompliance and the capacity of improved compliance to reduce health care expenditures. In *Improving Medication Compliance.* National Pharmaceutical Council, Reston, VA, 1985.

61. Berg, JS, Dischler, J, Wagner, DJ, et al. Medication compliance: healthcare problem. *Ann Pharmacother.* 1993;27:S5–S19,S21–S22.

62. Kier, KL, and Pathak, DS. Drug-usuage evaluation: traditional versus outcome-based approaches. *Top Hosp Pharm Manage.* 1991;11:9–15.

63. Sloan, NE, Peroutka, JA, Morgan, DE, et al. Influencing prescribing practices and associated outcomes utilizing the drug use evaluation process. *Top Hosp Pharm Manage.* 1994;14:1–12.

64. Rosman, AW, and Sawyer, WT. Population-based drug use evaluation. *Top Hosp Pharm Manage.* 1988;8:76–91.

65. Kelly, WN. Drug use control: the foundation of pharmaceutical care. In *Pharmacy Practice for Technicians*, 2nd ed. Delmar, Albany, NY, 1999, chap. 7.

66. Kelly, WN. *Prescribing medication and the public health: laying the foundation for risk reduction.* Haworth Press, Bingingham, NY. 2006.

67. Brodie, DC. Drug-use control: keystone to pharmaceutical service. *Drug Intell.* 1967;1:63–65.

68. Rucker, TD. Prescribed medications: System control or therapeutic roulette? In *Control Aspects of Biomedical Engineering.* International Federation of Automatic Control, Oxford, UK, 1987.

5

PHARMACY SUPPORTIVE PERSONNEL

Being a health care professional means being part of a team that is focused on one goal — helping the patient achieve better health. Pharmacists are a part of this health care team, and their part is to help the patients make the best use of their medication. This is a big job, and one that pharmacists cannot do alone. Thus, within their profession, pharmacists have developed other categories of pharmacy workers to help get the work done more efficiently and allow pharmacists to be more focused on the patient.

Some of the categories of supportive personnel within the pharmacy profession, starting with the less skilled, are couriers (delivery personnel), clerks (sales, purchasing, and billing), and data entry personnel (enter patient and drug information into the computer). In some states, these workers are called pharmacy assistants. The most skilled ancillary personnel in pharmacy are called pharmacy technicians. Pharmacy technicians work alongside pharmacists and are essential in providing comprehensive, quality, and cost-effective prescription and pharmacy services for patients.

This chapter is primarily about pharmacy technicians. It begins with defining supportive personnel and pharmacy technicians, and explaining where technicians work and why they are needed. Next is information on what pharmacy technicians do, what they know, how they become certified, how they are supervised, and what it means to be professional. Finally, the chapter covers earnings, working conditions, satisfaction, advancement, and job outlook.

LEARNING OBJECTIVES

After reading this chapter, you should be able to:

- Explain the categories of pharmacy supportive personnel
- Define the term *pharmacy technician*
- Explain the legal limits of pharmacy technicians
- Discuss what functions pharmacy technicians can and cannot perform in most states

THE PHARMACY TECHNICIAN

A *pharmacy technician* is an individual working in a pharmacy who, under the direct supervision of a licensed pharmacist, aids in the highest pharmacy tasks that do not require the professional judgment of the pharmacist. Basic, routine activities in the pharmacy, such as unpacking goods, stocking shelves, and delivering medication, may be carried out by someone less skilled than a pharmacy technician.

The occupation of the pharmacy technician is continually evolving. The role of the pharmacy technician is greatly expanding because of an emerging consensus on what knowledge, skills, and abilities are needed to be a pharmacy technician and what role pharmacists should play in overall pharmacy practice, including direct patient care. Consensus is also being reached on the functions, educational training requirements, proper supervision, and recognition of pharmacy technicians by state boards of pharmacy.[1] The recognition of pharmacy technicians and their status within the profession of pharmacy has increased because of the recent creation of a voluntary, national certification process.

EMPLOYMENT

Pharmacy technicians held about 258,000 jobs in 2004. About 7 out of 10 jobs were in retail pharmacies, either independently owned or part of a drugstore chain, grocery store, department store, or mass retailer. About 2 out of 10 jobs were in hospitals, and a small proportion was in mail-order and Internet pharmacies, clinics, pharmaceutical wholesalers, and the federal government.[2] Today, there are more pharmacy technicians than licensed pharmacists in the United States, and based on current employment projections, there is a need for many more.

WHY PHARMACY TECHNICIANS ARE IMPORTANT

The rising workload of prescriptions and drug orders could not be met without the services and help of pharmacy technicians. This increase in workload is expected to continue for the next decade as the "baby boomers" — those born after WWII (1946 to 1964) — attain their retirement years during the next few years.

Besides meeting the prescription and drug order demand, the contribution to patient care when pharmacy technicians are used to their fullest extent cannot be overemphasized. The pharmacist and pharmacy technician working together as a team can provide higher-quality patient care. There is a positive association between the use of pharmacy technicians and the extent of clinical services provided to patients.[3] With the proper use of pharmacy technicians, more of the pharmacist's time can be devoted to serving the patient rather than to the physical dispensing of the drug product.

Just within the dispensing and drug distribution roles, a pharmacist, using proper delegation and supervision, can consistently improve both the quality and quantity of the work by working as a team. The key is to have well-trained pharmacy technicians, pharmacists who recognize and know how to delegate and supervise technicians, and a pharmacy supervisor who recognizes, thanks, and rewards others for teamwork.

Pharmacy technicians can help achieve more work, free pharmacists to spend more time with patients, and can help keep pharmacists from making errors. The pharmacist should help pharmacy technicians learn, encourage pharmacy technicians to do more, and provide positive feedback and appreciation when pharmacy technicians do well. All of this advances teamwork, goodwill, and morale and enriches the workplace for everyone.

WHAT PHARMACY TECHNICIANS DO

Pharmacy technicians are trained to perform various functions within a pharmacy. These functions vary depending on the pharmacy. For example, what pharmacy technicians do in hospital pharmacies is different from what they do in community pharmacies. What pharmacy technicians do in mail-order pharmacies is slightly different from what they do in community pharmacies. What pharmacy technicians do in home care pharmacies is slightly different from what is done in hospital pharmacies. What pharmacy technicians do in pharmacies serving nursing homes is somewhat different from what they do in either hospitals or community pharmacies.

What a pharmacy technician is allowed to do in one state may not be allowed in another state because of differences in state laws and regulations. What a pharmacy technician may be allowed to do in one pharmacy may not be allowed in another pharmacy because of the policies and procedures of the owner or corporation, the institution, or the pharmacist under whom the pharmacy technician is working. All pharmacists are trained differently, and each pharmacist has biases about how the job should be done. Thus, pharmacy technicians need to be flexible and learn how each pharmacist wants things done. No matter what, a pharmacy technician should not be asked or allowed to do anything that would violate legal requirements.

Pharmacy technicians, if properly trained, can perform any of the dispensing and drug distribution functions of a pharmacist that does not involve professional judgment or is not restricted by law. The pharmacist must check all prescriptions dispensed before they leave the pharmacy's control (i.e., are given to a patient, caregiver, physician, nurse, etc.).

All pharmacy technicians may not be asked to do the same things. This will vary according to the ability and experience of the technician and whether the pharmacy is specialized or divides the work into specialized areas.

Functions of Pharmacy Supportive Personnel

Some specific functions performed by pharmacy supportive personnel are shown in Table 5.1, which lists functions by supportive personnel and what is typically performed in a community or hospital pharmacy. These functions will vary according to the size of the pharmacy, the number of people employed, and the direction of the pharmacist in charge.

The functions performed by hospital pharmacy technicians are different and more complex than those performed by technicians in community pharmacies. For example, after receiving training, hospital and community pharmacy technicians are allowed to compound some medications and add drugs to intravenous solutions (IVs) using aseptic technique by assuring that the solution remains sterile (not contaminated with bacteria or other infectious agents). This does not mean hospital pharmacy technicians are better than community pharmacy technicians, just different.

Pharmacy supportive personnel, especially pharmacy technicians, perform slightly different functions in specialty pharmacies, such as home health care, nuclear medicine, and consultant pharmacy (extended care). Pharmacy technicians in home health care pharmacies mostly prepare special IV additive solutions (for pain, infection, and nutrition) and medication for patients at home. These patients receive care from visiting

Table 5.1 Typical Functions of Supportive Personnel in Community and Hospital Pharmacies[a]

Supportive Personnel	Community Pharmacy	Hospital Pharmacy
Technicians	Receive the prescription	Interpret drug orders
	Verify patient information	Enter patient information and drug orders into computer system
	Read the prescription	Fill unit dose orders
	Enter information into computer	Prepare IV additive solutions and sometimes TPN and chemotherapy solutions
	Retrieve and return medication to stock	Prepackage drugs
	Count and pour medication	Order and inventory drugs
	Label the container	Compound medication
	Present to pharmacist for final check	Final check
Clerks and Assistants[b]	Wait on customers	Unpack medication
	Ring up sales	Stock shelves
	Unpack merchandise	Deliver medication
	Stock shelves	Perform clerical functions
	Prepare insurance forms	
	Other clerical duties	

[a] Functions vary by state law and may vary from pharmacy to pharmacy.
[b] And sometimes pharmacy technicians.

nurses and family as well as other health professionals — including pharmacists.

Pharmacy technicians working in nuclear pharmacies mainly help prepare low-level radioactive compounds that are injected into patients for use as diagnostic agents in nuclear medicine and radiology departments of hospitals. Pharmacy technicians working for *consultant pharmacists* prepare medications, according to a prescription, for patients in *extended care facilities* such as nursing homes, assisted-living centers and similar specialized nursing units.

WHAT PHARMACY TECHNICIANS NEED TO KNOW

Pharmacy technicians need various knowledge, skills, and abilities to help pharmacists and patients.[4] The basic knowledge, skills, and abilities for pharmacy technicians include:

- Communicating pleasantly and effectively with patients, prescriber offices, and coworkers
- Having good spelling and reading skills
- Having good math and pharmacy calculations skills
- Reading and understanding medical terminology, pharmacy jargon, and abbreviations
- Understanding and remembering generic and trade names of drugs
- Reading and interpreting prescriptions and drug orders
- Having good computer skills
- Selecting the correct drug
- Performing pharmaceutical calculations
- Counting and measuring medication
- Compounding drugs (hospital)
- Labeling medication containers
- Using aseptic techniques (hospital and home health care)

Successful pharmacy technicians need to be alert, organized, tidy, dedicated, good at communicating, responsible, and detail oriented. Although they should be able to work alone, they should also be willing and able to take directions from, and have their work checked by, *pharmacy interns* (who are pharmacy students in training and are registered by state boards of pharmacy) and pharmacists. They must appreciate the importance of always being precise and accurate. Candidates interested in becoming pharmacy technicians cannot have a prior record of drug or substance abuse.

HOW PHARMACY SUPPORTIVE PERSONNEL ARE TRAINED

In the past, most pharmacy supportive personnel were trained informally and on-the-job. Most of the on-the-job training was done by observing another worker. This is still true for pharmacy clerks and assistants, but it is less true for pharmacy technicians. Therefore, many pharmacy technicians have received some formal training either where they work, in an educational program, or both. Pharmacy employers prefer pharmacy technician applicants who have been formally trained, have experience as a pharmacy technician, and have strong customer service and communication skills.

Currently, there are some state, but no federal, requirements for training pharmacy supportive personnel. In Washington, the pharmacy technician must complete a state board of pharmacy–approved training program, which usually lasts 16 weeks.[5] After completion of the training program, the technician must pass a final test and complete 500 hours of training to receive a certificate.

Because there are still no legal requirements in most states to train pharmacy technicians, some employers elect to train pharmacy technicians informally and on-the-job. This is especially true in community pharmacies. Seeing the need to train community pharmacy technicians better, the National Association of Chain Drugstores and the National Community Pharmacy Association (representing independent retail pharmacies), developed *The Community Retail Pharmacy Technician Training Manual.*[6]

Formal education and training programs for pharmacy technicians are available at some hospitals, proprietary schools, vocational and technical colleges, and community colleges. Some common requirements to be accepted into a formal pharmacy technician program include a high school degree and a satisfactory working knowledge of English, mathematics, chemistry, and health education.

A model curriculum for formal pharmacy technician programs has been developed by the American Society of Health-System Pharmacists (ASHP; which is also the national accrediting body for pharmacy technician (PHT) educational programs).[7] The curriculum centers around 12 major areas of job responsibility and 18 knowledge and skill areas. The model curriculum contains 35 training modules. In addition, some technician training programs require clerkships or internships where students gain experience working in pharmacies. Students receive a diploma, certificate, or an associate degree, depending on the program.

Pharmacy technician training programs can receive *accreditation* — assurance that the program meets minimum standards as an acceptable program to most pharmacists. The main objectives of accreditation are to (a) upgrade and standardize the formal training that pharmacy technicians receive; (b) guide, assist, and recognize those health care facilities and academic institutions that wish to support the profession by operating such programs; (c) provide criteria for the prospective technician trainee in the selection of a program by identifying those institutions conducting accredited pharmacy technician programs; and (d) provide prospective employees a basis for determining the competency of pharmacy technicians by identifying technicians who have successfully completed accreditation.

In an article titled "Has the Time Come for National Standards on Technician Training," the issue arose as to whether the Accreditation Council For Pharmacy Education should establish uniform national standards for technician training. This issue was spurred on by the ASHP setting pharmacy technician training standards in eight areas:[8]

- Administrative responsibility for the program
- Qualifications of the training site
- Qualifications of the pharmacy service
- Qualifications of the program director and preceptors
- Qualifications and selection of the applicant
- The technician training program
- Experimentation and innovation
- Granting a certificate

To meet standards, technician training programs should provide a minimum of 600 hours of training over 15 weeks or more. A list of ASHP-accredited pharmacy technician programs is available from the ASHP or is available on the Worldwide Web.[9,10]

The issue of national standards for pharmacy technician training was also spurred on by "White Paper on Pharmacy Technicians 2002: Needed Changes Can no Longer Wait," which was endorsed by many pharmacy and pharmacy technician organizations.[11,12] This white paper is discussed later in this chapter.

TECHNICIAN CERTIFICATION AND COMPETENCY

Certification

In 1995, the pharmacy profession developed a voluntary, national *certi-fication* process for pharmacy technicians. Certification is a process by which a nongovernmental agency or association grants recognition to an individual who has met certain predetermined qualifications specified by that agency or association.[13] The Pharmacy Technician Certification Board (PTCB) was established to create one consolidated, national technician examination and certification process.

Certification helps pharmacy technicians formalize and even elevate their careers, including the feeling that they are truly part of a health care team. Employers know that individuals who pass the examination have a standardized body of knowledge. Passing the test increases the techni-cian's confidence, which increases the technician's performance in the pharmacy. Some pharmacists view the pharmacy certification process as comparable to completion of an associate degree. Certification also sets these technicians apart from uncertified technicians.[14] Many pharmacies are now requiring certification as a condition of employment. Such require-ments will help elevate the level of pharmacy practice.

The advantages of pharmacy certification to employers are decreases in the training time and cost of on-the-job training. Most of all, it indicates that the pharmacy technician has a certain knowledge about pharmacy practice. Eligible candidates must have a high school diploma or GED (general education development).

The Pharmacy Technician Certification Examination (PTCE) was initially based on the results of the 1991–1994 Scope of Pharmacy Project and was designed in collaboration with testing experts.[15] Today, a task force analysis by the PTCB serves as the basis for the test. The examination is a valid measure of the technician's knowledge and skill base for activities that are most commonly performed by a pharmacy technician, as determined by a national task analysis. The examination contains 125 questions, and candidates are given 3 hours to complete the test. The content of the examination covers tasks pharmacy technicians perform in various practice settings including community and institutional ones.[5]

The PTCE is administered three times a year at more than 120 sites across the nation. Pharmacy technicians who pass the examination (75 to 80% in 2005) earn the title of certified pharmacy technician. As of April 2006, 231,745 pharmacy technicians were certified.[16] The proportion of certified pharmacy technicians varies by type of pharmacy and geographical location.[17]

Renewal of certification is required every two years. A total of 20 hours of continuing education in pharmacy-related topics are required within the 2-year period. At least 1 hour shall be in the area of pharmacy law. A maximum of 10 hours may be carried out in practice sites (in-service projects) under the supervision of the pharmacist(s) for whom the certified pharmacy technician works. Certification will be removed if the pharmacy technician does not take steps to recertify. A state board of pharmacy can also suspend a pharmacy technician from working for breaking the law or for behavior not appropriate for pharmacy personnel.[16]

Pharmacy technicians who would like to apply for certification can contact the PTCB at 2215 Constitution Avenue, NW, Washington, DC 20037-2985 or http://www.ptcb.org/Exam/apply.aspx. The telephone and fax numbers are, respectively, (800) 363-8012 and (202) 429-7596.

The cost of the PTCE in 2006 was $120. A survey revealed that 33% of chain pharmacies, 40% of hospitals, and 50% of independent pharmacies pay for their technicians to take the PTCE.[17]

Books and other study guides are available to help in preparing to take the PTCE. A practice exam is also available online from the PTCB. Some of these resources are listed at the end of this chapter.

Competency

Successfully passing the PTCE only assures a certain knowledge level. It does not measure competency. Competency is defined as being capable, sufficient, or adequate in what you are required to do. In the spring of 2000, the National Association of Boards of Pharmacy (NABP) passed a resolution supporting a national program for assessing the competencies necessary for technicians to assist in the practice of pharmacy.[18] How the NABP will ultimately assess technician competency is unknown. The NABP is also considering defining several categories of pharmacy supportive personnel and is in communication with the PTCB regarding their plans.

PHARMACY TECHNICIAN ORGANIZATIONS

It is important for pharmacy technicians to network with other pharmacy technicians and to belong to a membership organization that will represent them. Some pharmacist organizations, especially local and state, have membership categories for pharmacy technicians and provide specific continuing education and newsletter articles.[19,20] Among the national organizations that have special members affiliation for pharmacy technicians are the American Pharmacists Association, the ASHP and the National Community Pharmacy Association.[9]

Pharmacy technicians also have their own professional organizations. The National Pharmacy Technician Organization and the American Association of Pharmacy Technicians are the two national organizations for pharmacy technicians, and both have state chapters and growing memberships. Each has an annual convention, continuing education programs, and other services.

SUPERVISION OF PHARMACY TECHNICIANS

Good sense and the law require that a pharmacist ensure that the medicine prepared and dispensed from the pharmacy is correct for the patient. The pharmacist must make sure all drug products prepared by pharmacy technicians are checked. For public safety, some state boards of pharmacy have regulations about the number of pharmacy technicians a pharmacist can supervise. A survey of state pharmacy rules concerning the supervision of pharmacy technicians in hospitals[3] revealed that 9 states required a technician to pharmacist ratio of 1:1, 6 required 2:1, three required 3:1, 9 did not specify a ratio (but required a sufficient number of pharmacists and supportive personnel as thought necessary by the pharmacy director), and 24 did not mention a ratio. Some states permit a higher technician to pharmacist ratio if the technicians are certified.

The same survey developed a technician-restriction score (TRS) as a way to decide which states were the most and least restrictive.[3] Technician to pharmacist ratios and the extent of supervision were considered when composing the TRS for each state. A pharmacy regulation requiring "immediate and direct" supervision of a pharmacy technician, meaning the pharmacist has to be within the sight or sound of a pharmacist, would contribute to a higher TRS than if the pharmacist were merely required to be within the same building but responsible for the technician. A low technician to pharmacist ratio would contribute to a lower TRS than a high technician to pharmacist ratio. Based on TRS scores, 26 states were classified as less restrictive and 25 states were classified as more restrictive.

A national survey of hospital pharmacy services found that the technician to pharmacist ratio on pharmacy department payrolls was consistently 1:1, even for states that had a higher ratio allowed by law.[21] This finding suggests that the employment of more pharmacy technicians may be limited more by pharmacists or for cost reasons rather than by state rules and regulations.

Technician to pharmacist ratios are also regulated for community pharmacy practice by many state boards of pharmacy. These ratios are controversial. In one survey, nearly 6 of 10 pharmacist respondents were satisfied with their state's technician to pharmacist ratio, which was 1:1 or 2:1.[17] More pharmacists working in chain pharmacies (43%) than pharmacists working in independent pharmacies (28%) believe more pharmacy technicians to a pharmacist should be allowed.

Some pharmacists believe there should not be any technician to pharmacist ratio restrictions. Since the pharmacist is ultimately responsible for everything that happens in a pharmacy, they should control what is safe, how many pharmacy technicians should be used, and how the technicians are supervised. However, other pharmacists and some state boards of pharmacy are wary of not having mandated technician to pharmacist ratios, because it may make it easier for a profit goal to supersede a safety goal.

Another safety feature being used in some states is the *registration* of pharmacy technicians, similar to the way pharmacists are registered. Registration is being officially enrolled on an existing list.[13] It is a mechanism through which states can monitor the individuals employed as technicians. State boards of pharmacy will be able to keep a record of any complaints or remedial actions about a pharmacy technician, which will help protect the public. Some states, such as Texas and Wyoming, require technicians to be certified, and some states differentiate between certified and noncertified technicians in permissable tasks.

BEING A PROFESSIONAL PHARMACY TECHNICIAN

Being a pharmacy technician can be a rewarding career. For those who seek such a career and would like fulfillment and job satisfaction, it will take more than just knowledge, skills, and abilities to do the job. It takes commitment, hard work, and being professional.

A *professional* is someone qualified to perform the activities of a profession, who has character, sensitivity to others, and the desire to fulfill ethical and professional standards. Pharmacy technicians must realize that they represent the time-honored profession of pharmacy. They also must respect the profession by their dress, their personal hygiene, their character, and how they serve and treat others.

All patients, pharmacists, and coworkers must be treated with respect. The pharmacy technician should be courteous, polite, and listen and communicate well. The pharmacy technician must also respect confidentiality, whether it involves a patient, a coworker, or the business for which the technician is working.

Pharmacy technicians should understand the impact — positive or negative, minor or major — they can have on the pharmacy service. Valuable technicians will make the pharmacy practice and business more successful in the areas of quality of care and economics. Part of the job of pharmacists and pharmacy technicians is to make the pharmacy service better and more successful. It is true that the more successful the pharmacy service, the more successful are the pharmacists and pharmacy technicians who work there.

Having a good attendance record and getting to work on time is important, as is getting along well with coworkers and volunteering to do extra work. This is what pharmacists like to see and hear from pharmacy technicians.

Earnings

Median hourly earnings of wage and salary pharmacy technicians in May 2004 were $11.37. The middle 50% earned between $9.40 and $13.85.[2]

Working Conditions

Pharmacy technicians work in clean, organized, well-lit, and well-ventilated areas conducive to doing professional work. Pharmacy technicians spend most of their day standing. There also may be some heavy lifting.

Pharmacy technicians work the same hours as pharmacists, and in organized health care settings, there are usually three shifts — days (7 a.m. to 3 p.m.), evenings (3 p.m. to 11 p.m.), and nights (11 p.m. to 7 a.m.). Most pharmacy technicians work 35 to 40 hours a week. There are many opportunities for part-time work in retail and hospital settings and some opportunities for overtime work.

Some pharmacies are busier than others. In fact, some are fast-paced and some experience a high level of distractions. In these settings, pharmacists and pharmacy technicians need to be vigilant and cautious about committing errors of commission and omission and have double-check systems employed.

Workflows vary from site to site, and pharmacy technicians need to adjust to changing conditions. This can be stressful.

Satisfaction

There have only been a few studies completed on pharmacy technician satisfaction. It is known that there is greater satisfaction when pharmacy technicians feel that they are a part of a care team or work in decentralized pharmacies in hospitals.[22,23] Other factors that improve satisfaction are positive relationships with coworkers, job variety, and training. Factors contributing to dissatisfaction are work procedures, workload, staffing, and lack of recognition.[24]

Advancement and Expanded Roles

Most pharmacy technicians start in an entry-level position and are supervised carefully even when doing the most basic functions. Once the pharmacist employer or supervisor has had an opportunity to observe and work with the pharmacy technician, the pharmacy technician may be given more leeway and less direct supervision. Some pharmacies have career ladder programs. These programs allow the pharmacy technician to advance to higher-level functions and receive more pay.[25] Some pharmacy technicians may become specialized, such as those working in special types of pharmacies (consultant pharmacies, nuclear pharmacies, etc.) or performing specific functions (i.e., inventory control, purchasing). Others may supervise other technicians as head or lead technicians.

In general, many pharmacy leaders and pharmacists are hoping that as more pharmacy technicians are certified, technician roles will be expanded so pharmacists can delegate dispensing functions and spend more time with patients. In some pharmacies, technicians are allowed to prepare medication with the pharmacist checking the computer entry versus the prescription or drug order and the medication to be dispensed against the prescription or drug order. In some hospital pharmacies, technicians are allowed to check other technicians for preparation of IVs and certain categories of drugs within the unit dose system. This reduces the number of pharmacists needed in dispensing, specifically, computer entry, drug selection, and labeling.

In dispensing, the ideal would be for pharmacists to take oral prescription orders, oversee the controlled substances, check the final product (including the prescription, drug labeling, and computer entry), and leave the rest to certified pharmacy technicians.

JOB OUTLOOK

The job outlook for pharmacy technicians is bright. The number of prescriptions dispensed yearly is expected to rise dramatically and exceeded four billion in 2006. This is mostly due to the rising number of senior citizens as well as changes in Medicare and other programs and the universality of prescription coverage in health insurance plans. In addition, a recent survey has shown that pharmacists spend two-thirds of their time in technical and nonjudgmental tasks, whereas they prefer to spend time making sure the drugs are prescribed and used correctly.[26] Almost all of these technical and nonjudgmental functions can be performed by pharmacy technicians or by using automation.

The recruitment of competent pharmacy technicians is already getting more difficult. Most chain store pharmacies are having a harder time recruiting pharmacy technicians, as are independent pharmacists and hospitals.[17] Perhaps because recruiting has gotten so difficult, many employers do not advertise specifically for certified pharmacy technicians. However, the most sought after pharmacy technicians will be those with certification, formal training, experience, and knowledge of automation.

WHITE PAPER ON NEEDED CHANGES

In 2002, 12 organizations authored a white paper on needed changes with pharmacy supportive personnel.[12] The white paper documented the history of pharmacy technicians in the United States and the need for more technicians based on the pharmacist's expanding scope of practice and the rising number of prescriptions. The paper then outlined 13 recommendations in 5 areas: vision (3); roles, responsibilities, and competencies (2); education and training (3); credentialing and accreditation (2); and the regulation (3) of pharmacy technicians in the United States. The most significant of these recommendations were the calls for standards for the education and training and for determining the competencies required for high-level performance at each level of pharmacy supportive personnel.

SUMMARY

Pharmacy technicians play an important role in providing efficient and quality pharmacy products and services for patients. The more education, training, and experience pharmacy technicians have, the more qualified they become. Coupled with national certification, a good work attitude and record can make for a successful career. For some people, starting as pharmacy technicians can ultimately enhance their careers as pharmacists – should they decide to continue their professional education.

The job market for pharmacy technicians is expected to grow with the increase in the number of prescriptions as the U.S. population grows older. In addition, the role of technicians is expected to expand as pharmacists expand their clinical role with patients. Well-trained pharmacy technicians who act professionally and seek a career as a pharmacy technician have bright futures.[27]

DISCUSSION QUESTIONS AND EXERCISES

1. Some state boards of pharmacy have technician to pharmacist ratios (e.g., 2:1 or 3:1) that set the number of technicians one pharmacist can supervise. Are these ratios a good or bad thing?
2. Make an appointment to interview a certified pharmacy technician and a technician who is not certified. Ask both technicians the same questions and record your answers. Compare your results.
3. Make an appointment with one community and one hospital pharmacist to find out how they feel about using certified pharmacy technicians versus uncertified pharmacy technicians. What are their opinions about mandatory technician to pharmacist ratios? Compare your results.
4. Which do you feel is more efficient: using three pharmacists and no pharmacy technicians or using two pharmacists and three certified technicians. Why?
5. Name three functions pharmacy technicians cannot perform in pharmacy.
6. Name three functions pharmacy technicians can perform in most states that will free pharmacists to spend more time with patients.
7. A patient receives the wrong medication. A pharmacy technician comes to you (the pharmacist) and says that he or she made the error but that you checked it and said it was okay. Who is responsible for this error?
8. Should pharmacy technicians be allowed to check each other's drug preparations so the pharmacist can spend more time with patients? Why or why not?
9. Who should greet and take the prescription from the patient: the pharmacy clerk, the pharmacy technician, or the pharmacist? Who should give the medication to the patient?
10. In the scenario in question 9:

a. Which is most cost-efficient?

b. Which will free the pharmacist to spend the most time with patients?

CHALLENGES

1. For the pharmacy student. It is important for pharmacists and pharmacy technicians to be "on the same page" to maximize benefits to patients and to have a harmonious working environment. For extra credit, and with the permission of your professor, prepare a concise report on working with pharmacy technicians. In doing this, interview a seasoned pharmacy technician about the pros and cons and pet peeves of being a pharmacy technician.

2. For the pharmacy technician student. Working in a community pharmacy and hospital pharmacy are very different. For extra credit, and with the permission of your professor, prepare a concise report on these contrasting environments from the point of view of a pharmacy technician. In doing this, you should make on-site observations in both settings.

WEB SITES OF INTEREST

National Pharmacy Technician Association: http://www.pharmacytechnician.org/

Pharmacy Technician Certification Board: http://www.ptcb.org/

Am. Association of Pharmacy Technicians: http://www.pharmacytechnician.com

Pharmacy Technician Educators Council: http://www.pharmacy.org/pharmtech.html

ADDITIONAL PHARMACY TECHNICIAN TEXTS AND RESOURCES

The Pharmacy Technician: Hogan, D, and Shrewsbury, R, et al: Perspective Press/Morton Publishing Company, 2004.

Pharmacy Practice for Technicians: Durgin, J, and Hanan, Z. Delmar Publishers, 2003.

Pharmacy Practice for Technicians: Ballington, D. EMC-Paradigm Publishers, 2003.

Pharmacy Technician Principles and Practice: Hopper, T. Mosby/Saunders/Elsevier, 2003.

Pharmacy Technician Workbook and Certification Review: Perspective Press/Morton Publishing Company, 1999.

The Pharmacy Technician Companion: Harteker, L. APhA, 1998.

Certification Review for Pharmacy Technicians: Reifman, N. ARK Pharmacy Consultants, 2003.

National Certification Technician Manual: Lile, J, Miller, D, and Pakkula, J. Michigan Pharmacists Association, 2001.

Ethics for Pharmacy Technicians: Buerki, R, and Vottero, L. AIHP, 2001.

ACKNOWLEDGMENT

The writing of this chapter was assisted by Harold L. Bober, R.Ph., Ph.D., Director of Pharmacy Technician Programs at Front Range Community College in Westminster, CO.

REFERENCES

1. American Society of Health-System Pharmacists. White paper on pharmacy technicians. *Am J Health-Syst-Pharm.* 1996;53:1793–1799.
2. U.S. Department of Labor, Bureau of Labor Statistics. Pharmacy Technicians. Available at http://www.bls.gov/oco/ocos252.htm. Accessed April 17, 2006.
3. Raehl, CL, Pitterle, ME, and Bond, CA. Legal status and functions of hospital-based pharmacy technicians and their relationship to clinical pharmacy services. *Am J Hosp Pharm.* 1992;49:2179–2187.
4. Stoogenke, MM. *The Pharmacy Technician.* Brady, Prentice Hall, Upper Saddle River, NJ, 1998.
5. Collins, PM. The pharmacy technician: a valuable asset in today's pharmacy. *Wash Pharm.* 1999;41(2):38–39.
6. Schafermeyer, KW, and Hobson, EH. *The Community Retail Pharmacy Technician Training Manual.* National Association of Chain Drug Stores and NARD, Alexandria, VA, 1999.
7. Model Curriculum for Pharmacy Technician Training. American Society of Health-Systems Pharmacists. Bethesda, MD, Available at http://www.ashp.org.
8. Durgin, JM, Sr., and Hanan, ZI. *Pharmacy Practice for Technicians.* Delmar, Albany, NY, 2004.
9. AK Harvey Whitney, ed. *Pharmacy Technician Education and Training: 1997 Directory.* Harvey Whitney Books, Cincinnati, OH, 1997.
10. American Society of Health-Systems Pharmacists. Pharmacy Technician Training Programs. Available at www.ashp.org/public/links.html. Accessed February 13, 2001.
11. Chi, J. Has the time come for national standards on technician training? *Drug Topics Arch.* January 26, 2004.
12. Rouse MJ. White paper on pharmacy technicians 2002: needed changes can no longer wait. *Am J Health-Syst Pharm.* 2003;60:37–51.
13. Gosselin, AG, and Robbins, J. Pharmacy technicians. In *Inside Pharmacy: The Anantomy of a Profession.* Technomic, Lancaster, PA, 1999, chap. 7.

14. Knowlton, HL. Benefits of a board-certified technician. *Am J Health-Syst Pharm.* 1997;54:2562–2565.

15. Anonymous. Summary of the final report of the Scope of Pharmacy Project. *Am J Hosp Pharm.* 1994;51:2179–2182.

16. Pharmacy Technician Certification Board. Available at http://www.ptcb.org/. Accessed April 17, 2006.

17. Conlan, MF. Tech's time. *Drug Top.* 1999;143:52–54, 59–60.

18. Landis, NT. NABP proposes national competence assessment for technicians: standard roles, requirement considered by task force. *Am J Health-Syst Pharm.* 2000;57:1204.

19. Kranz, BJ. The many aspects of pharmacy. *Fla J Hosp Pharm.* 1994;14(Nov): 16–18.

20. Jayne, J. Recognize technicians as part of pharmacy team. *Mich Pharm.* 1998;November:3–7.

21. Raehl, CL, Bond, CA, and Pitterle, ME. Pharmaceutical services in U.S. hospitals in 1992. *Am J Hosp Pharm.* 1992;49:323–346.

22. Trevarrow, BJ. Pharmacy technicians as members of care teams. *Am J Health-Syst Pharm.* 1998;55:1810–1812.

23. Rycek, WA, Kuhrt, MM, and Alexander, ML. Making the most of pharmacy technicians. *Am J Health-Syst Pharm.* 2000;57:2160–2162.

24. Braun, LD, Holloway, BA, Hoffman, RL, et al. Use of a pharmacy department employee survey to reduce employee turnover and improve job satisfaction. *American Society of Health System Pharmacists, Midyear Clinical Meeting;* 1990;25:392D.

25. Strozyk, WR, and Underwood, DA. Development and benefits of a pharmacy technician career ladder. *Am J Hosp Pharm.* 1994;51:666–669.

26. Cardinale, V. New chain study supports need for more ancillary personnel. *Drug Top.* 2000;144:54.

27. Whitney, HAK. A career as a technician. *J Pharm Technol.* 1987;3:169–170.

6

PHARMACY TECHNOLOGY
AND AUTOMATION

Technology has penetrated health care. The computer, like no other single instrument, has changed the way overall health care is practiced. Information technology and automation have also changed the way pharmacy is practiced, and it will continue to do so for some time.

Information technology and automation improve the medication-use process and can help advance pharmacy practice and pharmaceutical care. It is important that the use of technology and automation in pharmacy practice be well thought out and used correctly.

This chapter will discuss the difference between pharmacy technology and automation, the importance of each, and describe how each is used. The types of automation used in pharmacy will be presented. Steps in moving to a more automated approach to pharmacy and why information technology and automation are so important to pharmacy will also be covered.

LEARNING OBJECTIVES

After reading this chapter, you should be able to:

- Define information technology
- Define pharmacy automation
- State six benefits of using information technology and automation in pharmacy
- State some of the challenges of implementing and using pharmacy technology and automation
- State the three general types of pharmacy automation

- Name three specific types of automated dispensing devices used in the pharmacy
- Name three general types of automated dispensing devices used in patient care areas
- Discuss the pros and cons of using pharmacy automation from the standpoint of safety

INFORMATION TECHNOLOGY VERSUS AUTOMATION

Information technology refers to the storage, access, and use of information stored in a database (software) that can be accessed using computers. *Pharmacy automation* is an aggregate of two or more physical components and a set of procedures in the pharmacy medication process that function together.[1]

Pharmacy should use technology and automation for several reasons: (a) to improve medication safety, (b) to improve patient care, (c) to improve efficiency of the medication process, and (d) to improve the documentation of care.

IMPROVED SAFETY

Information technology and automation should improve patient safety by building into the medication process a system of checks and balances that would be humanly impossible to know, remember, and to perform. Computers can track and check hundreds of procedures and let the users know when possible problems are discovered.

IMPROVED PATIENT CARE

By incorporating various standards of practice and care plans, the computer system can track all orders and check patient results and thus track actual performance versus desired performance. The computer can also provide reminders to the users of how to improve performance.

IMPROVED EFFICIENCY

Computers work much faster than humans. Thus, when properly set up, computer systems can process medication orders, provide documents and information about patients, and help prepare medication for patients. Medication orders can be processed faster, and patients can receive their medication sooner.

IMPROVED DOCUMENTATION OF CARE

The use of technology and automation can provide details on what has taken place in the drug-use process — the processing, preparation, dispensing, and administration of medication. Such details and documentation cannot be provided by manual systems.

USE OF PHARMACY TECHNOLOGY AND AUTOMATION

Pharmacy technology and automation are relatively new in pharmacy. The first national survey to discover the use of pharmacy automation in the United States took place in 1996.[2] At that time, very little information technology and automation was being used in pharmacy, except for packaging and counting medication.

In 2002, the American Society of Health-System Pharmacists (ASHP) conducted a national survey of hospital settings to determine the status of dispensing and administration.[3] An estimated 8% (up from 4.5% in 1999) of hospitals use a robotic drug distribution system. This system automates the dispensing of unit doses to inpatients from a central pharmacy. The slow adoption of this beneficial system appears to be based on the cost.

The ASHP survey also discovered that a majority (58%) of hospitals are employing point-of-use automatic dispensing machines (ADMs) that work like bank ATMs in their decentralized areas (nursing units) of the hospital. In those hospitals using ADMs, 82.2% had pharmacists check the accuracy and integrity of the medications placed into the devices, either before or after replenishment. In 72.4% of cases, the ADM was linked to the pharmacy computer system.

The most notable use of pharmacy automation is in Veterans Administration (VA) Medical Centers.[4] The VA system has seven regional consolidated mail-order pharmacies (CMOPs) that use extensive automation to prepare medication for VA outpatients. Three more CMOPs are planned (see Mail-Order Pharmacy in Chapter 19).

The adoption of new pharmacy technology and automation to improve efficiency and patient safety is slow. The three most common reasons it is not going faster seem to be that automation costs too much, we are unable to justify buying the equipment to upper-level managers, and there is not enough space to house the equipment.

Although the use of technology and automation is not as developed in the retail pharmacy setting as it is in hospital pharmacy, chain store pharmacies are starting to use more and more pharmacy automation.[5] The use of pharmacy technology and automation in the retail practice setting is being fueled by a need for improved productivity, the increasing number of prescriptions to be filled, and the current pharmacist shortage.

INFORMATION TECHNOLOGY

Information technology stores, accesses, and uses information in a database that can be accessed by pharmacists using computers. This technology provides information to pharmacists about drugs, drug therapy, and patients. The information may be on the Internet, stored in a database at a remote location, or stored in the memory of the pharmacy's computer.

Hospitals and hospital pharmacists have recognized the need for, have embraced, and have moved quicker than community pharmacy in integrating and using information technology and automation.[5] However, community pharmacy's use of information technology and automation is changing.

Computers and databases of information have removed the need for paperwork, increased access to information, speeded up information processing, are being used to increase market share, and have freed up and made tools available for pharmacists to practice pharmaceutical care.

Less Paperwork

Pharmacies used to have a lot of paperwork. This included prescription records, manual patient profiles, controlled substance records, and insurance information. Insurance claims had to be written, copies made, and the original sent to the third-party payer. Computer storage has nearly eliminated these procedures.

Faster Access to Information

Pharmacies linked to the Internet now have information at their fingertips almost at lightening speed. Access to information about new drugs, old drugs, drug therapy, and diseases are available with only a few clicks of the computer mouse. Pharmacists can read articles, answer quizzes, and gain continuing education credit without leaving their pharmacies or their homes. All of this was impossible just a few years ago.

An example of new information technology is the National Institutes of Health's new alternative and complementary medicine database.[6] Pharmacists have a difficult time keeping up-to-date on these products. Thus, if a patient asks the pharmacist about an unfamiliar herbal product, the pharmacist can find the information at http://nccam.nih.gov with the click of the computer mouse.

Another example of information at your fingertips is Epocrates® — mobile pharmacy software for your handheld device. Handheld devices, like those made by Palm and others, can hold drug and formulary information that is updated routinely for the user. Many pharmacists and doctors carry these with them wherever they go.

Increased Speed in Processing Information

A major advantage of computers is their speed. This is important in pharmacy, where there is no end to the increased number of prescriptions to dispense and insurance claims to process. The increased processing of orders helps efficiency and we hope improves safety. The increased processing and electronic transfer of insurance claims improves cash flow for businesses.[5]

Hospital pharmacy computers are either linked to a total information system or linked to other computer systems within the hospital. Thus, they have access to patient information, including a patient's latest laboratory findings so that the pharmacist can help provide appropriate care. Some hospital pharmacies can receive order information directly from medical staff members' private offices.

A development in hospitals is the movement toward computerized prescriber order entry (CPOE) systems. These are systems in which prescribers order their medication, laboratory tests, and diets by entering them directly into a computer using keystrokes, light pens, touch screens, or voice activation.[7]

Unlike hospital pharmacies, community pharmacies are seldom linked to health care patient databases or physicians' offices. Thus, patient information has to be gained from the patient, and thus the information is limited. However, this is changing. One company is linking patients, physicians, pharmacies, other health care providers, and insurance carriers into a single system.[5] Patient confidentiality will need to be assured before such a system becomes operational. The system will start as a national claims and resolution center.

It will not be long before physicians will be able to order medication using a computer or by talking into a hand-held device and then transfering the prescription to the patient's pharmacy. This will save a lot of time in the pharmacy, should reduce medication errors from improved handwriting legibility, and free pharmacists to spend more time with patients.

Increasing Market Share

Community pharmacies are starting to use the computer in creative ways to increase market share. They have taken the lead from physicians, who have developed *telemedicine*. One telemedicine company helps improve patient care by bringing intensive care unit patients to intensivists, critical care physicians who are scarce and who are remotely located.[8] Patient information, on-time real-time transmission of electronic monitoring of the patient, and two-way pictures and conversations with patients, nurses, and physicians on the scene can take place.

Another example of telemedicine is how patients can buy on-line consultations with physicians over the Internet. Although this will never replace a physical examination by the physician, it can provide much needed information and advice on whether the patient should see a physician, go to the emergency room, or not worry about the problem.[9]

Pharmacy has now started down the road of *telepharmacy*,[10] which includes the dispensing of medications and information and the provision of pharmaceutical care to patients from a distance.[11] Some community pharmacies, especially some chain store pharmacies, are starting to use the computer to accept orders for prescription refills and to send prescription refill reminders to patients.[5]

Some on-line (Internet) pharmacies accept new prescriptions from patients. However, some of these may not be licensed pharmacies, and patients need to be cautious about this.[11] In addition, a recent survey of 300 adult on-line consumers revealed that most people would rather patronize their local pharmacy than a *virtual pharmacy*.[12] The reasons provided for not liking an on-line pharmacy included less comfort level with the pharmacist, insurance not accepted, physician not being able to enter the prescription on-line, and the service being more expensive.

Tools for Pharmaceutical Care

Computers and information technology can provide tools and help free up pharmacists to practice pharmaceutical care. Computers can store patient information to help pharmacists check patients and make recommendations to physicians on the appropriate use of medication. Computers can help screen patients and provide lists of patients who might benefit from the care of a pharmacist. They also can perform complex pharmacokinetic dosing calculations and check for problems in dosage, overlapping therapy, and drug interactions.

New information and patient monitoring technology is becoming available regularly. One example of a device that pharmacists can use to monitor patients is DynaPulse (PulseMetric Inc., San Diego, CA). DynaPulse is a noninvasive device that can be used to monitor blood pressure and 16 hemodynamic values in patients in less than a minute. These results can be stored in a computer for documentation and future reference and can be sent over the Internet to the patient's physician.

E-Prescribing

E-prescribing (electronic prescribing) is the use of an automated data entry system to generate and send a prescription to the community pharmacist, rather than writing it on paper and giving it to the patient. Automation of the outpatient prescribing process has many potential benefits, especially increased safety.

The challenges associated with E-prescribing are getting doctors to use it and settling who will pay for the equipment and software. In 2003, small groups of doctors in the Boston area started using and evaluating e-prescribing.[13] Investigators found that patients love it and recognize that it removes mistakes and decreases time spent in the pharmacy.

In 2005, SureScripts, a network provider of electronic prescribing services, announced an agreement with Epic Systems Corporation to connect the EpicCare EMR (electronic medical record) to the SureScripts network, enabling thousands of physicians to prescribe and transmit prescriptions electronically to more than 85% of retail pharmacies.[14] This, and the requirements for e-prescribing in the new Medicare Part D benefit, will soon make writing prescriptions by hand obsolete.

Computerized Prescriber Order Entry

One technique utilized to improve prescribing and transcribing accuracy is the use of computerized prescriber order entry (CPOE) systems. CPOE allows prescribers to enter their orders directly into the hospital information system, either on a terminal in the hospital, or sometimes from their handheld Palm devices or office computers.

Integrating *clinical decision-support systems* (CDSS) with CPOE is the key ingredient to improving prescribing practices and safety. CDSS is software that includes rule sets, and when these rules are violated, the prescriber sees an alert that something may be wrong (too much drug, a drug interaction, or a contraindication for the drug).

Summary

Information technology is improving pharmacy practice by improving efficiency, providing more and faster access to information, and helping free up pharmacists to do pharmaceutical care. This, in turn, is helping improve pharmacists' morale and professionalism.[5]

AUTOMATION

A Brief History

Pharmacy automation started in the late 1960s with the use of tablet-counting machines — units that held medication and had a dial for setting the number to be counted. The medication container was placed below an opening in the device that delivered the tablets into a container. During the 1980s, the first device to automate the preparation of *total parenteral nutrition* (TPN) solutions became available. The first automated unit-dose filling machine was available in the early 1990s. Many automated medication-use products are now available.

Since the first national survey on pharmacy automation in the United States in 1996, the use of automation has slowly increased and should dramatically increase over the next 10 years. With the growth projections for retail prescriptions showing no signs of slowdown, the current shortage of pharmacists, and the cost cutting going on in hospitals, automation in pharmacy may increase dramatically. Such growth should also reduce one of the barriers to using automation — cost.

Benefits of Pharmacy Automation

The benefits of using pharmacy automation are improved speed, accuracy, documentation, and efficiency and the ability to analyze, compare, and provide new information.

Improved speed: Microprocessors in automated equipment are able to process information at almost lightening speeds. This speed is needed in the medication process so the time from when the physician writes the medication order until the patient receives the first dose is the shortest possible.

Improved accuracy: Unless there is a human programming or intervention error, computers are flawless at computing and processing information. This is needed in the medication process to remove errors. When set up properly, computer-driven automated processes should substantially reduce medication errors.

Improved documentation: Without a doubt, a major advantage of computers and automated medication devices is their ability to document what has taken place in a clear format. Who ordered the drug, who dispensed it, who checked it, who gave it, how much they gave, and when it was given is automatically recorded. This improved documentation helps when a rare *medicolegal* problem arises and for finding out what happened and how the process can improve.

Improved efficiency: Pharmacy automation can do the work of many people, and salaries are the highest health care cost. Automation can save salary costs, can free pharmacy technicians to do other important tasks, and can free pharmacists to do pharmaceutical care.

Ability to analyze, compare, and provide new information: Pharmacy automation is starting to advance to the next level, which is to analyze and compare information, based on criteria set up by practitioners, and provide new information and recommendations to improve patient care. For example, automated pharmacy systems, based on data analysis and a decision tree, can elect not to dispense a medication until the information is reviewed by a pharmacist.

Challenges of Pharmacy Automation

Some of the challenges of automation include the cost, space, fear of being replaced, and one error becoming many errors.

Cost: Currently, the major challenge to using pharmacy automation is cost.[2] Pharmacy automation is expensive. Automated unit-dose dispensing equipment in a medium to large hospital can cost a half million to over a million dollars. Automated equipment for community pharmacies is also costly; thus, decisions to buy these devices must be carefully considered. The benefits must outweigh the costs. It must be remembered that other costs will be saved after using automation. In addition, equipment purchases can be amortized and depreciated, which produce savings over time. Automation will also bring more organization, and the pharmacist will have more control and hopefully more time to spend with patients.

Space: One problem with pharmacy automation is squeezing the equipment into pharmacies that are already too small to do what they do now. Some renovation of space may be needed to house some types of automation. The equipment manufacturers have been working to decrease the size of their equipment.

Fear of being replaced: When automation first arrived, pharmacy technicians and some pharmacists feared that they would be replaced when pharmacy automation became available. However, with time this fear has been reduced with the increasing volume of work and the shortage of pharmacists.[15]

One error can become many errors: Pharmacy automation can either decrease errors or make them worse.[16,17] If an automated preparation and dispensing device is not set up correctly, the same error can be repeated many times until the error is discovered. Soon after automated compounding devices that make TPN solutions became available, it was discovered that these devices, when set up incorrectly, can make repeated and potentially lethal errors.

Selecting Pharmacy Automation

Buying an automated dispensing system can be a daunting task. One can become easily overwhelmed by all the different types of equipment. The ASHP recently published some basic steps to help make the job easier in selecting an automated dispensing system.[18] First, identify the issues that need to be resolved by the equipment or system. Second, decide the system features you want. Third, compare your findings with what the current technology offers.

THE MARKET FOR PHARMACY AUTOMATION

Despite the slow adoption of pharmacy automation, there are estimations that the market for pharmacy automation in 2003 was $1.4 billion and that the annual growth would be 11.7% to reach nearly $2.5 billion in 2008.[19] It is estimated that in 2008, 80% of the market will be inpatient pharmacy automation systems, and 20% will be in ambulatory pharmacy automation systems.

If these estimations are correct, pharmacies will be acquiring much more automation from 2003 to 2008.

Types of Pharmacy Automation

There are three general types of pharmacy automation: (a) tablet counters, (b) intravenous (IV) compounders, and (c) dispensing machines.

Tablet Counters

These devices count oral solids (tablets and capsules). The first such device was the Baker Cell. Today there are many other kinds of these devices. Some pharmacies have as many as 100 to 200 counting cells to count and dispense their top 100 to 200 drugs. Once the medication order is placed into the computer, a message is sent to the counting device for the drug, and the device counts and dispenses the drug into a prescription container. A label is also created by the pharmacy computer, but it must be placed on the container manually.

IV Compounders

Most of these devices are for compounding TPN solutions. The machine is connected by separate lines to various bulk IV solutions (e.g., D5W, NS, and D50W), bulk electrolytes (e.g., KCl), vitamins (e.g., A, B, and C), and minerals (e.g., iron). The compounder must be programmed to know which line contains which bulk IV, electrolyte, vitamin, and mineral. When making a TPN solution, the pharmacy technician or pharmacist attaches a main IV line coming from the IV compounder into a sterile container that will contain the TPN solution. The compounder is then set to deliver the needed quantities of ingredients for the TPN solution, and the machine fills the container automatically.

Dispensing Machines

Dispensing automation is the largest category of equipment. Pharmacy automation is now categorized by where it is used: in the central pharmacy, in decentralized areas, or other pharmacy automation. Devices can be divided into two basic kinds: (a) systems that repackage medications from bulk and (b) systems that use overpackaged, manufacturer-wrapped unit-of-use.[16]

Some manufacturers do not provide their medication in *unit-dose* (single, unit-of-use) packaging for patients in hospitals or *blister packs* (cards with multiple unit-doses of a medication for patients in nursing homes). The medication in the blister pack can be pushed out of the card with a finger when needed. Most health system pharmacies and consultant pharmacists use various repackaging and labeling machines to put medications sold to them in multidose bottles into unit-doses or in blister packs. Pharmacy technicians load the bulk medications into the devices and package one medication at a time.

Some of the more advanced packaging and labeling devices stock multiple lines of medication in different containers that are hand filled by pharmacy technicians. Some of the systems automate the production of compliance packs (medication labeled for day of the week). Compliance packs are used for subacute, long-term care, and ambulatory patients. The packs can be labeled with the patient's name, drug name, and dose.

For community pharmacy practice, there are systems that can be connected to the pharmacy computer, which once selected, can dispense a specific medication from an automated counting device that has been manually filled with bulk tablets of a medication. It will then fill a prescription container and label the bottle based on information it receives from the pharmacy computer. Pharmacies usually will have a cell for each of the most popular drugs.

One community pharmacy is using robotics to dispense 450 prescriptions a day.[20] Because the pharmacists no longer have to spend so much time in the dispensing process, they can spend more time counseling patients on the use of their medication.

Some health system pharmacies and some consultant pharmacists serving many nursing homes will have the medication that is not available in unit-dose packaging repackaged by *repackagers*, which are companies that specialize in putting bulk medication into unit-of-use (unit-dose) or blister packs (overpackages).

Once each dose of medication is in a single, unit-of-use package, either by buying or by packaging equipment in the pharmacy, it must be dispensed to the patient, hopefully using the best way to do this, which is the *unit-dose system* (see Chapter 9, Hospital Pharmacy). In manual unit-dose systems, pharmacy technicians pick individual doses of medication ordered for a patient and place them into the patient's unit-dose drawer. In *centralized* (in the central pharmacy) automated dispensing systems, bar-coded unit-doses of medication, based on information from the pharmacy computer system, are automatically dispensed using robotics into a patient's bar-coded medication drawer going by on a conveyor belt.

All the automatic devices discussed so far are used in the pharmacy. Automated dispensing machines (ADMs) can also be placed on the patient care units of hospitals or nursing homes. One brand name of ADMs is Pyxis. These devices are sometimes referred to as ATM-type devices like those used by banks to dispense money. All of these devices need user names and passwords and sometimes swipe cards for entry. Some are networked to the pharmacy computer or health system computer system and some are not; the latter is a floor stock system.

Most ADMs hold limited amounts of medication and therefore are usually used for narcotics, STAT (emergency), or first-time doses to get the patient started on the medication. Some newer ADMs can dispense 90 to 95% of the medications used on a patient care unit.[16] Some devices limit what can be accessed to a single dose of a medication or a single line of medication. Others allow access to multiple doses or to multiple doses of a multiple line of medications. The greater the access, the greater will be the likelihood of error.

Safety of Automated Devices

Have automated devices made medication administration safer? This is a good question, but the jury is still out. Automated devices in pharmacy have their pitfalls. First, the devices need to be loaded properly with the correct medication in the correct location. This procedure is critical and deserves strict policies and procedures to ensure everything will be all right. Who can load the device and whether there should be a double check on loading the device should be spelled out in a policy and procedure statement.[18]

Devices that use a bar code to check that the medication going into the device is correct are safer than those that do not have this check. Automated dispensing devices in the VA's CMOP system will not release the top of the automated device's storage area for medication until the medication is run past the bar code reader linked to the pharmacy computer and the computer gives a signal that everything is correct.

Assigning and keeping an up-to-date file in the computer of who may enter automated systems is a must. There is a tendency to rely on automated systems as being safe, and thus education and reminders are needed for those using automated dispensing systems to double-check everything and to think about what is being done. All doses removed from an ADM need to be double-checked against what the screen on the device is showing.

Until now, automated dispensing systems have not been *closed-looped* — the entire process checked by the computer before a medication is administered. This is how a closed-looped (also called *point-of-care*) system would work: Before a nurse administers a medication, the nurse runs a portable bar code reader across the patient's bar-coded wristband and then runs the portable bar code reader across the nurse's name badge that has a bar code identifying the nurse. Last, the nurse runs the portable bar code reader across the bar-coded unit-dose medication.

The information in the portable bar code reader is transmitted to the pharmacy or health system computer system. The system now knows the patient, the nurse, the medication, and the time of day. It checks this information against what has been ordered. If everything is correct, the bar code reader lights a green light letting the nurse know that the correct medication is being administered to the correct patient at the correct time of day. If not, the portable bar code reader will light a red light. Once the medication is administered, the nurse lets the system know the medication has been administered and the medication is automatically charted (recorded) as administered.

Closed-looped, point-of-care systems are now being tested, and it is hoped that all hospitals will be using this kind of system as soon as possible.[21] Such a system, along with a CPOE system, is considered to be the safest available.

Community pharmacies and consultant pharmacists should also be using systems that are closed-looped. Computer systems that have bar code readers that read the bar code on the medication container before the medication is dispensed should be used. This and systems that allow physicians to transmit their prescriptions to the community or consultant pharmacist's computer system would be true closed-looped systems.

Community, hospital, and consultant pharmacists still need to check all orders for the eight medication-related problems, under the pharmaceutical care model, and until bar code checking is available, check the final product before releasing it for administration.

AUTOMATING THE PHARMACY

Automating the medication distribution system is not an easy task, and it is expensive. However, one tragic error can result in even more of an expense to an organization and bad publicity. Before automating, the pharmacist should start by reading ASCP's white paper on automation in pharmacy.[1]

For pharmacy automation to take place, the pharmacist must take charge and have a good plan supported by rationale and clear goals.[22] "To realize the full benefits inherent in automation systems, it is necessary to understand the basic ideas of automation and to realize that automation is simply a tool to help achieve safety, efficiency, and the goals of practice. The goal of pharmacy practice is pharmaceutical care."[23] To do this, the work must be redesigned to improve workflow, minimize distractions, and place the pharmacist at the front of the medication preparation process. The middle of the medication process is where the medication preparation and dispensing are done by pharmacy technicians and automation.

In community pharmacies, it is recommended, under the pharmaceutical care model, that the pharmacist greet the patient, review the medication for appropriateness — by reviewing the eight medication-related problems, check the final product, and counsel the patient. In the hospital, the pharmacist should review the medication for appropriateness and check the final product before releasing it for administration. In the future, terminal bar coding or closed-looped systems will remove the need for this final check by the pharmacist.

Independent community pharmacists and small chain store pharmacies have created a new special National Community Pharmacy Association committee on innovation and technology to help independent practitioners understand and use advances in systems, information technology, and new tools.[24]

FREEING PHARMACISTS FOR PHARMACEUTICAL CARE

Using pharmacy automation makes the medication process safer for patients and frees pharmacists to perform pharmaceutical care, which in turn improves the quality of drug therapy for the patient. Into this mix is added the pharmacy technician, who must understand the medication-use process and the goals of pharmacy practice.[25] With these in place, pharmacy technology and automation can be used more as a quality assurance tool.[26]

There are several success stories about hospital and community pharmacies using automation and freeing pharmacists to perform pharmaceutical care.[6,15,27,28] At the same time, it is disturbing to learn that the average independent pharmacist spends 62% and the average chain store pharmacist spends 66% of the workday using the computer rather then spending more time with patients.[29] Equally disturbing in this report was that pharmacists often overrode safety alerts from the pharmacy computer system.

EVIDENCED-BASED, SAFE SYSTEMS

The primary purpose of using pharmacy automation is to improve safety. Thus far, there is strong evidence that using CPOE with CDSS and bar coding all medication significantly improve safety. Other systems that may improve safety, but for which there is not enough evidence yet to make that claim, include E-prescribing, the use of ADMs and smart infusion devices, and point-of-care (closed looped) medication systems.

THE FUTURE

It is hoped that in the near future:

- All medication is bar coded by the manufacturer
- All pharmacies use bar code readers
- Most hospitals have CPOE with CDSS
- Patients' identification wrist bands are uniquely bar coded
- All the name badges of health care workers handling medication are uniquely bar coded
- All hospitals and long-term care facilities use bar code readers at the bedside
- Smart infusion devices are the only infusion devices used in hospitals
- Hospital computer systems use triggers to alert if a patient may be experiencing an adverse drug effect

SUMMARY

Information technology and automation are tools that should be used by pharmacists. These improve the medication process by making it safer and more efficient. It is also a way to free the pharmacist to perform pharmaceutical care and in turn improve the quality of drug therapy for patients. Pharmacists need to take responsibility for gaining information technology and automation. They must also see that these systems meet the needs of the pharmacy staff and other health care workers who use them and that it is improving the care of patients. Although expert systems are in the future, pharmacists can help make them arrive sooner than later.

DISCUSSION QUESTIONS AND EXERCISES

1. Find three Internet sites providing drug information.
2. Rate the quantity and quality of drug information at each of the Internet sites you found in question 1.

3. How do you know the information at the sites you viewed is accurate and complete?
4. How does the quality of drug information at Internet sites differ from the primary and secondary sources of drug information?
5. Today, there are hand-held electronic organizers (such as Palm Pilots) that can store and record information. Discuss how they can help a clinically oriented pharmacist.
6. How can pharmacy automation make the drug-use process safer?
7. How can pharmacy automation make the drug-use process more dangerous?
8. Discuss how a closed-looped pharmacy automation system in an organizational health care system (such as a hospital) would work — start with prescribing and end with charting and charging for the medication.
9. Discuss how pharmacy automation can advance and enhance pharmaceutical care.
10. The drug-use process may be totally automated in the future.
   a. Discuss how this may affect pharmacy
   b. What may happen if the drug-use process is totally automated and pharmacists do not practice pharmaceutical care?

CHALLENGES

1. For extra credit, and with the permission of your professor, visit a pharmacy that uses automation and prepare a concise report on the automation in the pharmacy. What effect did automation have on safety? Documentation? Freeing up the pharmacists? If time was saved, was it used for patient care? Include your observations and opinions in the report.
2. Many pharmacists are using handheld devices (such as Palm Pilots) to have ready-to-use drug information at their fingertips. For extra credit, and with the permission of your professor, investigate and prepare a concise report on these devices and identify the kinds of information available that would help a pharmacist practice better.

WEB SITES OF INTEREST

Epocrates: http://www2.epocrates.com/index.html
American Society for Automation in Pharmacy: http://www.asapnet. org/

Neuenschwander Report: http://www.pharmacyautomation.com/the-neuco.html

Pharmacy Infomatics: http://www.pharmacyinformatics.com/

Pharmacy Automation: http://www.pharmacyautomation.com/

Pharmacy Automation Systems: http://rxinsider.com/pharmacy_automation_dispensing_technology.htm

REFERENCES

1. Barker, KN, Felkey, BG, Flynn, EA, and Carper, JL. White paper on automation in pharmacy. *Consult Pharm.* 1998;13:256–293.
2. Williams, SJ, Kelly, WN, Grapes, ZT, and Haymond, JD. Current use of pharmacy automation in the United States. *Hosp Pharm.* 1996;31:1093–1101.
3. Pedersen, CA, Schneider, PJ, and Scheckelhoff, DJ. ASHP national survey of pharmacy practice in hospital settings: dispensing and administration — 2002. *Am J Health-Syst Pharm.* 2003;60:52–68.
4. Pueschel, M. Meds by mail works for VA patients. *US Med.* 2001;37(Jun):28–29.
5. Heller, A. New technology advances pharmacy productivity. *Drug Store News.* 1998;8:CP29–30.
6. Ukens, C. Technology update. *Drug Top.* 2001;145(5):86.
7. American Society of Health-Syst Pharmacists. General principles for purchase and safe use of computerized prescriber-order entry systems. Available at www.ashp.org/patient_ safety/cpoes.html. Accessed June 27, 2001.
8. Lieder, TR. Telemedicine company brings ICU patients to the physician. *Am J Health-Syst Pharm.* 2000;57:2246–2250.
9. Paul, PC. Is there a physician on the web? *Atlanta Journal.* December 21, 2000, p. E2.
10. Anonymous. Focus group on telepharmacy. *Am J Health-Syst Pharm.* 2001;58:167–169.
11. McKenna, MAJ. Drugstoreonline.com? Navigating the frontier of Web prescriptions. *Atlanta Journal-Constitution.* April 24, 2001, p. 1 (Living Section).
12. American Association of Colleges of Pharmacy. Real pharmacists beat out virtual ones. *AACP News.* 2000;December:10.
13. Anonymous. Boston area physicians embrace e-prescribing technology as a tool to improve healthcare: docs say paperless prescribing prevents errors. February 7, 2003. Available at http://newswatch.cnn.com.content.php?page=AllArticleXml&feed=bizwire&type=xml&s. Accessed February 7, 2003.
14. Anonymous. SureScripts: agreement connects electronic medical records system to e-prescription service. *Health Insurance Week.* June 12, 2005, p. 115.
15. Parks, L. Pharmacies look to technology to ease prescription boom. *Drug Store News.* 2000;22(18):19–20.
16. Personal communication with M. Neuenschwander, The Neuenschwander Company. September 27, 2001.
17. Institute on Safe Medication Practice. Placing limits on drug inventory minimizes errors with automated dispensing equipment. ISMP Medication Safety Alert. 1999. Available at http:/www.ismp.org/msaarticles/limits.html. Accessed December 6, 2000.

18. Wong, BJ, Rancourt, MD, and Clark, ST. Choosing an automated dispensing machine. *Am J Health-Syst Pharm.* 1999;56:1398–1399.

19. Elder, MA. B-190 U.S. market for pharmacy distribution automation. BCC Research. February 2004. Available at http://www.bccresearch.com/biotech/ B190.html. Accessed May 23, 2006.

20. Koutnik, E. The pharmacy of tomorrow. *Pharmacy Times.* 2003: ?:42-44.

21. Thielke, T. Automation support of patient-care. In *Issues in Pharmacy Practice Management.* Wilson, AL, ed. Aspen, Gaithersburg, MD, 1997, p. 108–114.

22. Somani, S, and Woller, TW. Automating the drug distribution system, in *Issues in Pharmacy Practice Management.* Wilson, AL, ed. Aspen, Gaithersburg, MD, 1997, p. 92–106.

23. Lee, P. Automation and the future practice of pharmacy — changing the focus of pharmacy. In *Issues in Pharmacy Practice Management.* Wilson, AL, ed. Aspen, Gaithersburg, MD, 1997, p. 79–91.

24. Fredrick, J. Independents, small chains collaborate on technology improvement issues. *Drug Store News.* 2001;23(4):100.

25. Miller, DA, Zarowitz, BJ, Petitta, A, and Wright, DB. Pharmacy technicians and computer technology to support clinical pharmacy services. *Am J Hosp Pharm.* 1993;50:929–934.

26. American Society of Consultant Pharmacists. Automation's emerging role as a new quality assurance tool for the long-term care pharmacist. Available at http://www. ascp.com/public/pubs/tcp/1998/sep/forum.shtml. Accessed December 6 2000.

27. Hooks, MA, and Maddox, RR. Implementation of pharmaceutical care-process for professional transformation. *South J Health Syst Pharm.* 1998;3(1):6–12.

28. Horiuchi, V. Hospital robot does work of three pharmacists in half the time. Health & Fitness. July 23, 1999. Available at http://www.idahonews.com/ 072399/health_a/42934.htm. Accessed December 7, 2000.

29. Ukens, C. Technopharmacy. *Drug Top Arch.* November 2, 1998. Available at http:www.drugtopics.com. Accessed July 20, 2001.

7

PHARMACEUTICAL CARE

Pharmacy practice has changed in the United States from making drug preparations from plants found in nature to helping physicians decide which drug to prescribe and helping patients make the best use of their medication. This evolution from apothecary to clinical practitioner has not been easy, but it has been based on an ethos of helping patients and love of the profession. Today, many pharmacists strive to practice pharmacy using the principles of pharmaceutical care.

This chapter begins with a short history of pharmacy practice in the United States and then moves into defining pharmaceutical care and showing how it differs from *clinical pharmacy*. The reader will learn what it means to deliver pharmaceutical care and why this new practice model is important. Last will be a section on the enablers and challenges to performing pharmaceutical care and some information on how the move to pharmaceutical care is going.

LEARNING OBJECTIVES

After reading this chapter, the reader should be able to:

- Define pharmaceutical care (PC)
- Discuss how pharmaceutical care evolved
- Contrast pharmaceutical care and clinical pharmacy
- Identify and explain the six elements of pharmaceutical care
- Identify the eight medication problems
- Discuss the importance of pharmaceutical care

THEORY OF PRACTICE

Every profession has three bodies: a body of knowledge, a body of practice, and a body of ethics.[1] A body of practice must have a mainstream purpose that provides a badge of identification to both the professional and to the client.

Donald C. Brodie, professor of pharmacy at the University of California at San Francisco was the first to suggest that the pharmacy profession needed a theoretical model to distinguish itself and to evolve and actualize its preferred destiny.[1] In 1967, Professor Brodie suggested that drug-use control should be pharmacy's societal purpose. Brodie defined drug-use control as those events that happen "from the time the specifications of a drug are determined until the time the nurse administers it" (the drug).

In 1981, Donald C. McLeod wrote a chapter in *The Practice of Pharmacy: Institutional and Ambulatory Pharmaceutical Services* titled "Philosophy of Practice," in which he builds on Brodie's premise by saying that "dispensing, while being controlled by the profession, must not control the profession. Pharmacy must seek to maximize its contribution to patient welfare, and it must do so by enhancing the contribution of the individual pharmacist.[2]

In 1989, at an invitational conference of national thought leaders in clinical pharmacy practice, Professor Charles Hepler provided the audience with a compelling argument that pharmacy's societal purpose was to ensure the safe and effective drug therapy of the individual patient.[3]

A BRIEF HISTORY OF PHARMACY PRACTICE IN THE UNITED STATES

The Apothecary

The first apothecaries in the United States used methods learned in Europe, primarily in England. The basis of most medicine was plant material and included sources in nature such as barks and roots of trees. The pharmacist prepared the medicine by incorporating the substances from nature into a tincture, syrup, tea, cream, ointment, suppository, or capsule. Pharmacists prided themselves on the *art of pharmacy* by making accurate, eloquent, custom-designed pharmaceutical products.

As pharmaceutical companies grew, the art of pharmacy dwindled. By the early 1960s, most of the drug products were made by drug companies. The emphasis of pharmacy practice shifted from drug preparation to drug dispensing. By the early 1980s, most pharmacy schools taught only the most basic steps in drug compounding. Today, pharmacy students are learning to achieve positive health outcomes in patients by assuring the provision of rational drug therapy.

Drug Dispensing and Distribution

During the 1960s and 1970s, hospital pharmacy focused on making drug distribution safer. It was found that delivering medication by the *unit-dose system* of drug distribution was much safer than traditional methods of drug distribution in hospitals.[4,5] This was followed by the discovery that centralizing the preparation of *IV admixtures* — adding injectable drugs to sterile intravenous (IV) solutions — in the pharmacy was better than having each nurse do it on the nursing unit.[6] Between 1960 and the present, pharmacy has made many improvements in the dispensing and distribution of drugs to patients.

In the mid 1960s, pharmacy started reflecting on and questioning its role in health care. The pharmacist's role until then was confined to preparing and supplying medication. The pharmacist was expected to supply the medication to the patient as ordered by the physician. Only the dose could be questioned, and pharmacists were not to interfere with the *physician–patient* relationship. Thus, there was minimal interaction between the pharmacist and the patient.

Clinical Pharmacy

Pharmacy schools and pharmacists became more patient-oriented during the 1960s. This practice was eventually termed *clinical pharmacy*.[7] Clinical pharmacists were defined as participants in drug therapy decisions and regarded as drug experts or specialists. Between 1960 and 1980, a growing number of pharmacists, most of whom had Pharm.D. degrees and had completed a pharmacy residency, were calling themselves clinical pharmacists and practicing clinical pharmacy in hospitals.

Some functions of these early clinical pharmacists were to be available when the drug was prescribed, make recommendations on drug selection and the dose and duration of therapy, and monitor the drug administration and effects of the drug. These clinical pharmacy pioneers were often questioned by physicians and nurses about their presence on the patient care unit, and they were sometimes rebuffed. However, the clinical education gained while earning the Pharm.D. degree and the patient care skills gained during their residency programs carried them through. Many physicians and nurses were gradually won over to clinical pharmacy. Physicians and nurses started to understand the benefits — to themselves and to patients — of having a clinical pharmacist available on the patient care unit.

In the early 1980s, concern evolved that clinical pharmacy was not being interpreted the same way by all pharmacists. In addition, some clinical pharmacists were becoming so specialized and their practices so different from other pharmacists that this practice may have become its own discipline. Thus, in 1985, the American Society of Health System Pharmacists (ASHP) and its Research and Education Foundation, conducted an invitational conference at Hilton Head Island entitled "Directions for Clinical Practice in Pharmacy."[3]

The objectives of the conference were to examine the extent to which the profession had established goals about clinical pharmacy, to assess the current status of clinical pharmacy practice and education, and to identify some practical ways for advancing clinical pharmacy.

Few, if any, of the 146 invited pharmacy practitioners and educators had any idea they were about to take part in something that would start the profession on its way to its true clinical potential. The keynote address by Charles D. Hepler, entitled "Pharmacy as a Clinical Profession," was the stimulus that encouraged the group to think about pharmacy's societal purpose.[8] Hepler's premise was that once pharmacy agreed on its societal purpose, building a plan to fulfill that purpose should be obvious. The invitees agreed strongly on several points[9]:

- Pharmacy is the health care profession most concerned with drugs and their clinical application.
- A fundamental purpose of the profession is to serve society by being responsible for the safe and appropriate use of drugs.
- A fundamental goal of the profession is to promote health, and pharmacists can best do that by working to promote the best use of drugs.
- In following the above goal, pharmacy should provide leadership to other health care professions; this implies that pharmacists should advocate rational drug therapy rather than just reacting to treatment decisions made by others.

The conferees went on to agree that pharmacists should continue to be responsible for drug distribution and drug control activities, but these functions should be carried out by well-trained pharmacy technicians under pharmacist supervision. This would free the major portion of the pharmacist's time for clinical services. It was also agreed that drug distribution should be automated to as great an extent as possible.

It was obvious after the conference that the greatest force for change in the profession lies within. The Hilton Head Conference on clinical pharmacy helped propel pharmacy toward its clinical destiny and planted the seeds for the next evolutionary step in pharmacy's clinical development — *pharmaceutical care.*

FROM CLINICAL PHARMACY TO PHARMACEUTICAL CARE

Between the Hilton Head Conference in 1985 and 1989, enthusiasm for a more clinical role was building among pharmacy's leaders. Pharmacy's educational curriculum needed to change, and pharmacy practice would need to do things much differently to become a true clinical profession. A conference on "Pharmacy in the 21st Century" was called by 17 national pharmacy organizations in 1989. Like the Hilton Head Conference, something dramatic took place. This time, Charles Hepler and Linda M. Strand delivered a paper entitled "Opportunities and Responsibilities in Pharmaceutical Care," at the second conference on "Pharmacy in the 21st Century"(1989).[10,11]

Hepler and Strand argued that clinical pharmacy represented a transition in pharmacists seeking self-actualization and the full achievement of their professional potential. "Many pharmacists are standing at the threshold of professional maturation; indeed many have crossed over that threshold into patient care." The problem, said Hepler and Strand, is that these self-actualizing functions are slow to develop, and the functions (like pharmacokinetic monitoring) were still focusing on the drug rather than the patient. Something was needed to rally pharmacists to serve a higher good.

It was suggested that the higher good for pharmacy to serve was to prevent *drug-related morbidity* (drug-induced disease) and *drug-related mortality* (drug-induced death). Both the incidence and cost of drug-related morbidity and mortality was unacceptable. Many of the incidences of preventable drug-related morbidity and mortality can be prevented by patient-focused pharmacists.[12]

Hepler and Strand appealed to pharmacists to accept the mandate of preventing drug-related morbidity and mortality, but they cautioned that the application of clinical knowledge and skill (then known as clinical pharmacy) was not enough for effective pharmaceutical services. There needed to be an appropriate philosophy of practice and organizational structure within which to practice. It was proposed that the necessary philosophy of practice be called *pharmaceutical care* and that the organizational system to facilitate the provision of this care be called a *pharmaceutical care system*. Thus, the mission of pharmacy practice, which is consistent with its mandate, is to provide pharmaceutical care.

The paper and presentation by Hepler and Strand galvanized the profession. There was little argument about the mandate. The definition and concept of pharmaceutical care were appealing. In contrast to clinical pharmacy, all pharmacists, regardless of educational degree or practice setting, could provide pharmaceutical care. The profession soon settled on the mission of pharmacy practice — to help patients make the best use of their medication.[13] It was agreed that the best way to fulfill pharmacy practice's mission was to practice pharmaceutical care.

WHAT IS PHARMACEUTICAL CARE?

The initial definition of pharmaceutical care by Hepler and Strand was "the responsible provision of drug therapy for the purpose of achieving definite outcomes that improve a patient's quality of life."[10,11] In 1993, out of concern that the original definition meant that pharmaceutical care could be delivered by anyone, and fear that other health care practitioners would misinterpret this to mean that pharmacists would practice independently, the ASHP drafted a new definition for pharmaceutical care:

> Pharmaceutical care is defined as the functions performed by a pharmacist in ensuring the optimal use of medications to achieve specific outcomes that improve a patient's quality of life; further, the pharmacist accepts responsibility for outcomes that ensue from his or her actions, which occur in collaboration with patients and other health-care colleagues.[13]

This definition was later revised to, "The mission of the pharmacist is to provide pharmaceutical care. Pharmaceutical care is the direct responsible provision of medication-related care for the purpose of achieving definite outcomes that improve a patient's quality of life."

In 1997, Linda Strand provided a newer definition of pharmaceutical care: "a practice in which the practitioner takes responsibility for a patient's drug-related needs and is held accountable for this commitment."[14]

There continues to be controversy about the term *pharmaceutical care*. Some pharmacists — mostly community pharmacists — feel the word *pharmaceutical* should be replaced with the words *pharmacy* or *pharmacist* (e.g., pharmacy care or pharmacist care). The rationale is the that word *pharmaceutical* is too associated with drug products, and by calling it pharmaceutical care, anyone can provide it. The term *pharmacy* or *pharmacist* care avoids these problems. However, most professional pharmacy organizations and schools of pharmacy are still using the original term *pharmaceutical care* or the term *patient care*.

Elements of Pharmaceutical Care

Regardless of which definition of pharmaceutical care is used, each definition encompasses six general principles or elements.

Responsible Provision of Care

The pharmacist should accept responsibility for the patient. The pharmacist should say "my patient" rather than "the patient."

A pharmacy professor recently asked his class of pharmacy students, "How can you tell if the pharmacist is accepting the responsibility for the patient?" The classroom became deadly silent. None of the 120 students raised a hand. The professor repeated the question and waited. Finally, one brave student said, "I think it has something to do with worrying." The professor was intrigued by this and asked the student to explain her answer. "Well," the student said, " if a pharmacist works all day and goes home and never worries about a patient, or about something the pharmacists did or did not do for a patient, then that pharmacist probably is not accepting responsibility for his or her patients." This is exactly right — without worry, there probably is little responsibility that has taken place.

How do you take responsibility for a patient? First, you see every new patient as an opportunity. Second, you do everything in your power to help the patients make the best use of their medication.

Direct Provision of Care

Pharmaceutical care is directly provided to patients. This means pharmacists must be in direct contact with patients. They must see and talk with patients.[15] The patient-pharmacist interface is critical to helping patients and to helping make pharmacy a true clinical profession. Pharmacists who work in a hospital pharmacy and never go to the patient care units to see patients, and pharmacists in community pharmacies who never get out from behind their dispensing counters, are not providing pharmaceutical care. The patient, rather than the physician or the drug, should be the pharmacist's primary concern. The factors important in becoming a good pharmacist are shown in Figure 7.1. The term *good pharmacist* is used in the context of the ideal or most admired, rather than technically proficient.

Caring

The virtue of caring, a key characteristic among nurses and physicians, has been the most understated aspect of pharmacy. It is the centerpiece of pharmaceutical care.

The same professor who asked his class about accepting responsibility for patients asked the class, "What does it mean to care?" Again, no students were brave enough to answer. At this point, the professor asked the class to close their eyes and think about the person they cared about the most — a husband, wife, girlfriend, boyfriend, mother, father, sister,

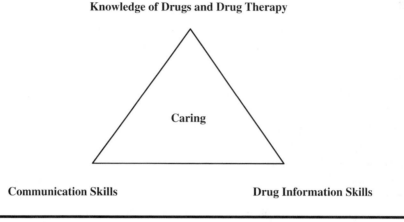

Figure 7.1 Important factors in being a good pharmacist.

brother, daughter, son, grandmother, grandfather, or grandchild. After a minute, the professor said, "Open your eyes and listen. Every time you interact with a patient, across the counter, or when they are in a hospital bed, pretend like that patient is the person you love the most." The professor then asked, "If you do this, what will happen?" Students started answering: "I would do my best." "I would do extra things." "I would make sure they understood everything."

What does it take to be a successful, patient-oriented pharmacist? There probably are different answers to this question, but most would agree on these four factors:

Up-to-date knowledge of drugs and drug therapy: Without this, it would be difficult to remain competent and be useful to patients or physicians.

Good drug information skills: Even if a pharmacist's knowledge base or memory are not as good as they need to be, these deficiencies can be overcome by knowing where to find information about drugs and quickly retrieving the information and then getting back to the person asking the question.

Communication skills: Even if you are knowledgeable about drugs or find the information when needed, it does not mean you will be able to communicate that information effectively. That means putting the patient and physician at ease, using terminology they understand, and not overwhelming them.

Caring: Even if you are not the most knowledgeable or do not have exceptional drug information and communication skills, you can be effective by caring for the patient. Patients are forgiving if they sense that you care. Turf battles with physicians often melt away if the physician feels you are working in the best interest of the patient. Caring is not less important than the other characteristics, but it is more powerful.

Achieving Positive Outcomes

Several positive clinical outcomes can occur as a result of taking medication: (a) cure of disease, (b) elimination or decline of a patient's symptoms, (c) arresting or slowing of a disease process, or (d) preventing a disease or a symptom. There are also negative outcomes from taking medication: (a) the medication fails to work as expected, (b) there are undesirable side effects, or (c) there are adverse drug reactions that cause moderate patient morbidity, a life-threatening or permanent disability, or death.

Besides clinical outcomes, there are also economic (cost) and humanistic outcomes (functional status, quality of life, and patient satisfaction). Under pharmaceutical care, it is the pharmacist's responsibility to do everything the pharmacist can to achieve positive patient outcomes and to avoid the negative effects of taking medication.

Improving the Patient's Quality of Life

Everyone has a certain, measurable *quality of life*. Many factors determine a person's quality of life, including social–economic status, educational background, social and business contacts, and health. Of these, health status is a major factor of a person's overall quality of life. A person's *health-related quality of life* represents the functional effects of an illness and its effects as felt by the patient. Most patients measure their health-related quality of life by what they can do versus what they could do before they were ill.

Under the pharmaceutical care model of delivering care, the pharmacist must, with the patient and the physician, set reasonable treatment goals for each drug prescribed that will improve the patient's functioning and health-related quality of life.

Resolution of Medication-Related Problems

According to Hepler and Strand, the task of pharmaceutical care is to resolve *medication-related problems* (MRPs).[10] MRPs are undesirable events a patient experiences that involve (or are suspected of involving) drug therapy that actually (or potentially) interferes with a desired patient outcome.

Pharmaceutical care involves identifying potential and actual MRPs, resolving actual MRPs, and preventing potential MRPs. There are eight kinds of MRP:[16,17]

Needed drug therapy: The patient has a medical condition that requires the initiation of new or additional drug therapy.

Unnecessary drug therapy: The patient is taking drug therapy that is unnecessary given his or her present condition.

Use of wrong drug: The patient has a medical condition for which the wrong or suboptimal drug is being taken.

Dosage is too low: The patient has a medical condition for which too little of the correct drug is being taken.

Dosage is too high: The patient has a medical condition for which too much of the correct drug is being taken.

Adverse drug reaction: The patient has a medical condition because of an adverse drug reaction or event.

Not receiving the drug: The patient has a medical condition for which the patient is not receiving the drug.

Drug interaction: the patient has a medical condition and there is a drug–drug, drug–food, or drug–laboratory test interaction.

Table 7.1 lists some of the common causes of MRPs.

PHARMACEUTICAL CARE VERSUS CLINICAL PHARMACY

As shown in Table 7.2, pharmaceutical care is not the same as clinical pharmacy, although it evolved from clinical pharmacy. Everyone's practice is different; thus, exceptions exist for the comparison of pharmaceutical care and clinical pharmacy provided in the table. However, in general, the comparison is valid.

The major difference between the two practice models is the primary recipient of the pharmacist's service. Under clinical pharmacy, the physician was the primary focus of the pharmacist's attention. The pharmacist provided the physician with drug information and performed drug and pharmacokinetic monitoring for the physician. The patients rarely, if ever, knew the pharmacist was involved with their care.

Providing services for the physician was a necessary step for the pharmacist to evolve clinically. It was necessary to establish credibility with physicians before pharmacists could begin to interact directly with patients. Until clinical pharmacy, the physician–patient relationship was sacred. Many physicians believed that no one else should have a similar relationship, particularly if that new relationship eroded the existing physician–patient relationship. Thus, it is important that pharmaceutical care

Table 7.1   Common Reasons for Medication-Related Problems in Patients

Needed Drug Therapy

A new medical condition
Preventative therapy needed
Return of an old medical condition

Use of Wrong Drug

More effective drug available
Drug not indicated for condition
Contraindication present
Dosage form inappropriate
Condition refractory to drug

Dosage Is Too High

Wrong dose
Frequency inappropriate
Duration inappropriate
Drug interaction

Not Receiving the Drug

Forgets to take drug
Cannot afford the drug
Side effects
Prefers not to take drug
Administration error

Unnecessary Drug Therapy

No medical indication
Nondrug therapy more appropriate
Duplicative therapy
Treating avoidable adverse reactions
Substance abuse

Dosage Is Too Low

Wrong dose
Frequency inappropriate
Duration inappropriate
Incorrect storage
Incorrect administration
Drug interaction

Table 7.1 Common Reasons for Medication-Related Problems in Patients (Continued)

Adverse Reaction

Allergic reaction
Unsafe drug for patient
Incorrect administration

Drug Interaction

Dose increased or decreased too fast
Drug causes decrease in second drug
Drug causes increase in second drug
Effect of two drugs are canceled
Drug–food interaction
Drug interference with laboratory test

Table 7.2 Comparison of Pharmaceutical Care and Clinical Pharmacy

Pharmaceutical Care	Clinical Pharmacy
More of a primary care model	More of a specialty, consultant model
Patient focused	Physician focused
Provided directly to patients	Usually provided indirectly to patients
Outcome directed	Process directed
Focuses on a variety of outcomes	Mostly focuses on clinical outcomes
Based primarily on caring	Based primarily on competency
Pharmacist responsible for patient outcome	Physician responsible for patient outcome
Quality-of-life role	Quality-of-care role
Practice in all settings	Practiced mostly in acute care settings
All pharmacists can provide	Some pharmacists provide

be done cooperatively with the other health professionals providing care for the patient.

Other major differences between pharmaceutical care and clinical pharmacy are that pharmaceutical care focuses on various patient outcomes, shows caring, and can be provided by all pharmacists regardless of educational background or training.

LEARNING ABOUT PHARMACEUTICAL CARE

Many new pharmacy students — those in their first professional year of pharmacy school — often have to complete an introductory pharmacy practice experience in patient care. This experience often involves "shadowing" an advanced practice experience student — a pharmacy student in his or her last professional year of pharmacy school — and see pharmaceutical care in action.

Introductory pharmacy practice experience students are scheduled or provided options for various shadow experiences. However, because of unfamiliarity with the terms used for these rotations, the first-year student may not know what to select or may feel unprepared for this experience. With this in mind, a description of the typical clinical rotations available for introductory practice experiences is provided here.

Medicine: These are hospitalized patients with acute and chronic illnesses treated by medical internists, and sometimes family physicians, who are members of the Department of Medicine. These are important rotations for students, as these patients usually have many medications prescribed and are excellent candidates for pharmaceutical care.

Ambulatory Care: These patients also have acute and chronic health care problems, but they are outpatients (not hospitalized). They are seen in hospital clinics and in physician's offices. Because of the environment, these patients often have different concerns and issues than inpatients (those in hospital beds).

Pediatrics: These patients are usually less than 12 years old, and they may be inpatients or outpatients. Pediatric patients have medication issues that are different from adults. Their medication is usually not complicated, but it is important.

Geriatrics and Long-Term Care: These patients are usually age 65 years or older. Rotations for students are usually at various long-term care facilities, but they also can be at geriatric inpatient units. These are good rotations for students. Geriatric patients usually use much medication and need counseling about their medication. These patients appreciate pharmaceutical care.

General Clinical: This rotation exposes the student to the broad-based daily activities of a patient-focused pharmacist and how pharmaceutical care should be practiced. This rotation may also expose the student to drug-use review, formulary management, patient medication history taking, pharmacokinetics, quality assurance activities, and the provision of drug information. The patient population may be mixed — medical and surgical.

Psychiatry: This pharmacy practice experience exposes the student to the area of mental health. The student will work with other members of the health care team to monitor drug therapy of patients with psychiatric diseases or drug abuse problems.

Surgery: These are hospital-based experiences designed to enable the student to gain ability in the basic principles of surgery and drugs used before, during, and after surgical procedures.

Cardiology: This practice experience is designed to help the student gain skills in treating and monitoring the therapy for cardiovascular disorders.

Infectious Diseases: During this practice experience, students learn about specific infectious diseases and about their prevention and treatment with drugs.

Home Health Care: More and more patients are being treated at home or are being released from the hospital to be treated at home. Pharmacy is responsible for providing and monitoring the use of these sophisticated infusion drugs (given intravenously).

Advanced Community Pharmacy Practice: This rotation is designed to introduce the student to pharmaceutical care in the community pharmacy. New, innovative, and billable pharmaceutical care services will be learned.

Drug Information: The student will learn how to research and answer drug information questions from physicians, nurses, pharmacists, and patients, as well as how to evaluate drugs and the drug literature.

Neonatology: This is a hospital-based practice experience designed to enable the student to acquire skills and knowledge about the basic principles of drug therapy in the neonate (less than 30 days of age).

Critical Care: This experience concerns the intense drug therapy of patients in critical conditions and confined to a critical care or intensive care unit of a hospital.

Hematology/Oncology: This is usually a hospital-based experience, but it could be an ambulatory experience or both. It concerns learning the treatment of patients with various blood disorders or cancer. The student learns the principles of pain therapy and cancer chemotherapy.

Substance Abuse: This experience is designed to expose the student to the problems of drug and alcohol abuse and the treatment most often used in the clinical setting.

Pharmacokinetics: This experience is designed to give the student hands-on experience in mathematically modeling the distribution and elimination of critical drugs in the body and determining the correct dosage of the drug based on these models. This practice is sometimes called *therapeutic drug monitoring* (TDM).

Poison Control: This experience will allow the student to gain experience in toxicology and the treatment of poisoning and overdose by working at a regional poison control center.

Emergency Medicine: This experience involves learning how to treat patients admitted to the emergency room for critical and acute conditions, including drug overdose.

Nutritional Support Pharmacy: This experience is a hospital experience designed to teach the student how to treat, prepare, and monitor intravenous nutrition therapy in patients unable to eat or to absorb nutrients from their gastrointestinal tract.

Nuclear Pharmacy: In this experience, the student will learn about the basic principles of nuclear medicine and how to prepare and monitor nuclear pharmaceuticals — drugs that are radioactive — and care for patients who receive these agents.

Health Outcomes Management: In this experience, the student will become well versed in the various health outcomes (clinical, humanistic, and economic) and be able to measure these to see if there is an association with specific drug therapy.

Other advanced practice experiences are available for students in pharmacy schools; however, these experiences have goals not specific to the practice of providing pharmaceutical care, for example, research, pharmacy benefits management, academic administration, and industrial pharmacy (sales, marketing, or medical information services).

All pharmacists are teachers, and they are taught that teaching (usually pharmacy students, but also patients, pharmacy technicians, nurses, and others) is a part of being a pharmacist. Students in advanced practice experiences learn by observing and listening to pharmacy practitioners who model correct behavior. Students also learn by doing pharmaceutical care, but always under the watchful eye and guiding hand of the pharmacist preceptor.

PROVIDING PHARMACEUTICAL CARE

Standard Process

No matter where a physician is educated or trained, the approach to the patient is the same, and as a patient, we recognize it when we see it. First, the physician asks for the patient's *chief complaint* (CC). Next are questions on *history of the present illness* (HPI), and then the *past medical history* (PMH). A physical examination is next, followed by a preliminary diagnosis. Last, laboratory tests are performed to confirm the diagnosis.

Like medicine, pharmacy needs a standardized approach to the patient, and one that patients recognize.[18] Thus, the following approach to pharmaceutical care is recommended:

1. Establish the patient–pharmacist relationship.
2. Collect and organize information about the patient.
3. List and rank the patient's medication-related problems.
4. After discussion with the patient, establish the desired outcome for each medication-related problem.
5. Determine feasible solutions for each medication-related problem.
6. Choose the best solution for each medication-related problem.
7. Discuss and negotiate the plan with the physician as needed.
8. Educate the patient about the plan and counsel the patient about the medication.
9. Design and implement an effective monitoring plan.
10. Follow up, measure, and document progress.
11. Bill for services as appropriate.

Selecting Patients to Monitor

Theoretically, all patients should receive pharmaceutical care. However, based on the numbers of patients, prescriptions, and drug orders, providing all the steps in the pharmaceutical care process is not possible for all patients, nor is it needed. One service that cannot be ignored is the pharmacist's offer to counsel patients about their medication. It is required by law.

Beyond this, certain patients may benefit more than others from pharmaceutical care. Thus, criteria can be established to select patients who will benefit from a pharmacist using all the recommended steps in the pharmaceutical care process. Some pharmacists select patients age 65 or over to monitor, as these patients usually take more than the average number of drugs. These patients should be monitored, because liver function (metabolizes or converts drugs so they can be eliminated) and renal (kidney) function (eliminates drugs from the body) diminish as patients get older.

Other criteria for selecting patients for pharmaceutical care are patients taking more than six drugs, patients with reduced liver or kidney function, and patients taking certain potent drugs.

Identifying, Resolving, and Preventing Medication-Related Problems

Once a process for identifying the patients who will benefit the most from pharmaceutical care is established, the next step is to follow the

Table 7.3 Ways to Identify MRPs in Patients

MRP	Rx or Drug	Patient's Computer Profile	Patient's Medical Record	Talk with the Patient
		Ways to Identify		
An untreated problem		X[a]	X	X
Wrong drug prescribed			X	X
Taking too little drug	X	X	X	X
Taking too much drug	X	X	X	X
Not taking the drug	X	X	X	X
Taking an unneeded drug				X
Experiencing a drug interaction	X	X		X
Experiencing an adverse drug reaction			X	X

[a] X = a good way to identify

recommended process for providing pharmaceutical care.[19] The heart of this process is to identify, resolve, and prevent MRPs. How is this best done?

Identifying Medication-Related Problems

As shown in Table 7.3, there are various ways to identify a patient's MRPs. One of the most efficient and comprehensive ways, and thus the best way, is by talking to the patient.

Every patient has a story. This story is real. In the patient's story will be the patient's MRPs. However, to gain clues about the MRPs, the pharmacist must win the trust of the patient and listen carefully. Trust begins in establishing the patient–pharmacist relationship. Trust is based on kindness, caring, empathy, honesty, justice, and confidentiality, and it is strengthened by actions of past caring — all virtues of a good pharmacist. Listening has to be done with the whole mind and heart and by trying to feel the patient's vulnerability. Listening carefully and asking probing questions will identify the patient's MRPs.

Resolving Medication-Related Problems

Once MRPs are identified, they need to be resolved. Some ways of resolving MRPs include adding a drug, canceling a drug, changing the dose, changing the way the drug is being given, or counseling the patient.

Preventing Medication-Related Problems

The best thing is to prevent MRPs before they begin. Some ways to do this are: (a) to educate, counsel, and listen to patients; (b) to educate physicians and nurses about drugs; (c) to program the computer to screen drug orders for problems; (d) to require the diagnosis or use of the medication on the prescription; (e) to require physician order entry of all drug orders; (f) the electronic transmission of prescriptions and drug orders to the pharmacist; (g) for the pharmacist to be present when the medication is ordered in the hospital or clinic; (h) to implement unit dose and centralized IV additive systems in all hospitals; (i) to reduce floor stock medication; and (j) to eliminate sound-alike and look-alike drug names.

Patient Problem List

A practical tool for assessing patients, used for years by the medical profession, is *SOAPing*, where S = subjective findings, the O = objective findings, A = assessment, and the P = plan. The subjective findings are the patient's signs (what can be seen) and symptoms (what the patient reports). The objective findings are what can be measured on physical examination or through laboratory measurement. The assessment is the working diagnoses based on the subjective and laboratory findings. The plan is a problem list in order of priority and what is to be done.

SOAPing can be used by pharmacists when identifying and resolving medication-related problems. For example:

S: Patient complains of being tired, thirsty, and sluggish. Patient states he has "sugar."

O: Blood glucose level is 220 mg/dL (high).

A: Diabetes is uncontrolled owing to poor compliance with taking insulin.

P: Determine why patient is not taking enough insulin. Remind the patient of why it is important for him to take the insulin and what may happen if he does not take it as prescribed.

Some pharmacists go through the subjective, objective, and assessment parts of SOAPing and then use a *problem list*. The list is a record of each MRP. After thinking of various solutions to each MRP, the pharmacist records the best solution and the goal or best outcome for that MRP. An example is shown in Table 7.4.

Table 7.4 Medication-Related Problem List for a Patient

Number	Medication-Related Problem	Solution	Goal
1	Theophylline toxicity	Reduce dose to 100 mg every 8 hours	Theophylline serum levels 10--20 µg/mL
2	Potential drug interaction	Smoking and oral contraceptive	Patient stops smoking or uses other methods of birth control
3	Rash on face and neck	Investigate penicillin allergy	Prove or disprove allergy
4	Antihistamine no longer needed	Recommend discontinuation	Stop order written

Pharmaceutical Care Plan

The problem list is part of something bigger — the *pharmaceutical care plan*. The plan documents the pharmaceutical care process and lists:

- Information about the patient
    - Demographics such as age and gender
    - Height and weight
    - Renal and liver function
    - Diagnoses
    - Quality of life
- Medication
    - Current medications
    - Medication allergies
- Problem list
    - MRP by priority
    - Recommended solutions
    - Goals for each drug and MRP
    - Status of recommendation (pending, followed, not followed)
- Patient outcomes (clinical, humanistic, economic)

Making Cents out of Pharmaceutical Care

Pharmacists have traditionally been paid for their knowledge and skill in dispensing medications correctly. Billing and payment for pharmaceutical care has been slow to develop, but this has been expected. Pharmacists have always given their advice and counsel away free. Thus, some pharmacists are uneasy with charging for these services. In addition, pharmaceutical care and its value are unfamiliar to patients and to payers such as insurance companies. In addition, most pharmacists are still learning what to charge for, how much to charge, and how to bill these services.

However, many pharmacists feel they are providing value-added, pharmaceutical care for patients and should be paid. Even pharmacists working for chain pharmacies feel they should receive a portion of the reimbursement earned by the chain because of their direct patient care services.[20]

Pharmacists are starting to request payment for *disease state management* — working closely with the patient and physician in the pharmaceutical management of the patient's chronic disease (diabetes, asthma, hypertension, high cholesterol levels), administering immunizations, and identifying and resolving MRPs.

There are various ways to be paid for pharmaceutical care services[21]

Charging patients up front: The best way to ensure payment is to require payment directly from the patient at the time the service is delivered. This is easier than one would think if the services are promoted, proposed, and delivered in the proper manner.[22]

Billing major medical payers for the patient: Some insurance plans cover pharmaceutical care services.[23] It is still best to require payment at the time of service and assist patients in submitting their own claims. If the pharmacist or pharmacy decides to bill an insurance company for pharmaceutical care services, it must be done properly by using one of two claim forms — the HCFA 1500 or Pharmacist Care Claim Form. The latter is the most user-friendly claim form for pharmacists to use. However, the HCFA 1500 claim form is the claim form most recognized by claims payment agencies across the nation. This claim form is not as easy to use, but once mastered will probably result in the most claims being paid.

Becoming a provider in a state or federal disease-state management program: These programs are usually administered through Medicaid (state) or Medicare (federal) agencies. States including New Jersey, Oklahoma, Texas, and Mississippi have disease state management programs that pay pharmacists to help manage the therapy of patients with certain chronic diseases. For example, in 1998, the Mississippi Medicaid program received a federal waiver allowing reimbursement to pharmacists for providing drug therapy management and patient education. Working under protocols drafted collectively with physicians, *credentialed* pharmacists in Mississippi are now eligible for reimbursement in the following clinical areas: diabetes, asthma, hyper-cholesterolemia, and anticoagulation therapy.

Contracting with major medical groups to manage specific patient populations: Major group health providers are starting to pay pharmacists to help manage certain patient populations taking certain categories of drugs to help improve patient compliance with taking the medication appropriately and to contain costs.

Some good texts are available containing details on what to bill, how to decide how much to bill, and how to bill for pharmaceutical care.[17,24,25] A study surveyed a convenience sample of 26 pharmacies in Georgia to find the extent of billing, the bills paid, and who was paying for pharmaceutical care. Of the pharmacies surveyed, 66% indicated they were providing pharmaceutical care to their patients, as defined in the survey instrument.[22,23] Twenty-six percent were documenting and billing for pharmaceutical care services. Copies of 86 claim submissions revealed that 52 were billed to major medical insurance companies and 34 were billed to patients. Of the claims submitted to insurance companies, 18 (about 35%) were paid. The average amount per claim was $57.24. All (100%) claims billed directly to patients were paid. The amount billed to patients ranged from $2 to $39, and the average was $14.

WHY PERFORM PHARMACEUTICAL CARE?

There are many reasons for pharmacists to expand their practices to perform pharmaceutical care: because of the patient, because the drug-use process is not perfect, because of drug morbidity and mortality, because it works, and because it may be pharmacy's salvation.

The Patient

The patient deserves pharmacy's best. Because drugs are so complex, and some so powerful, patients are often confused about their medication. Patients need to know their drug, what it is, how it works, how they should take it, why they should take it, what may happen if they do not take it, and what kinds of problems to be on the look out for when taking it.

Most patients feel vulnerable because of a lack of knowledge about drugs and drug therapy. What they need is a medication advocate. Physicians are usually too busy, and most of them are not interested in spending time with patients discussing this subject. Medication advice and counseling is not the central role of nurses. Pharmacists are in the best position to do this and are the best trained to fulfill this important role.

Problems in the Drug-Use Process

Although the drug-use process is well organized and has many checks and balances, it is far from perfect. Drugs are not always prescribed, dispensed, administered, and monitored correctly. There are even times when all of these steps are done correctly and the treatment fails because of misdiagnoses or physiological variations within patients. For example, in a well-publicized 1995 study, it was estimated that only 60% of treated patients have an ideal outcome.[26] In addition, 23.4% (±13.2%) of the cases resulted in treatment failure, and new medical problems developed in 10.5% (±5.4%) of the patients.

Drug-Related Morbidity and Mortality

Patients often experience unwanted effects of their medication. If these unwanted effects are more than mild side effects, and unexpected, they are called *adverse drug reactions* (ADRs). ADRs, drug interactions, medication allergies, and medication errors are sometime referred to as *adverse drug events* (ADEs) or *drug misadventures.*

A well-publicized report by the National Academy of Science's Institute of Medicine (IOM) estimated that between 44,000 and 98,000 hospital patients die each year in the United States because of medical errors.[27] This report estimates that at least 7000 patients die each year from medication errors. This is a modest number, as it does not include deaths from medication allergies, drug interactions, and adverse drug reactions, nor does it include patients outside the hospital.

About 0.2% of emergency room visits are because of the adverse effects of medication.[28] This results in roughly 125,000 visits, or 4.77 visits per 10,000 people per year. The prevalence of hospital admissions because of the adverse effects of drugs, based on a meta-analysis of 36 studies ranged from 0.2 to 21.7%; the median was 4.9% (range 2.9 to 6.7%), and the mean was 5.5% (±4.1%).[29]

The severity of drug morbidity varies. Bates et al. reviewed 4031 adults admitted to a hospital over a 6-month period.[30] During this time, 441 adverse drug reactions were identified. Of these, 1% were fatal, 12% life-threatening, 30% serious, and 57% significant. Table 7.5 lists some likely outcomes of drug misadventures based on the severity of morbidity and mortality.

Drug-related morbidity and mortality were estimated to cost $76.6 billion a year in the ambulatory setting in the United States. Even without the added cost of drug-related morbidity and morality for hospital and nursing home patients, the cost of $76.6 billion a year makes these adverse effects among the most expensive health problems in the United States.

Table 7.5   Range of Likely Drug Misadventure Outcomes

Morbidity and Mortality	Likely Outcome
Mild discomfort	None
Moderate discomfort	Physician visit
Severe discomfort	Emergency room visit
Life-threatening event	Hospital days
Permanent disability	Life-long care
Death	Invaluable

Table 7.6   Detection of MRPs in Hospital versus Community Patients by Pharm.D. Students (%)

MRP	Hospital[31] (n = 231)	Community[32] (n = 298)
Untreated indication	14.1	18.8
Drug used with no indication	13.7	2.3
Dose too low	31.5	3.0
Dose too high or duplicate Rx	17.4	15.8
Adverse drug reaction	6.4	25.8
Drug interaction	2.7	11.4
Improper drug selection	8.7	1.3
Failure to receive drug	2.3	7.3
Miscellaneous	3.2	9.0

Source: From Anderson, RJ, Nykamp, D, and Miyahara, RK. J. Pharm. Pract. 1995;8:83–88. With permission.

The good news is that many drug misadventures are preventable, and many can be prevented by pharmacists practicing pharmaceutical care.[12]

PHARMACEUTICAL CARE WORKS

Another good reason to practice pharmaceutical care is that it works — identifies, resolves, and prevents MRPs. Studies are being done to measure its impact on patient outcomes and quality of life. Table 7.6 lists the MRPs solved by Pharm.D. students while performing pharmaceutical care in a hospital and in a community pharmacy setting.[31,32]

Table 7.7   Significance of Pharm.D. Student Interventions

Classification[a]	Number (%)
Adverse significance	0 (0)
No significance	10 (4.6)
Somewhat significant	47 (21.4)
Significant	151 (68.9)
Very significant	10 (4.6)
Extremely significant	1 (0.5)
Total	219 (100)

[a] From Hatoum, et al.[33]

Source: From Briceland, LL, Kane, MP, and Hamilton, RA. *Am J Hosp Pharm.* 1992;49:1130–1132. With permission.

Four points can be made about these data.

- MRPs happen, and patients are not receiving the full benefit of their medication or are being harmed.
- If Pharm.D. students can find this many MRPs, think how many MRPs can be found and solved by experienced pharmacists.
- MRPs vary by patient — ambulatory versus inpatient.
- Pharmacists can identify, resolve, and prevent MRPs, and they should be recognized for these contributions to improving the health of patients.

A good model for pharmacy students to learn about pharmaceutical care is in the ambulatory care setting.[34] The Veterans Affairs medical centers have the premier model.[35] Pharmacists, especially those with a Pharm.D. degree and residency training, are delivering high-quality pharmaceutical care to veterans, especially in ambulatory care — the clinics. Another good model for pharmacy students to learn pharmaceutical care is in the U.S. Indian Health Service, which is part of the U.S. Public Health Service. Commissioned pharmacy officers deliver the most independent, high-level pharmaceutical care to populations of Native Americans. Their patient care services have been an inspiration to many pharmacists.[36]

The Economic Benefit of Clinical Pharmacy/Pharmaceutical Care

The first cost-benefit analysis of a clinical pharmacy service was published in 1979.[37] In a systematic literature search of economic studies published on the value of clinical pharmacy services between 1996 and 2000, the investigators found 59 controlled studies.[37] Sixteen studies included a benefit to cost ratio that ranged from 1.6 to 1 for a target drug program in a hospital-associated clinic to 17 to 1 for a disease state management program in a University hospital. Compared to a similar study by the same authors for the period 1988–1995,[38] a greater proportion of studies in the 1996–2000 review used more rigorous study designs. The investigators concluded the studies by saying "the body of literature from this 5-year period provides continued evidence of the economic benefit of the clinical pharmacy service evaluated."

It is clear that more research needs to be focused on documenting whether pharmaceutical care keeps patients out of their doctors offices, emergency rooms, and hospitals and whether adults return to work and children return to school earlier than without pharmaceutical care. These are the primary outcomes of interest to the majority payers of healthcare — business owners and the federal and state governments.

It May Result in Pharmacy Being a True Clinical Profession

Pharmacy has always been patient oriented, even when pharmacies were mostly corner drugstores and pharmacists were compounding most of the medication for patients. Pharmacists became less patient oriented when pharmaceutical companies supplied most of the drugs for the pharmacist to dispense. Pharmacists became even less patient oriented when insurance companies started paying for drugs and the amount of paperwork required to dispense and bill a prescription increased. Being tied to a product hinders the profession from being all it can be. It puts pharmacy more in the category of "retailer" than "professional" or "clinician."

Under pharmaceutical care, the patient is the central focus of the pharmacist, and there must be a patient–pharmacist relationship and interaction between the two parties. This and identifying, solving, and preventing MRPs and focusing on positive patient outcomes should substantially raise the practice of pharmacy to the level of a true clinical profession and help it achieve this status.

WHEN WILL ALL PHARMACISTS PRACTICE PHARMACEUTICAL CARE?

There are some barriers and challenges, but also some enablers and proven implementation steps to providing pharmaceutical care. Once most pharmacists practice pharmaceutical care, it will become the standard of practice. Those pharmacists not practicing pharmaceutical care will have to justify — in a court of law if sued — why they are not using this model of delivering care.

Barriers and Challenges

The barriers and challenges to pharmaceutical care have been identified.[23,39]

The Enemy Within

The number one barrier to the practice of pharmaceutical care may lie within the profession itself. Some pharmacists are reluctant to change, some lack confidence in their abilities to implement pharmaceutical care, and some fear increased liability. The key to overcoming this is formal education (external Pharm.D. programs) and continuing education programs that provide practicing pharmacists with advanced practice skills and increased confidence to practice pharmaceutical care. Pharmacists need to learn the full concept of pharmaceutical care and why it is important to practice in this manner.

Resource-Related Constraints

Freeing up enough time to perform pharmaceutical care is a major challenge to its implementation, especially in the community pharmacy environment, where the volume of prescriptions and paperwork is ever increasing. Unfortunately, the priority in most pharmacies is providing the medication to the patient, even if it is not the best medication (poorly prescribed) for the patient. Freeing up pharmacists' time for pharmaceutical care involves commitment, the increased use and expanded practice of pharmacy technicians, work redesign and automation, and an electronic medical record available to all licensed health practitioners.

Some pharmacists are under the misunderstanding that large sums of money are needed to provide pharmaceutical care. Changes are needed in space, equipment such as computer programs, and personnel, but these need not be expensive and can be phased in over time.

Lack of Support

Sometimes there is lack of support from owners, managers, and supervisors of pharmacists motivated to practice pharmaceutical care. It is frustrating when these doubters have business rather than pharmacy backgrounds. This is a difficult, but not impossible, barrier to overcome. Pharmacists in this circumstance often find it helps to dedicate themselves to patients and to prove that pharmaceutical care works by providing it whenever possible. Even if they can only work with two patients a day (i.e., 10 a week and over 500 a year), it will still have quite an impact.

Patients, nurses, and physicians are more easily impressed with pharmaceutical care, especially if it is obvious that the pharmacist is interested in helping patients and displays a caring attitude. It is also helpful if the pharmacist thinks of ways to help physicians and nurses in their prescribing and drug administration roles. Even from a business perspective, a pleased customer is likely to become a repeat customer.

Legal Barriers

Some laws and regulations made by state boards of pharmacy need changing to improve the pharmacist's clinical role. Here are a few changes that will help propel pharmacy's clinical role: (a) replacement of technician–pharmacist ratios with regulations that make the pharmacist accountable for the work of a safe number of technicians, (b) allowance of terminal dispensing by use of a bar code check, (c) electronic transmission of prescription and drug orders, and (d) allowing pharmacists to perform immunizations and some routine laboratory testing (such as finger sticks for drug level testing).

Studies Documenting the Value of Pharmaceutical Care

There is no question that well-designed studies documenting the value of pharmaceutical care will help advance its practice. Some pharmacists incorrectly believe there is a lack of such studies, when the truth is that there are plenty of such studies.[40] Thus, questions become, Why isn't this evidence being read, believed, or used? Why isn't it enhancing the pharmacist's image and advancing the payment of cognitive services at a faster rate?

Lack of Payment

Some pharmacists — a minority — believe they should not perform any pharmaceutical care or any new service without being paid first, whereas others believe the profession needs to demonstrate the value of the new service before it can request and be paid.

ENABLERS TO PHARMACEUTICAL CARE

Several trends enable pharmaceutical care to be the practice model of choice for all pharmacists.

Changes in Pharmacy Education

All colleges of pharmacy now have the Pharm.D. degree as the entry-level degree to practice pharmacy. This was a long time coming, but it has arrived. In addition, for pharmacists with B.S. degrees in pharmacy, there are now many nontraditional Pharm.D. programs that allow them to earn the advanced degree without having to go back to school full-time. Continuing education programs are available for all pharmacists to learn or to enhance their clinical skills.

Certified Pharmacy Technicians

Pharmacy technicians now have a means of being certified to verify they have certain knowledge about pharmacy. Using more qualified pharmacy technicians will allow pharmacists to spend more time with patients.

Function Analysis and Workflow Redesign

Pharmacists are starting to understand that major changes will need to take place in the workflow to free time for them to perform pharmaceutical care. What is less understood, and perhaps more important, is that an analysis of work function and responsibility needs to take place.

Many pharmacists are performing functions that can and should be performed by technicians. The problem is that many like it this way. However, these pharmacists are being overpaid for what they are doing, and they are wasting their knowledge and skills by not performing higher patient care functions. Excellent information is available on how to redesign workflow and perform a function analysis.[24]

Collaborative Practice Agreements

Many professional pharmacy organizations and state boards of pharmacy have been successful in achieving *collaborative practice agreement* legislation through state legislatures. These agreements establish a working relationship of a pharmacist or group of pharmacists working in a pharmacy with a physician or group of physicians whereby the pharmacist is able to manage the therapy of patients under a protocol or the umbrella of a physician.[41] Such agreements expand the pharmacist's scope of practice and will advance pharmaceutical care.

Pharmacy Automation and Information Technology

Automated equipment for drug dispensing, preparation, and distribution is a boon to pharmacists, as it is usually safer and frees up pharmacists to spend more time with patients. Automated systems are available for dispensing prescriptions, preparing IV admixture and total parenteral nutrition (TPN) solutions, filling patient's unit dose drawers, and dispensing floor stock, narcotics, and other controlled substances in hospitals.[42]

Medication Errors

Recent and broad publicity about the extent of medical and medication errors provides pharmacists and pharmaceutical care an opportunity to flourish.[27] Pharmacy needs to step forward proudly and boldly and prove it is ready to take a leadership role in decreasing this important health care problem.

IMPLEMENTING PHARMACEUTICAL CARE

Changing to a new practice style is not easy. It takes courage and commitment. However, some things have been learned that can be helpful to those starting to make the transition to pharmaceutical care.

Changes the Profession Needs to Make Happen

Many things need to happen to make it easier for pharmacists to implement pharmaceutical care. Pharmacy practice acts and the regulations that support them need to be reviewed and changed to use pharmacy automation and allow pharmacists to make decisions about the safe and effective use of pharmacy technicians. Pharmacy laws that say "the pharmacist must terminally check the prescription before it is dispersed to a patient" are outdated, as this check can now be done faster and more accurately by automation. The profession also needs to expand the use of collaborative practice agreements and expand laws allowing pharmacists to perform more laboratory testing. More work needs to be done about allowing pharmacists with proper training to gain provider numbers and bill for the clinical services they provide.

Freeing Up Pharmacist's Time to Provide Pharmaceutical Care

In general, four things are required to free pharmacists to provide pharmaceutical care:

> *Radically reengineer the drug dispensing and drug distribution systems:* Pharmacists need to do pharmacist-only and only pharmacist-only functions, and technicians need to do all the rest. Within each pharmacy, the pharmacists, as a group, should decide which functions they and only they will do. In a community pharmacy, this

should include greeting patients, accepting prescriptions, and counseling the patients about their medication. Depending on state law, it should also include taking verbal orders, overseeing controlled substances, and checking the final product dispensed. In the hospital, it will only include checking pharmacy technicians and probably taking verbal orders.

Use as many pharmacy technicians as possible: To have enough time to do pharmaceutical care, pharmacists should use all the certified pharmacy technicians the law allows and they feel comfortable supervising.

Automation: As much of the drug dispensing, preparation, and distribution process as possible should be automated, even if it means employing fewer people to free up money to purchase the equipment. There are multiple rewards for using automation — increased patient safety and more time for pharmacists to care for patients, which in turn makes for safer, more appropriate drug therapy for patients.

Increased use of information technology: Information technology, such as software programs to identify patients to monitor, providing up-to-date drug information, and treatment algorithms, can help the pharmacist provide the best pharmaceutical care for patients.

Leadership and Teamwork in Implementing Pharmaceutical Care

Strong leadership is needed to implement pharmaceutical care. The leader, whether it is the owner, the director of pharmacy, or a motivated pharmacist, needs to know how to lead. The leader must also remember that pharmaceutical care is a team effort that includes prescribers. Thus, it is important to work as a team when planning pharmaceutical care services. Everyone working in the pharmacy should know what pharmaceutical care is, why it is needed, and have input on how it will be implemented and provided. It is important to establish goals, develop an implementation plan, and provide necessary training and the resources to fulfill the plan.

Pharmaceutical Care in the Community and Hospital Environments

How pharmaceutical care is being implemented and provided in the community pharmacy and hospital environments is covered in Chapters 8 and 9.

DOCUMENTING PHARMACEUTICAL CARE

The pharmaceutical care plan documents the pharmacist's care. This documentation is needed for several reasons: (a) It is a way to put all the important information the pharmacist needs in one place. (b) It keeps the pharmacist from having to remember everything about the patient. (c) It helps the pharmacist to organize his or her thoughts. (d) It serves as a record of the pharmacist's recommendations and care. (e) It documents patient's outcomes that can be correlated with what the pharmacist has done for the patient. (f) It can be the basis for the pharmacist billing for the care rendered.

The ASHP has established guidelines on documenting pharmaceutical care in patient medical records.[43] The guidelines cover gaining approval to document pharmaceutical care and what documentation should include as a minimum. However, the guidelines seem limited in scope and might include documenting, when possible, the benefit of the pharmaceutical care consultation.

PROGRESS IN ESTABLISHING PHARMACEUTICAL CARE

It has been 17 years since the profession first learned of pharmaceutical care. Is progress being made? Is pharmaceutical care becoming the practice model of choice? The answers are yes and no.

The profession has fully embraced pharmaceutical care as noted by every national and most state pharmacy organizations making individual and joint statements and resolutions about pharmaceutical care. The profession has also taken some bold steps to see that pharmaceutical care becomes the practice model of choice. Examples of this boldness include adopting the Pharm.D. degree as the sole entry-level degree to practice pharmacy, the implementation of external Pharm.D. degree programs, the expansion of pharmacy residencies including community pharmacy, the certification of pharmacy technicians and various pharmacist specialties, and the arrival of collaborative practice agreements.

Despite all of these bold moves by the profession, pharmaceutical care is not happening at the pace pharmacy leaders had hoped. Although 84% of pharmacists support pharmaceutical care, many pharmacists are reluctant to make the leap of faith to pharmaceutical care without the safety net of their traditional dispensing role.[44] The increasing number of prescriptions and drug orders do not help, and although pharmacy automation can help, its use is perceived as expensive.

Patients who receive the services of a pharmacist practicing pharmaceutical care benefit from it, as they receive superior drug therapy. However, most patients do not receive this benefit. Therefore, pharmacy needs to find the key to making pharmaceutical care happen at a much faster rate.

Seeing this as a major need, the American College of Clinical Pharmacy (ACCP) issued a white paper entitled "A Vision of Pharmacy's Future

Roles, Responsibilities, and Manpower Needs in the United States."[45] Each of the major professional pharmacy organizations were asked to respond to this paper, and the responses were published. Although responses were slightly different, all pharmacy organizations that responded were in general agreement.

It is hoped this agreement may spark one clear voice for pharmacy on this important topic, help propel the implementation of pharmaceutical care, and speed pharmacy toward being a true clinical profession.

SUMMARY

The profession has moved from focusing on the drug to focusing on the patient. The pharmaceutical care model makes pharmacy a true clinical profession. However, pharmacists will need to relinquish the tasks of drug dispensing and distribution and just be accountable for these functions. If pharmacists focus on and are recognized for improving patient outcome, their likelihood of being paid for this will increase significantly.

DISCUSSION QUESTIONS AND EXERCISES

Approach 1: One pharmacist stays behind the counter all day. The pharmacy clerk greets the patient, accepts the prescription, and hands it to the pharmacist. The pharmacist types the label, retrieves the medication, counts out the medication, puts it in the bottle, and hands it back to the clerk. The clerk puts the medication into a bag, hands it to the patient, rings up the sale, and asks for the money. This happens 120 times in 8 hours.

Approach 2: Another pharmacist uses a certified technician rather than a pharmacy clerk. The pharmacist greets and introduces himself to the patient and accepts the prescription. The pharmacist asks the patient about the need for the medication, and hands the prescription to the certified pharmacy technician to fill. While the prescription is being filled, the pharmacist interviews the patient to determine if any of the eight MRP's are present. After checking the prescription, the pharmacist shows the medication to the patient, lets the patient know what the medication is for, how it is to be taken, and provides any precautions. The pharmacist thanks the patient for stopping in and lets the patient know that the pharmacist is always available to help. The pharmacy technician bags the medication and rings the sale.

Which of these approaches would:

1. Provide the highest quality of care? Why?
2. Be the most appreciated by the patient? Why?
3. Bring back the most patients to the pharmacy? Why?
4. Produce the most pharmacist satisfaction? Why?
5. Generate the most pharmacy revenue? Why?
6. Generate the most pharmacy profit? Why?
7. What would you call approach 1?
8. What would you call approach 2?
9. What do you feel are the two major challenges in providing pharmaceutical care?
10. List two solutions for each of the challenges you listed in question 9.

CHALLENGES

1. A common expression is that many pharmacists are superb pharmacy technicians. That is, they like spending most of their time performing the technical and clerical functions of pharmacy such as typing labels, counting drugs, making IV additives, and completing paperwork, all of which can be done by pharmacy technicians. These pharmacists minimize their face-to-face contact with patients. For extra credit, and with the permission of your professor, investigate this problem first hand and prepare a concise report documenting the problem, state why it is a problem, investigate its etiology, and suggest how best to resolve this problem.
2. For extra credit, and with the permission of your professor, outline, design, and describe how workflow in a community pharmacy would maximize pharmaceutical care. What are the functions? Which functions would be accomplished by pharmacy clerks? Pharmacy technicians? Pharmacists? What are the benefits of your recommended work flow to the patients? The pharmacy owner? The pharmacy clerks and technicians? The pharmacists?

WEB SITES OF INTEREST

Statement on pharmaceutical care: http://www.ascp.com/public/pr/policy/pharmaceutical.shtml
The American College of Clinical Pharmacy: http://www.accp.org/
Pharmaceutical care networking: http://www.aphanet.org/pharmcare/pharmcare.html

Payment for pharmaceutical care: http://www.ascp.com/public/pr/policy/payment.shtml

Pharmaceutical care discussion group: http://www.pharmweb.net/pwmirror/pwq/pharmwebq9.html

REFERENCES

1. Brodie, DC. Drug-use control: keystone of pharmaceutical service. *Drug Intell Clin Pharm.* 1967;1:63–65.
2. McLeod, DC. Philosophy of practice. In *The Practice of Pharmacy: Institutional and Ambulatory Services.* ed. McLeod, DC and Miller, WA. Harvey Whitney Books, Cincinnati, OH, 1981, chap 1.
3. ASHP Research and Education Foundation. Directions for clinical practice in pharmacy. *Am J Hosp Pharm.* 1985;42:1287–1306.
4. Barker, KN. The effects of an experimental medication system on medication errors and costs. Part 1: Introduction and errors study. *Am J Hosp Pharm.* 1969;26:342–343.
5. Black, HJ, and Tester, WW. Decentralized pharmacy operations utilizing the unit dose concept. *Am J Hosp Pharm.* 1964;21:345–350.
6. Zellmer, WA. Solving problems associated with large-volume parenterals. I: Pharmacist responsibility for compounding intravenous admixtures. *Am J Hosp Pharm.* 1975;32:255.
7. Francke, GN. Evolvement of clinical pharmacy. In Francke, DE and Whitney, HAK, Jr, eds. *Perspectives in Clinical Pharmacy; A Textbook for the Clinically-Oriented Pharmacist Wherever He May Practice.* Drug Intelligence Publications, Hamilton, IL, 1972, p. 26–36.
8. Hepler, CD. Pharmacy as a clinical profession. *Am J Hosp Pharm.* 1985;42:1298–1306.
9. Zellmer, WA. Achieving pharmacy's full potential. *Am. J Hosp Pharm.* 1985;42:1285.
10. Hepler, CD, and Strand, LM. Opportunities and responsibilities in pharmaceutical care. *Am. J. Pharm Ed.* 1989;53(winter suppl):7S–15S.
11. Hepler, CD, and Strand, LM. Opportunities and responsibilities in pharmaceutical care. *Am J Hosp Pharm.* 1990;47:533–543.
12. Kelly, WN. The potential risks and prevention. Part 4: Report of significant adverse drug events. *Am J Health-Syst Pharm.* 2001;58:1406–1412.
13. American Society of Hospital Pharmacists. Statement on pharmaceutical care. Available at http://www.ashp.org/bestpractices/statements.html.
14. Strand, LM. Re-visioning the profession. *J Am Pharm Assoc.* 1997;37(4):474–478.
15. Haines, ST. *The Patient-Pharmacist Interface. Pharmacotherapy Self-Assessment Program,* 4th ed. American College of Clinical Pharmacy. Kansas City, MO. 2001.
16. Strand, LM. Drug-related problems: their structure and function. *DICP Ann Pharmacother.* 1990;24:1093–1097.
17. Cipolle, RJ, Strand, LM, and Morley, PC. *Pharmaceutical Care Practice.* McGraw-Hill, New York, 1998.

18. American Society of Health-System Pharmacists. ASHP guidelines on a standardized method for pharmaceutical care. *Am J Health-Syst Pharm*. 1996;53:1713–1716.

19. Robertson, KE. Process for preventing, identifying and resolving problems in drug therapy. *Am J Health-Syst Pharm*. 1996;53:639–650.

20. Rochester, CD, and Curry, CE. Chain-community pharmacists' view toward practice in a reimbursement-based pharmaceutical care environment. Presented at the ASHP-Midyear Clinical Meeting, 1999, 34(Dec), P-236E.

21. Stasny, JA, and Marlow, M. Getting paid for pharmaceutical care. *ComputerTalk*. 1998;18:76–77.

22. Wickman, JM, Marquess, JG, and Jackson, RA. Documenting pharmacy care does make ¢ents (and dollars too). *GA Pharm J*. 1998; 20:12–14.

23. Wickman, JM, Jackson, RA, and Marquess, JG. Making ¢ents out of caring for patients. *J Am Pharm. Assoc*. 1999;39:116–119.

24. Rovers, JP, Currie, JD, Hagel, HP, et al. *A Practical Guide to Pharmaceutical Care*. American Pharmaceutical Association. Washington, DC, 1998.

25. Smith, MC, and Wertheimer, AI. *Social and Behavioral Aspects of Pharmaceutical Care*. Haworth Press, New York, 1996.

26. Johnson, JA, and Bootman, JL. Drug-related morbidity and mortality. *Arch Intern Med*. 1995;155:1949–1956.

27. Kohn, LT, Corrigan, JM, and Donaldson, MS. *To err is human: building a safer health system*. Institute of Medicine, Washington, DC, 1999.

28. Aparasu, RR, and Helgeland, DL. Visits to hospital outpatient departments in the United States due to adverse effects of medications. *Hosp Pharm*. 2000;35:825–831.

29. Einarson, TR. Drug-related hospital admissions. *Ann Pharmacother*. 1993;27:832–840.

30. Bates, DW, Cullen, DJ, Laird, N., et al. Incidence of adverse drug events and potential adverse drug events: implications for prevention. *JAMA*. 1995;274:29–34.

31. Briceland, LL, Kane, MP, and Hamilton, RA. Evaluation of patient care interventions and outcomes by Pharm.D. clerkship students. *Am J Hosp Pharm*. 1992;49:1130–1132.

32. Anderson, RJ, Nykamp, D, and Miyahara, RK. Documentation of pharmaceutical care activities in community pharmacies by Doctor of Pharmacy students. *J Pharm Pract*. 1995;8:83–88.

33. Hatoum, HT, Hutchinson, RA, et al. Evaluation of the contribution of clinical pharmacists: inpatient care and cost reduction. *Drug Intell Clin Pharm*. 1988;22(Mar):252–259.

34. Lobas, NH, Lepinski, PW, and Abramowitz, PW. Effects of pharmaceutical care on medication cost and quality of patient care in an ambulatory-care clinic. *Am J Hosp Pharm*. 1992;49:1681–1688.

35. Alsuwaidan, S, Malone, DC, Billups, SJ, and Carter, BL. Characteristics of ambulatory clinics and pharmacists in Veterans Affairs medical centers. *Am J Health-Syst Pharm*. 1998;55:68–72.

36. Sardinha, C. Indian Health Service: paving the way for pharmaceutical care. *J Managed Care Pharm*. 1997;3:36,41–43.

37. Schumock, GT, Butler, MG, Meek, PD, et al. Evidence of the economic benefit of clinical pharmacy services: 1996-2000. *Pharmcotherapy*. 2003;23(1):113–132.

38. Schumock, GT, Meek, PD, Ploetz, PA, and Vermeulen, LC. Economic evaluations of clinical pharmacy services: 1988-1995. *Pharmacotherapy.* 1996;16:1188–1208.

39. Implementing pharmaceutical care. Proceedings of an invitational conference conducted by the American Society of Hospital Pharmacists and the ASHP Research and Education Foundation. *Am J Hosp Pharm.* 1993;50:1585–1656.

40. American College of Clinical Pharmacy, and the European Society of Clinical Pharmacy. Proceedings of the first international conference on clinical pharmacy. Documenting the value of clinical pharmacy services. *Pharmacotherapy.* 2000;20:233S–346S.

41. Ferro, LA, Marcrom, RE, Garrelts, L, et al. Collaborative practice agreements between pharmacists and physicians. *J Am Pharm Assoc.* 1998;38:655–666.

42. Neuenschwander, M. Limiting or increasing opportunities for errors with dispensing automation. *Hosp Pharm.* 1996;31:1102–1106.

43. Ukens, C. Inside today's pharmacist. *Drug Top.* 1998;142:70–78.

44. American College of Clinical Pharmacy. ACCP White Paper: a vision of pharmacy's future roles, responsibilities, and manpower needs in the United States. *Pharmacotherapy.* 2000;20:991–1020.

45. American College of Clinical Pharmacy. ACCP manpower white paper: alternative viewpoints. *Pharmacotherapy.* 2001;21:116–127.

8

AMBULATORY (COMMUNITY)
PHARMACY

The practice of ambulatory (serving those who can walk or move about freely) pharmacy in the community is the oldest type of pharmacy practice, and it remains the first choice of roughly 60% of new pharmacy graduates. Of the different types of ambulatory practice settings, the most common is the community pharmacy. Community pharmacists serve patients by providing information and advice about health and drugs, provide medication, and refer patients to other sources of help and care, such as physicians, clinics, hospitals, and emergency rooms.

This chapter is about the different types of community pharmacies, what it means to provide service, and how pharmaceutical care is practiced in this setting. This chapter will provide an overview of the procedures most community pharmacies use in filling prescriptions and counseling patients. Next will be information about traditional and newer services offered by community pharmacies. It will also cover the different positions for pharmacists in community pharmacy, how pharmacists spend their time, and how satisfied they are with what they do. Last will be some predictions on what community pharmacy may soon be like.

LEARNING OBJECTIVES

After reading this chapter, you should be able to:

- Identify the four types of community pharmacies
- Explain how the four types differ
- Compare patient satisfaction with the types of pharmacies

- Discuss the extent of pharmaceutical care being provided in community pharmacies
- Discuss some of the real challenges to providing pharmaceutical care in this environment
- Discuss the types of dispensing errors
- Contrast traditional and newer patient services being offered in community pharmacies
- Explain how community pharmacists are billing for cognitive services
- Discuss how satisfied pharmacists are working in community pharmacy
- Identify two current trends in community pharmacy

TYPES OF COMMUNITY PHARMACIES

There are four types of community pharmacies: (a) independent, (b) chain store, (c) mass merchandiser, and (d) supermarket. For each type of community practice site, some things are the same, whereas other things are unique. Mail-order pharmacies also serve ambulatory patients, and some data is provided on these types of pharmacies in this chapter and in Chapter 19, Other Opportunities for Pharmacists.

As shown in Table 8.1, some things that differ among community pharmacies are prescription volume and the changing market share for prescriptions. Although Table 8.1 reflects 2003 and 2004 data, it is the latest and most comprehensive data available at this writing. What is important is not the specific numbers in the table, but the relationships and trends shown in the table. For example, chain store pharmacies filled the most prescriptions in 2004, followed by independent pharmacies. However, the prescription volume is growing the fastest in the supermarket pharmacies (1.1%) and growing the least in independent pharmacies (0.3%). Sales for prescriptions grew the most for mail-order pharmacies (17.9%) and the least for independent pharmacies (5.2%%). The number of independent pharmacies decreased by 4.9%, whereas the number of other pharmacies grew 0.7 to 6.1%.[1]

Independent Pharmacies

The *independent pharmacy* is where the profession began, and in many ways it remains the heart and soul of pharmacy. Many independent community pharmacies started as family-owned corner drugstores in towns both big and small. The town's pharmacist was a trusted professional and friend and an active member of the community. Although this nostalgic

Table 8.1 Prescription Activity in 2004 and Percent Change from 2003 in the United States

Activity	Independent Pharmacies	Traditional Chain Store Pharmacies	Supermarket Pharmacies	Mass Merchandiser Pharmacies	Mail-Order Pharmacies
Total Rxs[a]	728 (0.3%)	1,510 (1.1%)	470 (1.6%)	353 (2.4%)	214 (13.2%)
Number of outlets	17,931 (−4.9%)	20,849 (0.7%)	9,818 (3.9%)	6,777 (6.1%)	?
Rx sales[a]	$40.5 (5.2%)	$91.0 (6.2%)	$27.0 (6.9%)	$21.2 (7.6%)	$41.3 (17.9%)
Market share[b]	18.3%	41.2%	12.2%	9.6%	18.7%

[a] In billions
[b] Based on sales

Source: National Association of Chain Drugstores. Industry facts-at-a-glance. 2004 Community Pharmacy results. Available at http://www.nacds.org/wmspage.cfm?parm1=505. Accessed April 19, 2006. With permission.

part of Americana is fading, and the soda fountains are gone, independent community pharmacy is still alive and adapting to new competition.

The uniqueness of independent community pharmacy lies in the word *independent*. Independent community pharmacies are owned by pharmacists who can practice the way they choose as long as it is within the law.

Each pharmacy owner has the privilege of setting the rules and policies of his or her pharmacy. The success of the business is largely within the owner's hands, but it is getting more difficult to stay in business because of increasing competition and decreasing reimbursement. Between 1990 and 1998, over one-third of independent community pharmacies in the United States went out of business: from 31,879 to 20,641.[1] In 2004, the number of independent community pharmacies dropped to 17, 931, a decrease of 15% since 1998.

The typical independent pharmacy in 2003 filled 190 prescriptions a day (up from 152 a day in 1999), or 59,423 new and refill prescriptions a year (up from 47,000 in 1999).[2] In 2004, the average independent community pharmacy was open 6 days a week for 57 hours. In 1999, the average proprietor's total income (including salary and store profit) before taxes was $165,819. (Note: more up-to-date figures could not be found).

In 2004, the average independent pharmacy employed 10.6 full-time equivalent (FTE) employees, of which 2.6 were pharmacists and 3.5 were pharmacy technicians.[3] Generic drug utilization was 53%.

Independent community pharmacies provide various services beyond providing prescription medication. More than half of independent community pharmacies provide delivery, compounded prescriptions, nutritional products, durable medical products, and herbal medicines.[2]

Pharmacists who want to know their patients, are attracted by the possibility of owning their own business, or who want to find a job in their hometowns, or almost any town, will like independent community pharmacy practice. About 20% of new pharmacy graduates select independent community pharmacy as their first job as a pharmacist.

Chain Store Pharmacies

The dominant corporations in *chain store pharmacy* are Walgreens, CVS, and Rite Aid. The practice of pharmacy in chain stores is similar, yet different, from the practice of pharmacy in independent community pharmacies. What is similar is the dispensing. After that, everything is different. First, working in a chain drugstore means you are working for a large corporation rather than a small family business. Therefore, the pharmacist needs to be sensitive to the corporate culture and policies.

Positions for pharmacists in chain pharmacies are plentiful, as the chain store pharmacy industry is expanding rapidly. Signing bonuses are available, and salaries are generally higher than in independent and hospital pharmacies. Some large chain pharmacy companies also offer salary and stock bonuses. There is also job security and opportunity for moving up to management. About 40% of new pharmacy graduates select chain pharmacy practice for their first jobs as pharmacists.

Chain store pharmacy practice is fast paced, usually much more so than the practice in independent pharmacies, and it needs intense focus, organization, and efficiency. There is usually less opportunity to interact with patients because of the volume of prescriptions to be dispensed. It is important that there be enough pharmacy technician help so the pharmacist can properly practice pharmacy and counsel patients.

Working in a chain store pharmacy can be stressful because of the volume of work. In addition, the frustrations of patients complaining about prescription prices is worse in chain pharmacies, since the patients there are more often bargain shoppers.[4] Another frustration can be that managers within the corporation who have responsibility for the pharmacy often have business backgrounds and do not understand pharmacy and patient care.

Supermarket Pharmacies

The emergence of pharmacies within supermarkets, such as Kroger, Winn Dixie, SuperValu, Wegmans, and Publix, has occurred within the last 15 years. The concept supermarkets use to attract customers is convenience — one-stop shopping. Patients can drop off their prescriptions at the pharmacy and do their shopping rather than idly waiting for their prescriptions.

The concept is working. As shown in Table 8.1, *supermarket pharmacies* are one of the fastest growing segments of the retail prescription business. According to the Food Market Institute (FMI), there were 10,867 supermarket pharmacies in 2004 versus 9,919 in 2003.[5] However, the median number of daily prescriptions dispensed declined to 120 from 127 in 2003. During 2003, 87% of responding supermarket companies reported having a Web site where they averaged 25 prescription orders per day per Web site.

Supermarkets are trying to create an atmosphere that provides a sense of community and a shopping experience the new wellness consumer is seeking.[6] "Consumers are looking for stores, people, brands, and products they can trust." Obviously, supermarket pharmacies seem to be serious about connecting with consumers and are here to stay.

Some pharmacists feel that working in a supermarket is unprofessional. Others feel that it is a perfect blend between working in a chain store pharmacy and an independent community pharmacy. You still need to deal with a corporate structure and corporate policy, but there are opportunities to develop relationships with patients.[7]

However, not all supermarkets are progressive in offering pharmacists opportunities for professional growth and advancement. There is also the requirement to be flexible enough to work any hour of the day or night, as many supermarkets offer 24-hour pharmacy service.[8]

On the plus side, it appears that supermarket pharmacies are embracing pharmaceutical care and patient counseling more than chain store pharmacies, based on a recent push at improving customer service and satisfaction.

Mass Merchandiser Pharmacies

An even more recent development than supermarket pharmacies is the placing of pharmacies inside the stores of mass merchandisers such as Wal-Mart, Kmart, Target, Ames, Sams, and Costco. These stores are capitalizing on a major shift in the buying practices of the public. Today, consumers are consolidating their shopping trips and are spending more money for life's basics — such as prescriptions — at discount stores.[8]

Not much has been published about the pros and cons of practicing pharmacy inside these commercial enterprises. How much pharmaceutical care and patient counseling will be practiced in *mass merchandise pharmacies* is yet to be determined.

PATIENT SERVICE AND SATISFACTION

No matter where a pharmacist chooses to practice, the success of the pharmacy service is largely dependent on good service and patient satisfaction. Both of these factors are dependent on two other factors: the pharmacist's attitude toward patients and management's (the corporation or owner) attitude about how the pharmacy and pharmacist should function. When both the pharmacist and management agree that service and patient satisfaction are supreme, then more pharmacists and, in turn, more patients will be satisfied. More patient satisfaction means more patients will return and more patients will recommend the pharmacy to friends.[9,10]

Pharmacy technicians, pharmacy interns, and pharmacists owe their employer a good day's work, the provision of good service, and doing everything possible to make their employer successful. The more successful the employer, the more likely the employees will succeed as well.

A major study on customer satisfaction with pharmacy services was conducted by Ortho Biotech as a service to the pharmacy profession.[11] This study revealed that the chain store pharmacy was the most often used pharmacy as cited by 64% of the respondents. Supermarket pharmacies

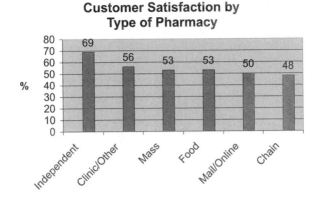

Figure 8.1 Customer satisfaction by type of pharmacy. (*Source:* 2005 Wil-sonRx™ Pharmacy Survey Report, © 2005 Wilson Health Information, LLC, New Hope, PA. For more information contact info@WilsonRx.com or visit www.Wil-sonRx.com. With permission.)

were used by 15% of the respondents, followed by independent pharmacies (12%) and mass merchandiser pharmacies (11%).

The most often cited reasons for using a specific pharmacy were location, accepting an insurance card without problems, the ease of getting prescriptions refilled, and store hours. Pricing was seventh, and unfortunately, pharmacists were ninth (of 10 responses).

As shown in Figure 8.1, independent pharmacy customers are the most satisfied, and chain store and mail-order pharmacy customers were the least satisfied. Similar results were found in a survey by *Consumer Reports*.[12] Courteousness of staff is the leading predictor of pharmacy customer satisfaction, followed by ease of getting prescriptions filled, satisfaction with substitute medication(s), and prescriptions being filled accurately with no errors. The pharmacist being available to answer questions about drugs was sixth, and the pharmacist's interest in the customer's health and well-being was seventh (of 10 different responses).

A 2005 national survey found Valu-Rite to be the highest-rated pharmacy overall.[11] "Value-Rite's customers are most likely to report that they are on a first name basis and have known their pharmacists for a long time." The survey also found, for the third year in a row, Publix to be the number one rated supermarket pharmacy nationally. "Publix's customers are particularly satisfied with their pharmacy's convenience, including store hours and parking." Costco Pharmacy was rated the number one mass merchant/discount pharmacy, and Medco was the top-rated mail/online pharmacy. Walgreens was the number one chain pharmacy overall and the top drive-thru pharmacy.

PHARMACEUTICAL CARE

One of the principles of pharmaceutical care (PC) is that it can be practiced in any practice site, not only in organized health care settings such as hospitals. One big question has been, Will pharmaceutical care flourish in community pharmacies? Or is the environment too business oriented — too product related — for pharmaceutical care to survive? Many community pharmacists believe pharmaceutical care is the right direction for pharmacy, but some feel they are just too busy to practice it.

Extent and Growth

In 1999, *Drug Topics* discovered that there was support for pharmaceutical care in community pharmacies.[13] Only 9% of pharmacist respondents working in independent pharmacies and 19% of chain drugstore executives said they are not involved with pharmaceutical care. Table 8.2 shows the extent and growth of pharmaceutical care in independent and chain store pharmacies between 1999 and 2000.[14] The information was gathered by survey and thus self-reported. No new information was available at the time of this writing (2006).

Table 8.2   Community Pharmacy Involvement in Pharmaceutical Care, 1999 to 2000

Question	Independent Pharmacies		Chain Drugstores	
	1999 (n = 216)	2000 (n = 276)	1999 (n = 31)	2000 (n = 58)
Involvement in Pharmaceutical Care?				
Very	24%	20%	16%	24%
Some	67%	66%	65%	62%
None	9%	14%	19%	14%
Will Increase Involvement?				
Will	48%	44%	68%	72%
Will not	24%		13%	
Not sure	28%		19%	

Source: Adapted from Ukens, C. *Drug Top.* 1999;143(23):93 and Conlan, MF. *Drug Top.* 2000;144(23):70.

The information showed that most independent pharmacies and chain store pharmacies were involved in pharmaceutical care and that each type of pharmacy had plans to do more, especially chain stores. How much pharmaceutical care is being practiced in mass merchandiser and in supermarket pharmacies has not been published and thus is unknown.

Bright Spots

There are a few bright spots for pharmaceutical care in community pharmacy. One is the Ashville Project in North Carolina, where in 1994 a group of pharmacists, an employer, a health-care system, and two universities decided to try to help.[15–18] A group of pharmacists would help manage patients' diabetes. "They would meet with the patients each month, talk to them about their blood-sugar and other lab values. This experiment was supposed to last just 6 months. Today, the Asheville Project has grown from 46 participants with diabetes to 700 people with 4 different chronic diseases. It is history now, and famous among pharmacists."

In this project, each patient met with a pharmacist for an initial 60-minute consultation. Patients were trained by pharmacists to make sure they knew how to monitor their blood sugar correctly. Then patients met with their pharmacists monthly to review blood-sugar results, discuss their condition, and set goals. After 6 months, 75% of patients showed at least some improvement in blood sugar. Sixty-three % of them showed blood sugar in the optimal range, compared to 38% of patients before the intervention. Total medical costs decreased by $1622 to $3356 per patient per year. This freed money for preventive medications and reduced the need for emergency room and hospital care.

Another bright spot has been demonstration projects in the Iowa Medicaid program and one between Wellmark Blue Cross and Blue Shield of Iowa, the Iowa Pharmacy Association, and the Outcomes Pharmaceutical Health Care network of pharmacies.[19,20] In the latter project, patients with asthma, hypertension, diabetes, or ischemic heart disease were identified and enrolled by pharmacists to participate in the project. Community pharmacists identified resolved medication problems in these patients and were encouraged to utilize a health outcomes management documentation system.

Pharmacists were reimbursed for patient care services based on a resource-based relative value scale calculation. "Depending on the complexity of the patient's medical needs, the number of current medications, and the number of drug therapy problems identified and resolved, quarterly payments ranged from $14 to $105."[20]

During the project, 9517 patient care encounters were documented, with 14% of encounters resulting in the resolution of drug therapy problems. What pharmacists encountered most were inappropriate adherence to therapy, adverse drug reactions, and missing medication therapy. The majority of drug therapy problems were resolved through pharmacist intervention with the patient.

After deducting the administrative costs of the program, the unadjusted cost per patient of the intervention group was $3675, compared to $3907 per patient in the control group, or $232 lower per patient in the intervention group. After adjusting these figures for severity of illness, the per-patient cost of the intervention group and the control group were very similar ($3,762 vs. $3705). The authors concluded that the implementation of a model to reimburse pharmacists for their patient care services is feasible.

Disappointments

The results of one of the first randomized controlled studies to examine the effectiveness of outpatient pharmaceutical care programs found that patients enrolled in a pharmaceutical care program had only slight improvements in their medical conditions and were more likely to visit emergency rooms or be hospitalized than patients not in the program.[21,22] Investigators commented that one of the limitations of the study was that, despite their efforts to design a pragmatic program and reinforce its use, the program was not consistently used by the pharmacists. It is clear that "the right incentives and systems need to be in place in busy practices before the value of pharmacy interventions can be demonstrated."[21] On a positive note, patients in the pharmaceutical care program reported being more satisfied than other patients with the pharmacists and health care received.

A survey of the literature on pharmaceutical care and community pharmacy reveals less success in the United States than in Europe.[23,24] This may be because many countries in Europe have one electronic medical record for each patient and community pharmacists have access and may add their history to the patients record.

Future Studies

It is clear that future research needs to include cross sectional and cohort studies measuring the extent of pharmaceutical care in community pharmacies by type of practice setting. Future outcome studies need to investigate the motivation, consistency, and strength of pharmacist interventions. They also need to measure health outcomes and if adults return to work sooner and children return to school sooner because of the pharmacist interventions, rather than only measuring differences in cost and clinical indicators.[25]

Challenges

The growth of pharmaceutical care in community pharmacy may be inhibited by several factors. First, there is a misconception that it is expensive to practice pharmaceutical care; that is, you need to remodel, buy new computer software, and add personnel. This impression may have resulted from a study published on the costs of implementing pharmaceutical care when pharmaceutical care was just getting started in community pharmacy.[26] The study reported high start-up costs and low revenue for pharmaceutical care. This may have done more harm than good. The study suffered from some design flaws, as reported by the investigators, and the timing of the study was unfortunate.

The truth is that little money needs to be spent to start practicing pharmaceutical care. If it goes well, money can be spent over time to make improvements in performing, documenting, and billing for pharmaceutical care.

Another challenge to implementing pharmaceutical care in the community pharmacy environment is providing practicing pharmacists with the knowledge and skills to provide pharmaceutical care. Most pharmacists have some understanding of pharmaceutical care and support it, but they lack the necessary tools to practice it effectively. Continuing education programs, certification programs, and nontraditional Pharm.D. programs have taken time to develop, but are now in place to provide the skills for community pharmacists to practice pharmaceutical care.

Another challenge is generating revenue for pharmaceutical care. However, as previously discussed, charging for pharmaceutical care seems like the obvious answer to this challenge.

The last challenge, and perhaps the most difficult one, is increasing workload and the need for more pharmacists. At least, this is how it appears on the surface. There is no doubt that pharmacists are having to fill more prescriptions, which is well documented, and will be fueled by an increasing aging population. The controversy is about how to solve this problem. Many, especially chain store pharmacy management (most of whom are not pharmacists) are pressuring colleges of pharmacy to graduate more pharmacists. However, this may not be the best solution.

Even if the colleges of pharmacy increase their enrollments by 50% over the next 10 years, this may still not be enough to handle the large increase in the number of prescriptions expected over the next 25 years;

that is, if prescriptions are filled the way they are now, which demands pharmacist time and is not conducive to practicing pharmaceutical care.

CATALYSTS

It is becoming clear that pharmaceutical care will not happen in community pharmacies without catalysts such as (a) improving the pharmacist's clinical skills and knowledge about evidenced-based pharmaceutical care techniques that work, (b) freeing the pharmacist for pharmaceutical care by using more pharmacy technicians and automation, (c) reimbursement for pharmaceutical care, (d) more privacy for pharmacist–patient interaction, (e) access to the patients' medical records, and (f) a closer relationship with patients' doctors.[24,27]

Pharmacy organizations, schools of pharmacy, and programs offering community pharmacy residencies are doing their part to facilitate pharmaceutical care. There are also books that can help pharmacists implement pharmaceutical care in the community pharmacy setting.[28]

DISPENSING PROCEDURES TO IMPROVE PHARMACEUTICAL CARE

The following are the ideal steps in dispensing a prescription that will improve pharmaceutical care.

Accept the Prescription and Establish the Pharmacist–Patient Relationship

Ideally, the pharmacist should be the person greeting the patient and accepting the patient's prescription, not a clerk. Patients appreciate this practice. After establishing the pharmacist–patient relationship, the pharmacist should note the date of the prescription, verify the full and correct name of the patient, and get the patient's address and telephone numbers. If it is the first visit, the patient should complete a form that gathers demographic, insurance, and clinical information, such as drug allergies, about the patient.

Review the Prescription and Patient Information

Traditionally, and routinely, the pharmacist reviews the prescription and patient information from a safety standpoint. Some questions are:

1. Have I read the prescription correctly? Could I be misreading the name of the drug because of poor handwriting?

2. Does this prescription make sense for this patient? For the patient's age? For the patient's condition?
3. Is the dose correct?
4. Does this drug interact with other drugs or foods the patient is taking?

Pharmacy is in the process of expanding its role beyond review of prescriptions for safety to include review of drug and cost effectiveness. There is also more of a focus on patients rather than on the drug. All pharmacy students are taught how to review a patient's drug regimen. Older pharmacy practitioners are attending continuing education (CE) programs to learn the eight-step drug order review process.

The beauty of the pharmacist's comprehensive review of the prescription is that it represents half of a check and balance system for drug safety. If the pharmacist detects something amiss in the prescription, he or she will call and discuss it with the prescribing physician.

Data Entry and Review of the Patient's Medication Profile

Each patient should have a patient record or profile in the pharmacy's computer system. The basic information for this profile is gathered on each new patient using a form, and this information should be updated at least once a year on active patients.

Before a prescription is filled, the pharmacists should check the patient's profile for drug duplication, allergies, and potential drug interactions (some computers do this automatically). In order to do this properly, the patients must be asked what medications they are presently taking from *any source* (prescriptions from this pharmacy, other pharmacies, or samples). Each time a prescription is filled, it is added to the patient's profile by entering the information into the pharmacy computer system, which is a pharmacy technician function.[29]

Review of Insurance Coverage

Most patients do not pay for their own prescriptions or only pay a portion (a *copay*) of their medication. The balance is paid by a *pharmacy benefits manager* (PBM) or an insurance company contracted by the patient's employer. The problem that sometimes occurs when trying to fill a prescription is that the medication or total quantity ordered is not covered under the employee's insurance plan. This slows the prescription process. The bureaucracy and paperwork associated with filing claims seems to be getting worse, which is one of the chief concerns of many pharmacists. A way to deal with this is to pull these prescriptions out of the routine processing procedure and into an "exception area" where someone works on them separately. In this way, the remaining prescriptions to be filled can move along without delay.

Retrieve the Drug or Ingredients from Storage

Once the pharmacist is confident that a prescription is in the best interest of the patient and the insurance information is verified, the prescription needs to be filled. The first step in this process is for the pharmacy technician to retrieve the correct medication or the ingredients to prepare (mix) or compound (make) the medication. The locations of the drugs and ingredients for prescriptions are carefully planned for safety, efficiency, and inventory control.

To be safe, drugs that can be easily confused should be stored at a distance from each other. Another safe practice is to store potent, potentially dangerous drugs and drugs known to be associated with errors in a separate, special location. Putting this area under lock and key or making the area distinct will serve as a reminder to be extra careful when handling these drugs.

Some pharmacies store their medications by product, such as oral medication, ointments and creams, *ophthalmics* (for the eye), and *otics* (for the ear). The drugs in each category are placed alphabetically. Class II controlled substances must be stored separately and be under lock and key. Some pharmacies store their medications by company, especially if they are ordering those drugs directly from the pharmaceutical manufacturer. This makes it easier when taking stock of what needs to be ordered.

No matter how the drugs are stored in a pharmacy, all must be kept under ideal storage conditions in which they are protected from extreme temperatures and excessive sunlight. Others must be refrigerated. In addition, all the medication in stock must be up to date. Although some drug wholesalers and pharmaceutical manufacturers will take back and credit outdated stock, they do not like to see this happen often. Thus, the stock needs to be checked on a routine basis for outdated drugs, which is often the job of a pharmacy intern.

When retrieving medication or ingredients to prepare or compound a medication, the rule is to check it four times:

1. When it is taken off the shelf
2. During preparation
3. When putting the stock container or ingredients back on the shelf
4. When presenting the medication to the patient

Preparation or Compounding

Some medications need to be counted (tablets and capsules) or poured out (liquids such as tinctures, syrups, and suspensions). Other medications need to be prepared. An example is reconstituting antibiotic suspensions for pediatric patients. The drug comes in a powder or is freeze-dried and needs to be made into a liquid for the patient to use.

Compounding a prescription is more complex than preparation and involves physical chemistry and *secudum artem* — the art of pharmacy. *Secudem artem* involves the careful measurement of ingredients and knowing in what order to make the preparation and what technique to use to make an elegant final product.

In the past, most medications were prepared by compounding, and in parts of Europe and Asia are still made this way. About 1% of the prescriptions in the United States are compounded by the pharmacist, most of which are ointments and creams.[30]

Compounding prescriptions one patient at a time is considered to be the practice of pharmacy. The pharmacist may also compound products in anticipation of immediate needs; for example, enough for the next 24 hours. However, making more than is needed for immediate needs is considered by the U.S. Food and Drug Administration (FDA) to be manufacturing rather than the practice of pharmacy. If this is the case, the pharmacy would need a manufacturing license and would be required to follow *current good manufacturing practice* (CGMP) as set forth by the FDA.

When compounding a prescription, the pharmacist use implements such as an analytical balance to weigh ingredients, graduates for measuring liquids, spatulas for making ointments and creams, and mortars and pestles for particle reduction. All ingredients must be ±5% of the amount intended to be in the product or they are considered to be "misbranded," which is a violation of federal law.

Label the Prescription

Once the product is counted, prepared, or compounded and checked, it needs to be labeled. The basic requirements of the label are dictated by state law; however, these requirements do not vary much from state to state. Most labels are computer generated and contain a prescription number unique to that patient, product, and pharmacy. It will also have the date of dispensing, the patient's name, the physician's name, directions for use, and usually the name and amount of the drug, refill information, and the initials of the pharmacist who did the terminal check of the medication. It may also have lot number information and an expiration date. Preprinted information on the label will contain information about the pharmacy: its name, address, and telephone number.

Check for Proper Dispensing

Once the medication has been prepared and labeled, it needs to have a terminal check before it can be dispensed to the patient. The pharmacist must do this. After checking, the pharmacist's initials are added to the label and the patient's record. *Note:* This law needs to be changed to allow the terminal checking of the prescription with bar coding or similar technology, as it takes up time the pharmacist can be using to work with patients. Some states have changed their laws, whereas others have not.

Terminal checking is a safety and legal requirement. Although pharmacy technicians or other pharmacists may be involved in getting the prescription ready, only one pharmacist is accountable to see that the product is terminally checked and approved to be dispensed to the patient. Even if bar coding is used to terminally check the prescription, a pharmacist usually (in most states) must initial the label and patient record to show accountability.

Drug Use Review and Dispensing

Under the pharmaceutical care practice model, the pharmacist must check the medication for the eight medication-related problems sometime before it is dispensed (see Chapter 7, Pharmaceutical Care). In addition, other questions are: Is there anything that will interfere with achieving a positive patient outcome? Is there any abuse going on? What does the patient need to know to be compliant with taking the medication as prescribed?

Medication Delivery and Patient Counseling

It should be the pharmacist who delivers the medication to the patient, not the pharmacy technician or clerk. In addition, under OBRA 90 and good pharmacy practice, pharmacists, not technicians or clerks, must make an offer to counsel all Medicaid patients about their medication. Most state boards of pharmacy consider doing one thing for one class of patient and not doing it for another class unethical. Thus, most state boards of pharmacy have passed regulations that pharmacists must offer to counsel *all* patients.

Some pharmacists take counseling patients seriously, and some pharmacies have added private counseling areas for patients.[31] Several companies, such as Medicap and Eckerds, have experimented with counseling-only options. Medicap provides counseling and health screenings, such as bone density measurements, on an appointment basis. There is a charge for these services based on the service provided.[32]

A project by a pharmacy student at a school of pharmacy revealed that most patients do not understand the law that requires pharmacists to offer to counsel patients about their medication.[33] In the location where the study was performed, patients are often asked to sign something before they receive their medication. When asked what they were signing, 30% (of 80 patients at eight different sites) said that it was to document that they picked up the medication; 21% were unsure; 18% said they did this for insurance reasons; and, 6% said it was because certain drugs require a signature. Twenty percent (20%) were never asked to sign anything, and only 5% knew they were signing to document that they were offered counseling by the pharmacist.

A survey of 306 pharmacies in eight states revealed that 87% of patients were given some written information by community pharmacists about their prescriptions. However, the quality of the information varied considerably.[34]

Pharmacists often are too busy to counsel patients — yet it is the law. Some faculty members from the University of Toledo College of Pharmacy performed a study to discover the influence of prescription volume, pharmacy staffing patterns, the availability of resources, and practice setting on the pharmacist's perception of compliance with the law to counsel patients.[35] In the 21 pharmacies surveyed, in three different types of practice sites, the proportion of patients counseled varied from 5% to nearly 100%. The amount of counseling and the time spent per patient also varied. Prescription volume and type of practice site did not correlate with the frequency or extent of patient counseling despite the perception by pharmacists that these are major barriers to counseling. What did correlate with the extent of counseling were: (a) closeness of the current site to a perceived ideal, (b) the availability of medical and pharmacy references, and (c) a private counseling area.

The three Cs of effective patient counseling are communication, comprehension, and compliance:[36]

Communication: To communicate effectively with patients, pharmacists need to remove any barriers to good communication, be good listeners, and use open-ended questions.

Comprehension: To counsel patients properly, pharmacists should select only a few key counseling points and verify that patients understand what they need to know.

Compliance: Unless counseled, most patients will not take their medication exactly as prescribed. It is important to stress how often to take the medication and what may happen if the patient does not take it as prescribed.

Pharmacists in the Indian Health Service of the U.S. Public Health Service have developed a standardized, effective process for counseling patients.[37] Three prime questions that form the foundation for the medication consultation are: (a) What did your doctor tell you the medication is for? (b) How did your doctor tell you to take the medication? (c) What did your doctor tell you to expect? Each question probes the patient's knowledge of a specific area of understanding needed to self-medicate. The pharmacist can reinforce what the patients know and fill in the gaps in what they need to know.

AVOIDING ERRORS IN THE DISPENSING PROCESS

The first principle of pharmacy practice is *primum non nocere*, or "first, do no harm." Pharmacists are trained and pride themselves on being accurate.

Types of Medication Errors

There are many types of medication errors, and some are more dangerous than others. The most dangerous medication errors are those involving the wrong dose, when a patient receives the wrong drug, when the frequency of taking the medication is incorrect, and some drug interactions. All of these can result in significant harm to the patient. Other errors, such as dispensing the wrong form of the drug (a tablet instead of a liquid), misspelling the patient's name, and not labeling the container with the drug name and number of refills are also errors, but these will seldom result in patient harm.

Reasons for Medication Errors

Errors happen because of human failing, but they most often occur because of flaws in the medication-use process: the prescribing, dispensing, administration, and monitoring of medication. Said another way, errors are usually not the result of physicians, nurses, and pharmacists making an error, but of good people working in a bad system. Pharmacists have built safety net systems to catch errors; however, as work volume increases, or someone bypasses a certain step in the process, these safety nets may not catch the error in time.

Medication errors are based on a knowledge deficit or a performance deficit. *Knowledge deficit errors* are also called *mistakes*. In the case of a mistake, the person committing the error does not possess the knowledge to avoid the error. For example, if a pharmacist dispenses an overdose of a medication and did not know that amount of medication was an overdose, this will be classified as a knowledge deficit error or a mistake. *Performance deficit errors* are also called *slips*, as the person committing the error knew better but did not perform as expected. Slips are often caused by inattentiveness or distraction.

Some of the major contributors to errors are (a) not reading labels, (b) the oral prescribing of medication, (c) being too busy, and (d) sloppy handwriting.

Not reading the label is perhaps the number one cause of errors. The problem is often compounded by the way manufacturers label their drugs. Many drugs are labeled similarly. Many drugs look similar to the company's other drugs (same shape container, same color label, same label format, same print) except for a small detail such as the drug name or the strength. Many drug names look similar, for example, quinine and quinidine, prednisone and prednisolone, vincristine and vinblastine.

The rule for dispensing is to read the label at least three times: when the drug is retrieved from storage, before it is counted or measured, and just before it is dispensed. Some pharmacists use a fourth check when the drug is being put back into storage.

It is common for physicians to prescribe medication orally, usually over the telephone. It is also common practice for physicians to allow their nurses to communicate a prescription over the telephone to a pharmacist or pharmacy intern. Although verbal orders are legal, they can be dangerous if not handled carefully.

The first consideration when handling verbal orders is to make sure the caller is legitimate. Do you recognize the voice as a physician or the nurse of the physician? Second, each part of the prescription must be put into writing immediately — the physician's name, the patient's name, the drug, its strength and dosage form, the amount, the directions, and the number of refills. Third, it is critical that the details of the prescription, as heard, are repeated to the sender with a request for confirmation.

This procedure, sometimes called *echoing*, is an important safety practice that can catch errors, especially for drugs that sound alike. Examples of sound-alikes are Lodine and codeine, Lopid and Slo-bid, and Preven and Preveon. This practice confirms the dose and how often the medication is to be taken, which are two factors that can contribute, if incorrect, to significant morbidity or mortality.

There is no question that being too busy contributes to medication errors. All pharmacies have their busy times and their slow times. During the busy times, everyone in the pharmacy works harder to be efficient and to not have patients wait too long for their medication. It is during these busy times that errors have an increased likelihood of occurring, because of distractions and cutting important steps in procedures designed to prevent errors. Thus, the busier the pharmacy gets, the more diligent everyone needs to be.

The occasional busy time in the pharmacy is understandable, is usually not predictable, and is difficult to avoid. What is not understandable, and is unacceptable, is a pharmacy that is too busy almost all the time. Such pharmacies are time bombs for errors, and sooner or later a major error will occur. Unfortunately, it will be the pharmacist on duty who will get in trouble, not the management that was negligent in allowing unsafe conditions.

Sloppy handwriting by prescribers contributes to errors in prescriptions, but only if the pharmacist tries to guess what is written. Pharmacists must always call the prescriber when in doubt about what the prescription says. The ultimate answer to this problem is computerized physician order entry (CPOE).

There is no excuse for pharmacists to have to work without enough help or the resources to practice safely.[38] Pharmacists, bound by their code of ethics, are obligated to bring unsafe working conditions that may jeopardize patient safety to the attention of their employers. If these conditions do not improve, it would be wise for the pharmacist to seek other employment and to consider bringing the unsafe conditions to the attention of the state board of pharmacy.

COMMUNITY PHARMACY SERVICES

Community pharmacies provide various services for patients. These services can be divided into traditional services and newer, innovative services.

Traditional Services

Most people are familiar with the traditional community pharmacy services offered to patients: prescriptions, over-the-counter (OTC) drugs, and perhaps home delivery. The pharmacy services may also provide medications for nursing homes, and some pharmacists prepare intravenous products for home health care patients.[39] If the pharmacy is in a full-service store, greeting cards, cosmetics, magazines, and other sundry items may be available. The heart and soul of each community pharmacy is the prescription service and the OTCs.

Prescription Services

Not every pharmacy will choose to stock every drug. This is a physical challenge, because it takes space and is fiscally unwise to do. Drugs are

Table 8.3 The Top 10 Drugs, Total Prescriptions Dispensed, 2004

Rank	Product (Company)	Prescriptions[a]
1.	Hydrocodone W/APAP	92.7
2.	Lipitor	69.8
3.	Lisinopril	46.2
4.	Atenolol	44.2
5.	Synthroid	44.1
6.	Amoxicillin	41.4
7.	Hydrochlorthiazide	41.3
8.	Zithromax	37.1
9.	Furosemdie	36.5
10.	Norvasc	34.7

[a] In millions

Source: From NDCHealth Pharmaceutical. http://www.rxlist.com/top200.htm.

expensive, and each day a drug remains on the shelf unsold increases inventory cost. Most pharmacies choose to stock the most popular drugs. Table 8.3 lists the top 10 drugs by prescription volume in 2004.[40] Most pharmacies can obtain any drug within 1 day from a drug wholesaler if they need it or within an hour if they borrow it from another pharmacy.

Some pharmacies will make a business decision not to compound prescriptions (many corporate community pharmacies), whereas others (several independent community pharmacies) will elect to make compounding a high priority or even a specialty.

Over-the-Counter Drugs

The pharmacist is uniquely qualified to advise patients about OTC medications. From a business perspective, OTCs are an important source of income.

Patients seeking OTCs as the answer to their health concerns offer a unique opportunity for pharmacists to display their knowledge and caring attitude. Properly counseling OTC patients involved several steps:[41]

- Assess the patient's physical complaint, symptoms, and medical condition.
- Determine if the condition is self-limiting or needs medical intervention.

■ Advise the patient on the proper course of action, that is, no treatment with drug therapy, self-treatment with nonprescription products, or referral to a physician or other health care provider.

If self-treatment with one or more nonprescription drugs is appropriate, the pharmacist should:

■ Assist in product selection
■ Assess patient risk factors
■ Counsel the patient regarding proper drug use of the OTC
■ Note the use of the drug in the patient's profile
■ If possible, provide follow-up
■ Discourage the use of fraudulent and "quack" remedies
■ Prevent delays in seeking appropriate medical attention
■ Assess if a nonprescription drug is masking the symptoms of a more serious condition

Patients have the highest awareness of cold remedies, vitamins, and dental products and patients are usually satisfied with the selection and pricing of these items.[11]

Newer Services

The emergence of managed care has placed new emphasis on primary and preventive care and reduced some health care costs. At the same time, it has reduced reimbursement rates for dispensing prescriptions. This has caused many pharmacists to look beyond preparing prescriptions to a larger role in patient care — one that pharmaceutical care can make happen. Besides being the most trusted health care professional, the pharmacist is also the most assessable health care person.

Types of New Services

In the past 5 years, pharmacists have started to offer new patient care services in community pharmacies. Examples of these services are providing immunizations; blood pressure, cholesterol, and osteoporosis screenings; smoking cessation programs; bone scans; and analysis of weight and body fat. In addition, many pharmacies are getting involved in *disease state management* (DSM) programs. These programs involve the systematic review of a chronic disease (e.g., asthma, diabetes, high blood pressure, hypercholesteremia, depression), the available treatment options, and the outcomes that those treatments are expected to produce.

DSM programs may use protocols, guidelines, or algorithms that take the pharmacy practitioner through a series of questions leading to a decision about the best care for the patient. Of course, this is with the approval of the patient and his or her physician. It is paid for by the patient or the patient's insurance program. Well-designed DSM programs improve care, are cost effective, and use pharmaceutical care in their delivery.

Extent of New Services

New services are being tried in all settings. Table 8.4 shows new patient care services in independent and chain store pharmacies for 1999 to 2000. The data show that independent pharmacies, and especially chain store pharmacies, were aggressively pursuing these new services and there has been a significant increase in the use of *collaborative practice agreements* (defined in Chapter 7, Pharmaceutical Care) to set up new patient care services. Newer figures were not available at the time of this writing (2006).

Supermarket pharmacies are also implementing these services. In 1999, 40% of supermarket chains had pharmacies that offer DSM in at least some of their stores.[5] Over 60% offered consumer health programs or services such as flu shots and blood pressure testing. The extent of these new patient care services in mass merchandiser pharmacies is unknown.

Are Patients Using These New Pharmacy Services?

A study revealed that education about the patient's medical condition and testing for hypertension were the two services patients were most likely to receive.[11] Analysis of body fat, vision testing, nutritional counseling, bone density tests, and influenza vaccines were received by more than 15% of survey respondents. Between 14% and 31% of patients not offered preventive services would have liked to have them made available at their pharmacies. Testing for hypertension and hypercholesteremia were the two most wished for services by patients.

Examples of How New Services Are Being Offered

Two examples — one in a chain store pharmacy and one in an independent pharmacy — will explain how these new services are being offered.

Chain Store Pharmacy

Most chain store pharmacy corporations are experimenting with providing pharmaceutical care, offering new patient care services, and suggesting

Table 8.4 Extent of New Patient Care Services in Chain and Independent Pharmacies, 1999 to 2000

	Independent Pharmacies		Chain Store Pharmacies	
	1999 (n = 216)	2000 (n = 276)	1999 (n = 31)	2000 (n = 58
Specialize in Specific Disease				
Yes	71%	27%	39%	53%
No	29%	73%	61%	47%
If Specialize – Disease States				
Diabetes	81%	63%	88%	84%
Hypertension	31%	13%		13%
Asthma	19%	25%	41%	26%
Cholesterol		9%	12%	29%
Osteoporosis		2%		19%
Collaborative Practice Agreements	6%	6%	3%	18%
Pain management		21%		
Diabetes		21%		29%
HIV		14%		
Hormone replacement therapy		14%		
Immunizations				43%
Asthma				14%
Other Services				
Counseling/consulting	29%	24%	16%	26%
Teaching/education/screening	29%	28%	42%	55%
Wellness/vaccination			37%	45%

Source: Adapted from Ukens, C. *Drug Top.* 1999;143(23):93 and Conlan, MF. *Drug Top.* 2000;144(23):70.

claims for the reimbursement for the cognitive services performed. One such chain is Walgreens.

Walgreens has implemented a few patient care centers that are in-store clinics separate from the prescription department. The patient care center is a comfortable area for individual and group education, individual screenings, and individual consultations. Computerized DSM modules are used in diabetes screening and counseling, and there are women's health programs in osteoporosis, menopause management, and breast cancer risk assessment. In addition, there is heart disease risk analysis and cholesterol screening. Walgreens has provided sophisticated and automated equipment to do patient testing.

Payment for services include cash payment, third-party payment, and employer payment. Reimbursement includes the cost of testing plus the pharmacist's time. Fees are charged for the screening and for patient improvement based on improvements in certain baseline tests. The program is in its initial stage and results will not be known for some time.

Independent Pharmacy

One independent pharmacy, Lowell's Pharmacy in Artesia, New Mexico, has been a family-owned business since 1958.[42] It is a professional store with 1900 square feet of space and only two aisles of OTCs. The store has recently and successfully expanded into compounding specialty products for physicians and patients. They also started doing immunizations by providing flu shots in the store and at local businesses. New services recently added have been asthma testing, osteoporosis bone density scans, and fat analysis to determine a person's ideal weight, and the pharmacists can provide diet and exercise suggestions.

Do These New Programs Work?

It is still too early to judge the success of these programs in any formal fashion. What would be the criteria? Would it be clinical improvement as judged by clinical testing? Patient satisfaction? Reduction of health care costs? It may depend on who is paying the bill. Pharmacists are just starting to learn how to measure results and bill for their patient care services.

The first results are encouraging. For example, the American Pharmaceutical Association(APhA) Foundation recently reported that over a 2-year period, 900 high cholesterol patients were part of a collaborative pharmacy care program. The patients had a 90% compliance rate with their medication, and 60% achieved their desired cholesterol levels.[43] These figures are double anything else reported in the literature.

Payment for Community Pharmacy Care

For pharmacists to be paid for the cognitive services they perform, which are those services not associated with a product, they must show what they do is value added.[43] Options for getting paid include collecting money from the patient, billing the patient's insurance company, and billing the patient's employer. Most pharmacies that bill for cognitive services bill the patient's insurance company.

Drug Topics reported that 39% of chain store pharmacies were getting some payment for nondispensing services, whereas 15% of independent pharmacies said those services helped their cash flow.[13] In that same year, *Drug Topics* reported that supermarket pharmacies were being reimbursed 20% of their time for DSM programs.[5]

A study surveyed a sample of 26 pharmacies in Georgia to determine the extent of billing, the bills paid, and who was paying for pharmaceutical care. Of the pharmacies surveyed, 66% indicated that they were providing pharmaceutical care to their patients, as defined in the survey instrument;[44,45] 26% were documenting and billing for pharmaceutical care services. Copies of 86 claim submissions revealed that 52 were billed to major medical insurance companies and 34 were billed to patients. Of the claims submitted to insurance companies, 18 (about 35%) were paid. The average amount per claim was $57.24. All claims billed directly to patients were paid. The amount billed to patients ranged from $2 to $39, and the average was $14.

Pharmacists at 126 pharmacies participating in Iowa's Medicaid pharmaceutical care management (PCM) program receive payment for monitoring drug therapy of high-risk patients.[46] PCM was authorized by Iowa's state legislature in 1999.

Pharmacists must meet certain requirements to participate in the PCM program, and patients who are monitored must have at least 1 of 12 disease states, be using at least four nontopical medications, and be receiving those medications from a PCM-eligible pharmacy. Pharmacist–physician teams work with patients to improve the patients' health outcomes. Both providers are paid the same rate: $75 for initial assessment, $40 for new problem assessment, $40 for problem follow-up, and $25 for preventive follow-up assessment.

Of course, not all community pharmacies perform pharmaceutical care, and not all that are performing pharmaceutical care bill for their services. A study was performed to discover the influence of payment, pharmacy setting, pharmacist demographics, practice setting, and attitudinal characteristics on whether cognitive services (CS) were performed by pharmacists and the volume of CS performed.[46]

Documentation of CS was more likely if the pharmacist was an owner or manager, if documentation was not perceived as being burdensome, and if the pharmacy had a low ratio of prescription to total sales. Higher documentation rates were associated with study group status, lower pharmacy prescription volume as a percentage of total sales, and a higher percentage of prescriptions billed to Medicaid. Among pharmacists, two setting variables, medical center location and rural location, were associated with higher documentation rates.

COMPETITION WITH MAIL-ORDER PHARMACIES

As shown in Table 8.1, mail-order pharmacies had the most growth (17.9%) in prescription sales between 2003 and 2004. This growth is in large part due to insurance companies forcing the employees of companies they insure into mail-order by allowing the employee to obtain a 90-day supply (and one copay) of chronic medication, but allowing only a 30-day supply of that medication (and charging for three copays over three months) if the covered employees go to their local pharmacists.

A survey in late 2003 showed that 72% of respondents opposed or strongly opposed a plan from their employer that would require them to obtain their medication through the mail.[47] "Additionally, 83% of respondents would choose community pharmacy over mail-order if a 90-day supply of their prescription were available to them for one co-pay." The good news is that the new Medicare prescription drug benefit (started January 1, 2006) has leveled the field and allows beneficiaries to obtain a 90-day supply of medication (if authorized by their prescriber) at any pharmacy. In addition, in 2005, the growth in mandatory mail prescription programs leveled off as employers realized the advantage of offering their employees choice.[48]

COMMUNITY PHARMACIST SATISFACTION

How satisfied are community pharmacists? Most community pharmacists still like the possibility of interacting with and helping patients, and the pay is above average. However, there is concern about job stress secondary to the prescriptions to be filled.[49,50] In 1996, a study revealed that across all settings, the range was 9.8 prescriptions per hour (independents) to 13.2 prescriptions per hour (chain stores).[51] In 2003, independent pharmacies were filling an average of 180 prescriptions per day and supermarket pharmacies 120 to 170 prescriptions per day.[52,53] No figures could be found for chain stores, but rumor has it that these stores fill even more prescriptions per day. It is also unknown how many prescriptions per day are being filled by mass merchandiser pharmacies.

What is known is that pharmacists and state boards of pharmacy are becoming increasingly concerned about pharmacists dispensing too many prescriptions per hour and pharmacists not getting enough breaks. The North Carolina State Board of Pharmacy has set as a safe limit, 10 to 20 prescriptions per hour per pharmacist and a maximum of 150 prescriptions per pharmacist per day.[54] Because of heavy prescription workloads, pharmacists are not able to spend as much time as they would like with patients, or do what the law requires in regard to patient counseling.

A 2000 study sanctioned by the National Association of Chain Drug Stores (NACDS), and performed by Arthur Anderson research firm, revealed that chain store pharmacists spend less than one-third of their time on activities that require a pharmacist's expertise.[55,56] One-fifth of the pharmacist's time was spent on "third-party–related" activities, such as entering information from the patient's identification card and resolving conflicts related to restrictions on insurance coverage. The paperwork problems and the rising workload is frustrating, and some community pharmacists feel that their clinical skills are not being put to good use.

POSITIONS FOR PHARMACISTS IN COMMUNITY PHARMACY

Various positions are available for pharmacists in community pharmacy.

Pharmacy Interns

The first possibility is a *pharmacy intern*. A pharmacy intern must be a pharmacy student and registered by the state board of pharmacy in the state of employment. Pharmacy interns must work under the direct supervision of a licensed pharmacist.

Community Pharmacy Residents

New pharmacy graduates may want to do a 1-year residency in *community pharmacy* practice. Community pharmacy residencies teach the resident how to manage a community pharmacy and how to provide and bill for innovative pharmacy care services. The resident learns by doing but is closely mentored by a preceptor.[57] If the community pharmacy residency program is accredited, a residency project will be required and the results presented at a regional residency conference.

Most people feel that a 1-year residency is like gaining 2 to 3 years of practical experience and boosts the resident's confidence to practice. It also has been shown that those choosing to do a pharmacy residency often get the best career opportunities, and many go on to be leaders in the profession.

Staff Pharmacists

Most new graduates who do not do a community pharmacy residency will start by working as an entry-level pharmacist, but at an attractive wage based on supply and demand for pharmacists. Some like the role of a staff pharmacist and continue working in that capacity, whereas others will want to advance into management.

Store-Level and District Managers

Once experience is gained at the staff pharmacist level, some pharmacists will move up to supervisory or management positions within a pharmacy.[58] These pay more and require more skill in managing resources and people. They also are more stressful. The next step after this is a district manager over many stores.

Corporate Management

Some pharmacists move into the management structure of their corporation. These can be high-level positions that offer opportunities to improve how pharmacy is practiced within the company. For this to happen, many pharmacists seek added education in management, and some earn a master's of business administration degree (M.B.A.) from a school of business.

Pharmacy Ownership

Some pharmacists may want to own their own pharmacy. Nowadays, it is wise to have a good understanding of what this entails before purchasing a store. It is recommended that pharmacy students take an elective course in pharmacy ownership while in pharmacy school if this is something the student thinks he or she may want to do some day. Also, staff pharmacists who think they might like to be pharmacy owners should consult with a community pharmacy consultant or a faculty member specializing in community pharmacy ownership before buying a store.

FUTURE OF COMMUNITY PHARMACY PRACTICE

No one knows for sure what community pharmacy practice will be like in the future; however, there are some trends that will help shape this future.

> *Rising prescription volume:* Prescription volume is projected to rise dramatically over the next 25 years owing in part to the aging population. Pharmacists should carve out a niche for these older patients.[59] At least one pharmacy chain is preparing a strategy to capture baby boomers as patients retire and move into old age.[60]
>
> *Not enough pharmacists:* Based on projections of an aging population and a rising number of prescriptions, there will not be enough pharmacists even if pharmacy schools dramatically graduate more students; that is, if pharmacy is practiced in community pharmacies the way it is today.

Technology and automation: For pharmacy to fill all the prescriptions that will be generated over the next 25 years, and for community pharmacists to practice pharmaceutical care, there will need to be more use of pharmacy technicians, technology, and automation.[61–63]

Expansion of the community pharmacist into public health: It may be that pharmacists will expand their role, be recognized, and be paid for helping achieve national health care goals in immunization, smoking, HIV prevention, weight reduction, and exercise.

Payment for achieving positive patient outcomes: It is hoped that in 25 years, community pharmacists will be known more for their role in helping patients achieve positive outcomes from their drug therapy than for providing the medication, and that they will be paid accordingly.

IMPLEMENTING CHANGE IN COMMUNITY PHARMACY PRACTICE

A white paper, co-written by the NACDS, the (APhA), and the National Community Pharmacists Association(NCPA), was recently released. This is a historic event for these three organizations to agree on what steps need to be taken to move community pharmacy into the twenty-first century.[64,65] Three major challenges were outlined: (a) pressures on drug distribution and volume, (b) the impact of prescription benefit programs, and (c) workforce and education issues. A solution was offered for each challenge, and 25 steps were outlined to move community pharmacy forward.

SUMMARY

Community pharmacy is the heart and soul of pharmacy practice. About 60% of pharmacy graduates work in one of four types of community pharmacy practice sites after graduation. Each type of practice site has its pros and cons as a place to practice pharmacy. Based on the aging population and increased use of medication to improve health, community pharmacy practice will continue to grow rapidly over the next 25 years. To meet this growth and to practice pharmaceutical care, pharmacies will need to use more pharmacy technicians, use more automation, and make sure pharmacists only do pharmacist-only functions. It is hoped that by the year 2015, community pharmacists are known more for the care and counseling they provide than for providing medication.

DISCUSSION QUESTIONS AND EXERCISES

1. Based on what you know and have read thus far, record what you feel are the pros and cons of practicing pharmacy in:
   a. Community pharmacy
   b. Chain store pharmacy
   c. Mass merchandiser pharmacy
   d. Food store pharmacy
2. Based on what you know and have read thus far, what do you feel are the pros and cons of owning your own pharmacy?
3. List three things community pharmacists can do to improve patient satisfaction and three things they can do to improve patient safety.
4. Make an appointment to interview a pharmacist who is:
   a. An owner of a community pharmacy
   b. Working in a chain store pharmacy
   c. Working in a mass merchandiser pharmacy
   d. Working in a food store pharmacy
5. List three ways community pharmacists can improve their patient satisfaction, in order of priority, and explain why these methods will work.

CHALLENGES

1. Table 8.2 provides important information about the growth of pharmaceutical care in community pharmacies. However, the table needs updating that was not available at the time of this writing (2006). For extra credit, and with the permission of your professor, do a literature search, update Table 8.2, and send your results to the author.
2. Residencies in community pharmacy are relatively new. For extra credit, and with the permission of your professor, write a concise report about community pharmacy residencies. Include what they are, how many there are, how many residents are in these programs, and the advantages and disadvantages of doing this type of residency from the students, rather than the profession's point of view.
3. One of the most critical issues in filling a prescription order is the frequent inability to read the presciber's directions. Some medical schools have gone so far as to require mandatory courses in handwriting. Some experts think the answer lies in computerized origination of the prescription. For extra credit, and with the permission of your professor, prepare a concise paper probing the complex dimensions of solving this problem for the nation.

4. Pharmacy is often criticized because pharmacists spend an inordinate amount of time on technical functions — counting, pouring, labeling, and so on. For extra credit, and with the permission of your professor, construct methods that purport to minimize the negative social consequences with professional performance of this more restricted and yet prominent role of the pharmacist.

WEB SITES OF INTEREST

National Community Pharmacist Association: http://www.ncpanet.org/

National Association of Chain Drugstores: http://www.nacds.org

Career guide: http://www.ncpanet.org/students/independent_pharmacy_career_guide/index.shtml

Grocery store pharmacy jobs: http://www.rxrecruiters.com/grocery-store-pharmacy-jobs.htm

Food Market Institute: http://www.fmi.org/

REFERENCES

1. National Association of Chain Drugstores. Industry facts-at-a-glance (final 1999 figures). Available at http://www.nacds.org/industry/fastfacts.html. Accessed March 19, 2001.
2. National Community Pharmacy Association. Independent pharmacy today. Available at http://www.ncpanet.org/about/independent_pharmacy_today. shtml. Accessed April 19, 2006.
3. 2005 NCPA-Pfizer Digest. Executive Summary. Availabl at http://www.ncpa-net.org/pdf/2005digest.executivesummary.pdf. Accessed April 19, 2006.
4. Anonymous. *Career Planning: Practice Areas in Pharmacy, in Pharmacy Cadence*. PAS Pharmacy Association Services, Athens, GA, 1992, p. 40.
5. Anonymous. Supermarket pharmacies reports ups, downs in '04. *Drug Topics*. October 10, 2005. Available at http://www.drugtopics.com/drugtopics/content/printContentPopup.jsp?id=184093. Accessed April 19, 06.
6. Levy, S. What wellness consumers want, pharmacists should deliver. *Drug Top*. 2000;144(10):47.
7. Levy, S. Supermarkets: pharmacy's best-kept secret. *Drug Top*. 2000;144(5): 50–58.
8. Anonymous. Food for thought: discount stores eat into supermarket, drug store sales. *Chain Store Age*. 2000;76(5):49–52.
9. Hagerman, PR. Finding success in pharmacy's roots. *Mich Pharm*. 1996;34(Aug):27.
10. Hesterlee, EJ. Building a better profession. *Missouri Pharm*. 1991;65 (Dec):12–14.
11. Wilson, J. *2001 WilsonRx™ Pharmacy Survey Report*. Wilson Health Information, LLC, New Hope, PA. http://www.wilsonrx.com.
12. Anonymous. Relief for the Rx blues. *Consumer Rep*. 1999;64(10):38.

13. Ukens, C. Community pharmacy embraces pharmacist care. *Drug Top.* 1999;143(23):93.

14. Conlan, MF. Community pharmacies do more than dispense Rxs. *Drug Top.* 2000;144(23):70.

15. Spivey, A. The Ashville Project. Available at http://research.unc.edu/endeavors/win2004/asheville.html. Accessed April 19, 2006.

16. Cranor, CW, and Christensen, DB. The Ashville Project: short term outcomes of community pharmacy diabetes program. *J Am Pharm Assoc.* 2003;43:149–159.

17. Cranor, CW, and Christensen, DB. The Ashville Project: factors associated with outcomes of a community pharmacy diabetes care program. *J Am Pharm Assoc.* 2003;43:160–172.

18. Cranor, CW, Bunting, BA, and Christensen, DB. The Ashville Project: long-term clinical and economic outcomes of community pharmacy diabetes care program. *J Am Pharm Assoc.* 2003;43:173–184.

19. Carter, BL, Chrischilles, EA, Scholz, D, et al. Extent of services provided by pharmacists in the Iowa Medicaid Pharmaceutical Case program. *J Am Pharm Assoc.* 2003;43:24–33.

20. Anonymous. Impact of pharmaceutical care delivered in the community pharmacy setting: results of a two-year demonstration project. Available at http://www.iarx.org/Documents/Pharmacy%20Practice%20Initiatives%20-%20Wellmark%20Demonstration%20Article.doc. Accessed April 19, 2006

21. Weinberger, M, Murray, MD, Marrero, DG, et al. Effectiveness of pharmacist care for patients with reactive airways disease. *JAMA.* 2002;288:1594–1602.

22. Chi, J. Study's unintended results setback pharmacy? *Drug Top.* 2002;20:20.

23. Eickhoff, C. Pharmaceutical care in community pharmacies: practice and research in Germany. *Ann Pharmacother.* 2006;40(4):729–735.

24. Krska, J, Veitch, GBA, and Calder, G. Developing pharmaceutical care in community pharmacies. *Pharm. J.* 2000;265(7114). Available at http://pjonline.com/Editorial/20000916/practiceresearch/r33.html. Accessed April 19, 2006.

25. McLean, WM. When does pharmaceutical care impact health outcomes? A comparison of community pharmacy-based studies of pharmaceutical care for patients with asthma. *Ann Pharmacother.* 2005;39(4):625–631.

26. Norwood, GJ, Sleath, BL, Caiola, SM, and Lien, T. Costs of implementing pharmaceutical care in community pharmacies. *J Am Pharm Assoc.* 1998;38:755–761.

27. Amsler, MR, Murray, MD, Tierney, W, et al. Pharmaceutical care in chain pharmacies: beliefs and attitudes of pharmacists and patients. *J Am Pharm Assoc.* 2001;41(6):850–855.

28. Tindall, WN, and Millonig, MK. *Pharmaceutical Care: Insights from Community Pharmacy.* CRC Press, Boca Raton, FL, 2002.

29. Felkey, B. Latest technology can set you free. *Am Drug.* 1998;215(May):54–55.

30. Terrie, YC. Pharmacy compounding is flourishing once again. *Pharm. Times.* November, 2005. Available at http://www.pharmacytimes.com/article.cfm?ID=2780. Accessed April 21 2006

31. Slezak, M. New look for a new age. *Am Drug.* 1997;214(Jan):20–25.

32. Fleming, H, Jr. Medicap ready to launch counseling-only option. *Drug Top.* 2000;144(Feb 7):116.

33. Marcellino, K. What do Georgia's patients expect from their pharmacist? *Ga Pharm J.* 2001;23:22–23.

34. Potter, SB, and Black, CD. Feasibility of compliance with OBRA 90. Presented at the APhA Annual Meeting. 1994;141:102.

35. Ukens, C. Patients getting written information on their Rxs. *Drug Top.* 2000;144(4):41.

36. Kroon, L. Communication, comprehension, and compliance: three Cs of effective patient counseling. *Calif J Health-Syst Pharm.* 1999;11(May–June):24–25.

37. Gardner, M, Boyce, RW, and Herrier, RN. *Pharmacist–Patient Consultation Program PPC-Unit 1.* Pfizer, National Healthcare Operations, New York, 1993.

38. Breu, J. It's time for research to focus on patient safety in community setting. *Drug Top.* 2001:145(1):25–26.

39. Bagley, JL. Consultant services appeal to some drug chains. *Am Drug.* 1986;194(Oct):148–153.

40. NDC Health Pharmaceutical. The top 300 prescriptions for 2004 by number of US prescriptions dispensed. Available at http://www.rxlist.com/top200.htm. Accessed April 21, 2006.

41. *Handbook of Nonprescription Drugs.* American Pharmaceutical Association, Washington, DC, 2000.

42. Bailey, R. Generations treat generations at Lowell's Pharmacy. *Commun Pharm.* 1999;91(5):12–14.

43. Bouldin, AS, Bentley, JP, Huffman, DC, and Garner, DD. Independent pharmacy: rising to meet the challenge of the future. *J Pharm Market Manage.* 1996;10(2–3):149–166.

44. Wickman, JM, Marquess, JG, and Jackson, RA. Documenting pharmacy care does make ¢ents (and dollars too). *Ga Pharm J.* 1998;February:12–14.

45. Wickman, JM, Jackson, RA, and Marquess, JG. Making ¢ents out of caring for patients. *J Am Pharm Assoc.* 1999;39:116–119.

46. Christensen, DB, and Hansen, RW. Characteristics of pharmacies and pharmacists associated with the provision of cognitive services in the community setting. *J Am Pharm Assoc.* 1999;39:640–649.

47. NACDS. Attitudes about mandatory mail-order pharmacy. Available at http://www.nacdsfoundation.org/user-assets/Documents/PDF/Mail_Research_November_2003.pdf. Accessed April 21, 2006.

48. Edlin, M. Retail pharmacies fill 90-day prescriptions to compete with mail. *Managed Care Executive.* 2006;16(4):46–49.

49. Alvarez, NA. Searching for utopia. *J Am Pharm Assoc.* 1997;37:632–634.

50. Ortmeir, BG, and Wolfgang, AP. Job-related stress: perceptions of employee pharmacists. *Am Pharm.* 1991:31(9):27–31.

51. Shondelmeyer, SW, and Seone-Vazquez, E. Pharmacists are working harder. *Am Drug.* 1997;214(Aug):34–39.

52. Kirsche, ML. Gross margins, net profits up for independents. *Drug Store News.* July 19, 2004. Available at http://www.findarticles.com/p/articles/mi_m3374/is_9_26/ai_n6122106/print. Accessed April 21, 2006.

53. Food Marketing Institute. Supermarket pharmacy expansion continues as food retailers increasingly become a whole health solution for consumers, according to new study. Available at http://www.fmi.org/media/mediatext.cfm?id=564. Accessed April 21, 2006.

54. North Carolina Board of Pharmacy. Statement on pharmacist workload. March 26, 1997. Available at http://www.usalaw.com/a-mp-NC-Pharmacy-Board-workload.html. Accessed April 21, 2006.

55. Landis, NT. Non–patient-care activities dilute pharmacists' time, NACDS study shows. *Am J Health-Syst Pharm*. 2000;57:202.

56. Fleming, H, Jr. Time bomb. *Drug Top*. 2000;144(4):70.

57. Anonymous. The NACDS/NCPA community pharmacy practice residency guidelines. Available at http://www.nacds.org/resources/cppr.html. 2001. Accessed February 20, 2001.

58. Weber, L. Chain pharmacy practice: a career with endless opportunities. *Pharm Bus*. 1993;4(3):31–32.

59. Anonymous. The elderly increasingly depend on the guidance of pharmacists. *Calif Pharm*. 1998;45(3):14–15.

60. Anonymous. Walgreen cashing in on aging consumers. *Atlanta Journal-Constitution*. May 21, 2001, business section.

61. Ukens, C. Auto motion. *Drug Top*. 1998;142(18):78.

62. Sanz, F, Silveira, C, Diaz, C, et. al. Information technology in community pharmacies for supporting responsible self-medication. *Am J Health-Syst Pharm*. 2000;57:1601–1603.

63. Heller, A. New technology advances pharmacy productivity. *Drug Store News Chain Pharm*. 1998;8:CP29.

64. Anonymous. Implementing effective change in meeting the demands of community pharmacy practice in the United States. *Infusion*. 1999;5(Nov):43–48.

65. Anonymous. Organizations outline challenges, actions for community pharmacy. *Am J Health-Syst Pharm*. 1999;56:1915.

9

HOSPITAL PHARMACY

The health care team (physicians, nurses, pharmacists, and other health care workers) is most obvious in the hospital. Hospitals are also where the newest drugs, some of which are still being investigated, are used. Because of this, hospitals can be exciting places for pharmacists to work.

This chapter will explore the hospital, the patient, the health care team, and what it is like to practice pharmacy inside a typical hospital. It will cover pharmacy's mission within a hospital — control of drugs, their proper use, avoiding medication misadventures, and education and training. The role of the pharmacist and other members of the pharmacy department will also be covered. The chapter will end by discussing some trends that may shape the future of pharmacy practice in hospitals.

LEARNING OBJECTIVES

After reading this chapter, you should be able to:

- Provide a brief history of hospitals
- Discuss the types of hospitals
- Discuss how hospitals vary
- Explain how hospitals are accredited
- Explain how hospitals are organized
- Discuss the feelings of the hospitalized patient
- Explain the mission of the hospital pharmacy department
- Discuss how the hospital pharmacy goes about accomplishing its mission
- Discuss how the hospital pharmacist fits into the health care team
- Explain the drug-use process in the hospital
- Explain how most hospital pharmacy departments are organized

HOSPITALS

Hospitals have changed from small beginnings to becoming major health care centers of excellence.

How Hospitals Started

In ancient times, hospitals were shelters for travelers and pilgrims.[1] During the early Christian era, hospitals were places for Christian travelers in the Holy Land. In Europe, during the 1600s, "poor houses" were established to provide food and shelter for the downtrodden. In the early years of the United States, hospitals were infirmaries for the poor. In the late 1700s and early 1800s, hospitals were charitable places for the ill. It was not until the late 1800s and early 1900s that hospitals became safe and effective treatment centers. During the 1930s and 1940s, hospitals became known for their diagnostic skill, new treatment methods, and special care.

Modern Hospitals

Today's modern hospital is a sophisticated, high-technology center for the diagnosis and treatment of general or specific medical conditions — both acute and chronic. An *acute illness* is a medical condition that needs immediate attention, which if properly treated, is self-limiting. A *chronic illness* is one of long duration, which can perhaps last for a lifetime. The eight major chronic illnesses treated today are asthma, hypertension, diabetes, arthritis, obesity, depression, congestive heart failure, and hypercholesterolemia.

Besides diagnosing and treating these illnesses, hospitals also diagnose and treat rare and unusual conditions, perform surgery if needed, and educate patients about their health and how to manage and improve quality of life.

Types of Hospitals

There are three types of hospitals: general (about 83%), special (about 11%), and rehabilitation (about 3%).[2]

- *General hospitals* have emergency rooms, x-ray departments, and surgical suites and they care for general medicine and surgical patients.
- *Special hospitals* care for special populations of patients, such as pediatric, geriatric, or psychiatric patients. These have specialized equipment and health care providers with specialized expertise.

- *Rehabilitation hospitals* specialize in rehabilitating patients with orthopedic (bone and joint) or central nervous disorders.

Hospital Ownership

Hospitals are classified by whom they are owned — privately or publicly owned (city, county, state, or federal) — and whether they are *for-profit* or *not-for-profit*. All public hospitals are nonprofit. Many of the private hospitals are run by religious organizations and are not-for-profit, whereas other private hospitals are for-profit.

Hospital Size

Sixty percent of hospitals have less than 200 beds. In addition, the number of beds in hospitals have been dropping due to a major shift from acute to ambulatory care and declining lengths of hospital stays. These shifts are driven by the need to reduce cost.

Hospital Type

Table 9.1 shows the types of hospitals in the United States in 2004. Most of the hospitals were based in the community, and of these, most were urban (59.2%).[2]

Table 9.1   Types of Hospitals in the United States, 2004

Total number of all U.S. registered hospitals	5,759
Community hospitals	4,919
U.S. not-for-profit community hospitals	2,967
Investor-owned (for profit) community hospitals	835
State and local government community hospitals	1,117
Federal government hospitals	239
Nonfederal psychiatric hospitals	466
Nonfederal long-term care hospitals	112
Other	23

Source: Fast facts on U.S. hospitals from *AHA Hospital Statistics.* American Hospital Association, Chicago, 2004.

Table 9.2   U.S. Hospitals, 1990, 1995, and 2003

Item	1990	1995	2003
Total hospitals	6649	6291	5764
Total beds (1000)	1213	1081	965
Average daily census	844	710	657
Outpatient visits (millions)	368.2	483.2	648.6
Personnel (1000)	4063	4273	4650
Total expenses (billions)	$234.9	$320.3	$498.1

Source: Statistical Abstracts of the United States: The National Data Book. Health and Nutrition. U.S. Census Bureau, U.S. Department of Commerce, Washington, DC, 2006.

Hospital Statistics

Table 9.2 compares the statistics for hospitals in 1990, 1995, and 2003.[3] The number of hospitals, the total number of beds, the total admissions, and the average daily census all dropped during this time frame. Although these numbers indicate that there are fewer patients in hospitals, and those who are in the hospital are sicker.

At the same time, there has been a shift to treating more outpatients. Outpatient care is much less costly than inpatient care. Despite these savings, the cost of care in hospitals rose 36.4% between 1990 and 1997 and 55.5% between 1995 and 2003.

Hospital Accreditation

Hospitals receive *accreditation* — confirmation that they meet certain minimum standards of care — from the Joint Commission on Accreditation of Health Care Organizations (JCAHO). The JCAHO is a nonprofit, nongovernmental organization that inspects hospitals every 2 to 4 years. Some of the standards concern the pharmacy and the medication-use process in the hospital. Three surveyors complete the survey over a 2- to 3-day period. Although hospital accreditation is strictly voluntary, some governmental reimbursement (such as Medicare and Medicaid) is tied to JCAHO accreditation. However, nonaccredited hospitals can comply with federal conditions of participation and still qualify for Medicaid and Medicare.

Internal Organization

The typical hospital is organized into two distinct, but related, parts: the medical staff structure and the hospital structure.

Medical Staff Structure

The medical staff, the physicians, who are either private or on staff, have their own rules and regulations (bylaws), their own officers (president, vice-president, treasurer, and secretary), and governing board (executive committee). The medical staff is organized by departments, such as medicine, pediatrics, and radiology, and each department has a chief (e.g., the chief of surgery). The medical staff also has an extensive set of committees in the hospital to get its work done. Some examples of committees important to pharmacy are the pharmacy and therapeutics (P&T) committee, patient care committee, and ambulatory care committee.

The *P&T committee* (the director of pharmacy is usually the secretary) selects the drugs to be used in the hospital and approves policies and procedures that guide the appropriate use of drugs within the institution. Drugs selected for the *hospital formulary* must be effective, safe, and cost effective. A drug under review is compared to similar drugs in the formulary. A drug being considered for formulary status must be better than a drug that is currently being used (or equal and cheaper), and if it is better, will either replace the older agent or be given a trial period to see how it performs. After the trial period, a final decision is made about which of the drugs will have formulary status.

The pharmacy is responsible for writing the *P&T background* (the evaluation) of a drug being requested for formulary status. Formulary requests usually come from members of the medical staff, who must state the reasons a drug is being requested. P&T backgrounds are extensive, comparative evaluations based on the clinical studies and pharmacoeconomic evaluations (cost effectiveness) published in the medical and pharmacy literature.

Other important committees of the medical staff where pharmacists can contribute are the patient care committee and the ambulatory care committee. These committees often deal with issues of interest to the pharmacy.

Hospital Structure

Hospital employees other than physicians work in various departments of the hospital. The chief executive officer, the chief operating officer or president, the chief financial officer, and various vice-presidents of the hospital work in hospital administration. Reporting to the various vice-presidents are the directors of various hospital departments, for example, pharmacy, nursing, laboratory, and anesthesia.

PATIENTS

Patients entering the hospital, either as outpatients or as inpatients, come to this experience from different points of view. Some patients look forward to finding answers to their health care problems. Others are afraid the experience will be a bad one, in that they may discover they have a major illness or a poor prognosis. Some may be afraid of surgery. Others come trusting health care professionals, whereas others are leery. Some have language or cultural barriers. Some are afraid the cost of hospitalization will ruin them financially, whereas others are afraid a medical error will harm them.

A survey revealed what errors people fear the most. The top four "very concerned" items are about health care. They are: (a) errors associated with receiving health care in general (47%), (b) going to a hospital for care (47%), (c) going to a physician's office for care (40%), and (d) filling a prescription at a pharmacy (34%). Overall, 6% of the respondents felt they had suffered an injury or harm because of a medical error during the previous 12 months.[4]

Hospitals can be busy and confusing places for patients. Because of this confusion and respect for health care professionals, many patients turn themselves over to the health care team rather than become a partner in their health care. Patients have rights and need to be members of the health care team. They also need to understand their health situation, know their rights and duties, understand their alternatives, look for something that may not be correct, and continually work to improve their health.

Pharmacists need to understand the patient, who is usually not feeling well and is seeking better health. The pharmacist, a caregiver, should try to fill the patient's needs through knowledge and a caring attitude. The covenant relationship between the patient and pharmacist goes like this: "If you help me (the patient) make the best use of my medication, I will give you (the pharmacist) my respect, trust, and cooperation."

However, being successful at this covenant relationship is not always so easy, because every patient has a different set of circumstances and comes from a different background. The pharmacist must start with the facts, ask probing questions, be understanding, and show a caring attitude. Success usually comes with experience; however, the fundamental principles of respect for human dignity and feeling the patient's vulnerability lie at the core of a fruitful pharmacist–patient relationship. Yet, the short length of hospital stays (down from 7.8 days in 1970 to 4.8 days in 2003) for most patients makes it difficult for the hospital pharmacist to implement the covenant relationship.

HEALTH CARE TEAM

The health care team is never more obvious and visible than it is in the hospital. Physicians, nurses, pharmacists, dieticians, laboratory, and radiology (x-ray) personnel, to name a few, work together for the good of the patient. The health care team runs smoothly when each person on the team understands and respects each other's roles, communicates well, and always has the patient's best interest at the center of their attention. Including the patient in their care makes the team function even better.

How the pharmacist fits into the health care team is changing for the better. In the past, pharmacists were relied on to make sure the right drug was given to the right patient at the right time. This is still a key role for pharmacy from a drug distribution standpoint. However, to fulfill the first part — the correct drug — the pharmacist needs to know that the patient is diagnosed correctly and that the best drug for that patient has been prescribed. To do this, the pharmacist needs to be on the patient care unit after the patient has been evaluated and diagnosed and when the drug is being selected.

The pharmacist also needs to advise the nurse about the important job of administering medication. It is also the role of the pharmacist to be the patient's adviser when it comes to medication.

The goal should be that most patients say "yes" when asked if they talked with a pharmacist during their hospital stay. It is even better if the patient remembers the pharmacist's name. However, how many patients in hospitals do not even know there are pharmacists in the hospital?[5]

PHARMACY DEPARTMENT

The pharmacy department is considered to be an important department within every hospital. Whether it is viewed as a hospital department or a clinical department varies from hospital to hospital, and this is often dependent on how the pharmacy department views itself.

Pharmacy's Mission

The mission of most pharmacy departments in hospitals is the safe, effective, timely, and cost-effective use of drugs. It involves drug control, overseeing the drug-use process, being involved in the appropriate use of drugs, and avoiding medication misadventures. It also includes education and training.

Control of Drugs

The pharmacy, by law and JCAHO standards, is responsible for the control of medication throughout the hospital facility. The director of pharmacy is held accountable for this control. Control involves more than keeping supplies secure.[6] Control includes knowing where all drugs are stored, that there is enough (not too much nor not too little), and that all drug products are fresh and potent.

Inventory Control

Drug control starts with good inventory control. Good inventory control means keeping accurate records of what is used and how often it is used. Drugs must be stored properly in areas with correct temperature and light. Narcotics and other controlled substances must be stored properly. Schedule II controlled substances (substances with high addiction and abuse potential) must be stored under lock and key. Schedule III–V controlled substances are either spread throughout the stock or also kept under lock and key (see Chapter 4, The Drug-Use Process). Strict inventory and security requirements need to be followed for these drugs both in the pharmacy and when they are used on the patient care units.

Drug Samples

Other drugs needing strict control are *drug samples*. Drug samples are small quantities of drugs provided by drug manufacturers to physicians for starting a patient on a new drug to see how it works or if there are adverse effects before writing a prescription. Because physicians often see ambulatory patients in hospital clinics, samples sometimes show up there. Because the director of pharmacy must exercise control, the JCAHO states that there must be a hospital policy for drug samples. The policy of many hospitals is to not use drug samples.

Investigational Drugs

Another category of drugs that needs strict inventory control is *investigational drugs*. These drugs are used in clinical research trials where some patients receive the active (investigational) drug, whereas other patients receive a look-alike, nonactive drug (placebo). The pharmacy keeps records of which patient receives which drugs.

Overseeing the Drug-Use Process

There is a well-defined process to decide how drugs are used in the hospital:

Policies and Procedures: The pharmacy drafts policies and procedures on the important steps in the drug-use process (prescribing, preparation, dispensing, and administrating) for discussion by the P&T committee. The director of pharmacy is usually the secretary of this committee, and there is usually a nurse and a hospital administrator on this committee along with several members of the medical staff. The drug-use policies and procedures are discussed, changed, and approved for use by the committee. These policies and procedures should be regularly reviewed and updated.

Documenting Medication Use and Allergies: When admitted to the hospital, patients are asked what medications they take regularly and what allergies they have to medication. The answers to these questions are documented in the patient's record (paper or electronic medical record) and sent to the pharmacy electronically or by a copy (NCR paper) of the information.

Prescribing and Transmission of Orders: Physicians prescribe medication for patients using double-copy order forms (NCR). The original stays in the patient's record and the copy is sent to the pharmacy. There are various methods by which the pharmacy can receive the order: courier, fax, pneumatic tube, or electronically, which is the best way. The JCAHO standard states that the pharmacy must review a copy of what the physician has ordered; thus, transcriptions (rewriting orders) by nursing personnel are not permissible.

Drug Preparation and Distribution: National standards have been developed by the American Society of Health-System Pharmacists (ASHP) that pharmacists use as the basis for their policies and procedures to prepare and distribute drugs in hospitals. The use of these standards is critical in protecting patients and helping the pharmacy service to be up-to-date on what it is doing.

Three primary systems are used for distributing drugs in hospitals and other organized health care settings: floor stock, unit-dose, and centralized intravenous (IV) additives.

Floor Stock

Medication can be stored on the patient care units in the form of *floor stock*; however, this is not recommended. If this is done, medication should be limited. The caution for storing medication in this manner is because of safety. Floor stock offers more opportunity for error; there is no check and balance system to avoid mistakes. The nurse can go to floor stock where the medication is stored, usually on a shelf or in a drawer, take out what is needed and provide it directly to the patient.

The most common drugs in floor stock are narcotics, which should always be under lock and key with strict counting requirements, various IV solutions, and emergency drugs (usually in a kit). Some patient care units, such as the emergency room, intensive care units, the operating room, and recovery room, have more floor stock than others.

Unit-Dose

The second method of drug distribution is called *unit-dose*. A unit-dose is one dispensed from the pharmacy that is ready to be given to the patient, which means that no further dosage preparation, calculation, or manipulation is required.

The earliest attempts at unit-dose drug distribution were documented nearly 40 years ago in community hospitals by Simpson and Carver in Long Beach, California, and by Schwartau and Sturdivant in Rochester, Minnesota.[7] Unit-dose systems are safer than other drug distribution methods, because there is less opportunity for error and there is a built-in check and balance system.

In the unit-dose system of medication distribution, there are two medication drawers for each patient. One drawer is always in the pharmacy being filled, whereas the other is always on the patient care unit being used by the nurse to give medication to that patient. Each drawer is usually divided into two sections — one for regularly scheduled medication, and the other for PRN (as needed) medication. The pharmacy places enough medication for the patient for the next shift (7 a.m. to 3 p.m., 3 p.m. to 11 p.m., or 11 p.m. to 7 a.m.) or for the next 24-hour period. At the end of the shift or 24-hour period, the drawers are exchanged.

The built-in check and balance system in the unit-dose system is based on three sets of medication records: the doctor's orders in the patient's record, the patient's pharmacy profile, and the nursing Kardex (a card for each patient in a folder). In electronic systems, the Kardex is a printout produced by nursing.

The pharmacy receives a copy of the patient's medication orders. Ideally, pharmacy technicians, rather than pharmacists, enter the medication orders into the patient's profile, which is part of the pharmacy computer system. If the hospital has a total information system, the orders flow directly from the physician's electronic orders into an electronic version of the patient's pharmacy profile in the computer system. On the patient care unit, the unit clerk transcribes (copies) the medication orders into the nursing Kardex. The nurse must check and initial these transcriptions. The nurse uses the Kardex as a reminder of what, when, and to whom to administer medication. In an automated system, the nurse receives a printed list showing what to administer, to whom, and when.

There are two sets of medication records for each patient — the pharmacy patient profile and the nursing Kardex. They should be identical. The best procedure for checking a patient's unit-dose drawer is for the pharmacist to check the contents of the drawer against the nursing Kardex rather than the pharmacy patient profile from which the drawer was filled. If the drawer is not correct, it means one of three things happened: (a) the drawer was filled wrong, (b) there was a computer entry error made in the pharmacy, or (c) there was a transcription error made between the physician's order and the nursing Kardex. Which error occurred? The answer can be found by checking the physician's order in the patient's record.

An alternative method of unit–dose is to use automated dispensing machines (ADMs) instead of medication carts (see Chapter 6).

IV Admixtures

The third drug distribution system is for *IV admixtures*. IV additives are drugs added to IV solutions. Such medication is administered to patients intravenously (into their vein) and must be *sterile* (free of any germs that can cause infection — bacteria, viruses, and fungi). The technique of adding medication to IV solutions should be done carefully and under ideal conditions. In the past, nurses prepared the IV solution on the patient care unit, which is a place full of germs. If this is still allowed in the hospital, there must be a policy on how nurses should do this.

ASHP and JCAHO standards now recommend that IV admixtures be prepared in the pharmacy using aseptic (germ free) technique and a laminar flow hood. In 1997, 81.1% of hospital pharmacy survey respondents indicated that their hospital had a complete, comprehensive IV admixture program.[8] A *laminar flow hood* is an aseptic work area with positive-pressure airflow that filters the air. Pharmacists and pharmacy technicians are trained to properly prepare IV admixtures, and they should be recertified on how to do this.

Once the IV additives are prepared, preferably by a certified pharmacy technician, rather than a pharmacist, they are checked by a pharmacist.

When an IV admixture is contaminated during preparation, the bacteria grows exponentially with time and temperature. Therefore, IV admixtures should be prepared just before they are needed and refrigerated between the time they are prepared and the time they are used. Distributing IV admixtures to the patient care units is usually done by a courier or a pneumatic tube system.

Sterile Compounding

Sometimes physicians request injectable medication that is not available commercially, so hospital pharmacists must make the injections from scratch. This takes patience and expertise. Calculations need to be made carefully, and like IV admixtures, the injectable medication must be prepared in a laminar flow hood or clean room using aseptic technique. The USP has new standards (Chapter 797) for preparing sterile preparations that must be followed.

Decentralized Pharmacies

Drug preparation and distribution can be done from a large central pharmacy (66% of hospitals) or from a central pharmacy and smaller, decentralized satellite pharmacies (34% of hospitals).[8] Decentralized pharmacies are located in strategic locations in the hospital and serve several patient care units. Central pharmacies are more efficient, need less inventory, and use less personnel. The advantages of decentralized, satellite pharmacies are faster, more personalized service, and more opportunity for staff pharmacists to deliver pharmaceutical care on the floors.

Today, the drug preparation and distribution system in many hospitals uses various types of automation. Current and future automation used in pharmacies is discussed in Chapter 6, Pharmacy Technology and Automation.

Drug Administration

Drugs are administered to inpatients by registered nurses (RNs) or in some states by licensed practical nurses (LPNs) who have taken a course in medication administration. The nursing Kardex (manual system) or the *medication administration record* (MAR), an automated system, serves as a reminder to the nurse of when medication is to be given to the patient. In hospitals using general nursing care procedures, there may be a medication nurse who is responsible for administering all of the medication on a patient care unit for one shift. In *primary care nursing*, one nurse performs all duties for four to six patients, including the administration of medication.

After the first dose of medication is administered, which should be as soon as possible after the order is written, it is usually scheduled according to the hospital's standard dosing schedule. For example, all medication ordered "every 6 hours" is usually administered at 6 a.m., 12 noon, 6 p.m., and 12 midnight. A medication ordered q.i.d. (four times a day) is usually administered at 10 a.m., 2 p.m., 6 p.m., and 10 p.m.

The important questions to ask before administering medication are (a) Is this the correct patient? (Check the patient's arm band ID.) (b) Is this the correct medication? (c) Is the dose correct? (d) Is this the correct dosage form? (e) Is it the correct time to give the medication? Fortunately, the correct medication for the patient in the correct dose and in the correct dosage form should be in the patient's unit-dose drawer. However, the nurse needs to be careful about taking medication from the correct patient's drawer at the correct time.

Once the medication is administered, the nurse must "chart," or record, the medication administered to the patient by documenting what was given, how much, and when. This is done on the MAR.

Ensuring Rational Drug Use

Achieving rational drug therapy (the appropriate use of drugs) in the hospital is the goal of every pharmacy department and the medical staff. Achieving this goal is difficult, as is overcoming several challenges that make rational therapy less possible.

Challenges to Rational Therapeutics

The first challenge to rational therapeutics is the modest education and training on pharmacology and rational drug therapy that physicians receive in medical school. Second, because of the number of new drugs approved for use each year by the U.S. Food and Drug Administration (FDA), there is "information overload." Third, drug companies' marketing information about their drug products emphasizes the benefits of the medication. The drug companies are skillful in stating the best features of their drug products to increase sales. Fourth, there is a large gap between what clinical studies show works (evidence-based medicine) and how the medication is used in everyday practice.

An example of the gap between what is known and what is done is how peptic ulcer disease is treated. For years, peptic ulcers where thought to be caused by stress and aggravated by spicy foods. The long-standing treatment of peptic ulcers was the use of antacids, and, more recently, H2 antagonists such as cimetidine. We know today that most peptic ulcers are associated with the presence of the bacterium *Helicobacter pylori* and therefore should be treated with antibiotics. Yet today, many patients are still being treated the old way. This is what happens when physicians are too busy to keep up-to-date with the medical literature.

Pharmacy's Input into Rational Therapeutics

The challenges to achieving rational therapeutics represent real opportunity for pharmacists and pharmaceutical care. Pharmacy educators and some practitioners started noticing these opportunities in the mid to late 1960s. This spawned the *clinical pharmacy* movement.

Clinical pharmacy was first practiced by a handful of pharmacists in a few hospitals, mostly on the West Coast. With expanded education in the areas of pathophysiology, pharmacokinetics, laboratory medicine, therapeutics, and clinical pharmacy, new pharmacy graduates and pharmacy residents began to work directly with physicians, mainly the house staff (medical residents), to improve drug therapy. Acceptance of the pharmacist in this new clinical role was slow but moved forward methodically.

Today, pharmacists practicing in hospitals have moved forward to practicing pharmaceutical care, and many are well accepted for their expertise and help in effecting rational and safe drug therapy.

Drug Formulary

Rational therapeutics begins with having an effective *drug formulary*, which is a compilation of pharmaceutical agents (and often related products) authorized or recommended for prescriber selection and patient use in a given health care environment.[9] Selection of the the drugs of choice to be listed in the formulary is done by a P&T committee composed mainly of physicians, with representation from nursing and pharmacy. In addition, this committee approves the rules and regulations for administering the drugs listed in the formulary.

Formularies may be used as a compulsory control over drugs that may be prescribed (often accompanied by a protocol for requesting a nonformulary drug product) or as a voluntary guideline under a companion quality assurance program called a *drug utilization review* (DUR) or a *drug-use evaluation* (DUE).

The primary goals of a formulary fall under one or more of the following: (a) therapeutic objectives designed to improve patient health outcomes by means of certifying *drugs of choice*, (b) economic objectives aimed primarily at limiting purchases for drug products (cost control), and (c) realizing certain administrative ends such as ideal inventory control or easing claim processing.

Table 9.3   Top 20 Drugs ($ Volume) Used in Hospitals during 2005

Rank	Drug	Primary Uses
1	Procrit	Anemia of chronic renal failure
2	Lovenox	Prevention of deep vein thrombosis
3	Rocephin	Infection
4	Epogen	Anemia of chronic renal failure
5	Zofran	Prevention of nausea and vomiting from cancer chemotherapy
6	Levaquin	Treatment of respiratory tract infections
7	Remicade	Crohn's disease
8	Zocor	Hyperlipidemia/prevention of cardiovascular events
9	Rituxan	Non-Hodgkin's lymphoma
10	Neupogen	Reduce the incidence of infection in nonmyeloid malignancies
11	Zosyn	Infection
12	Neulasta	Reduce the incidence of infection in nonmyeloid malignancies
13	Paraplatin	Cancer
14	Integrilin	Reduce the risk of acute cardiac ischemic events
15	Propofol	Intravenous anesthetic
16	Aranesp	Anemia of chronic renal failure
17	Prevacid	Duodenal and benign gastric ulcers
18	Aciphex	Erosive or ulcerative esophagitis
19	Zyprexia	Psychotic disorders
20	Diprivan	Intravenous anesthetic

Source: Wolters Kluwer Health, Source Pharmaceutical Audit Suite, January 2005–December 2005. Dollars reflect wholesale acquisition cost (WAC).

Although many physicians contend that, by itself, a formulary restricts their ability to order any marketed pharmaceutical product, the major substantive issue is that formularies may make therapeutic goals less desirable than other objectives.[10]

Leading Drugs

Although every hospital's formulary will have different drugs, many of the drugs will be the same based on their efficacy, side effect profile, and cost. Table 9.3 lists the top 20 drugs used in hospitals during 2006.[11]

Pharmaceutical Care

Pharmacists in hospitals have led the way to the clinical practice of pharmacy. The hospital is the ideal environment to practice pharmaceutical care and for pharmacy students to learn about disease and treatment. Every hospital is at a different stage of development of pharmaceutical care. Some are just starting, some are far along, and some are still doing drug preparation and distribution only.

Pharmaceutical care in hospitals revolves around ensuring ideal drug therapy. As shown in Figure 9.1, *quality drug therapy* is safe, effective, timely, and cost effective. From a pharmaceutical care prospective, ideal drug therapy must be delivered so that the patient knows that the pharmacist is involved and cares. If ideal drug therapy is evidence based, then it is also rational.

For pharmacists to help deliver ideal drug therapy, they must be involved in prescribing, dispensing, administering, and monitoring the drugs used in the hospital, which is a big job. The basis for this involvement is *evidence-based medicine* — published clinical studies and the drug-use policies and procedures set up by the P&T committee.

Historically, pharmacists approached the clinical use of drugs by carrying out various clinical pharmacy functions. Clinical pharmacy residents and clinical pharmacists (usually those with the Pharm.D. degree and having completed a pharmacy residency) in the mid to late 1960s started working with willing physicians to help improve drug therapy for patients.

Certain useful clinical roles emerged from these pioneer clinical pharmacists. One role was to provide useful drug information and input to the drug therapy of specific populations of patients — those with pain, cancer, and those needing intravenous nutrition. This was first called

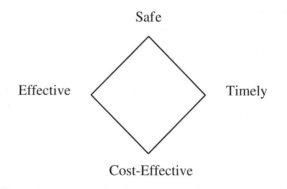

Figure 9.1 Quality drug therapy.

hyperalimentaion, but it is now called *total parenteral nutrition* (TPN). About the same time, it was discovered that the pharmacist could also be useful during a cardiac arrest, which occurs when the patient's heart stops and is sometimes called a code blue. The pharmacist's role on the cardiac arrest team is to draw up the drugs, make sure they are given in the correct order and in the correct dosage, and record what and when the drugs are given.

A breakthrough for clinical involvement by the pharmacist working in a hospital was monitoring drugs that have therapeutic plasma levels close to their toxic plasma levels. These drugs are usually effective, but they need to be used cautiously because of their potential toxicity. Because of the pharmacist's educational background in *biopharmaceutics* and *pharmacokinetics*, they are suited to working out the mathematical modeling needed to dose these drugs scientifically and safely. Pioneer clinical pharmacists in academic medical centers and community hospitals not only proved pharmacists could dose and oversee these drugs better than most physicians, but several started billing and receiving hospital reimbursement for this service.[12,13]

The ASHP conducts national surveys of pharmacy practice in acute care settings about prescribing and transcribing practices.[14,15] Table 9.4 shows the proportion of acute care hospitals offering various patient care

Table 9.4 Percentage of Hospitals and Health Systems with Pharmacist Consultations

Type of Consultation	Consultation Provided %		Adoption Rate for Recommendations % with >80% Adoption Rate	
	1998	2004	1998	2004
Drug information	93.1	90.0	51.3	94.3
Dosage adjustments	83.1	92.6	65.3	93.3
Pharmacokinetics	80.6	82.9	71.2	95.4
Antibiotic	80.5	82.7	52.6	86.7
Nutritional support	53.0	51.1	68.3	91.6
Patient teaching	51.3	43.0	74.2	91.3
Pain management	38.9	37.8	62.0	91.6
Anticoagulation	33.8	41.7	66.5	87.3
Compliance and medical history	20.2	14.2	62.0	95.7

services by pharmacists during 1999 and 2004. Also included in Table 9.4 is the proportion of pharmacists' recommendations about drug therapy that were accepted by physicians.

Pharmacists in some hospitals are able to prescribe drugs to patients under a written protocol, or a *collaborative drug therapy* management agreement that comprises guidelines of the medical staff. Pharmacists with a Pharm.D. and having completed a pharmacy residency, may apply for prescribing privileges in the Veteran's Affairs Medical Centers (VAMCs). A survey revealed that in 68% of the 50 VAMCs surveyed, ambulatory care pharmacists had prescribing privileges.[16] Thirty percent of all ambulatory clinics were managed by pharmacists, and 75% had at least some pharmacist involvement.

Pharmacist prescribing is also happening in some community hospitals. At Good Samaritan Hospital, a 200-bed hospital in Puyallup, Washington, pharmacists have received prescribing authority from the P&T committee for aminoglycoside antibiotics, theophylline, and pain control in ambulatory patients.[17]

Raehl et al. have studied the extent of pharmaceutical care in hospitals.[18] They discovered that comprehensive pharmaceutical care programs were established in 64% of hospitals affiliated with Pharm.D. programs, 42% with B.S. pharmacy programs, and 33% not affiliated with a pharmacy school. Two clinical pharmacy services — drug therapy protocol management and clinical pharmacokinetics consultations — increased substantially.[19] These researchers also discovered that as staffing for clinical pharmacists increased, drug costs decreased.[20] Continuing research is needed to discover factors associated with high pharmaceutical care indexes.

Clinical Pharmacy versus Pharmaceutical Care

Most of what has been written about pharmaceutical care above pertains to clinical pharmacy services. The differences between clinical pharmacy and pharmaceutical care are explained in Chapter 7, Pharmaceutical Care.

One of the major differences between clinical pharmacy and pharmaceutical care is the focus of the pharmacist's care. Under clinical pharmacy, the focus has mainly been the physician, whereas the focus under pharmaceutical care is the patient. Another major difference is that most clinical pharmacy service has been provided by pharmacists with a Pharm.D. degree and residency training (*clinical specialists*). Under the pharmaceutical care model, all pharmacists, including staff pharmacists and those with a B.S. degree in pharmacy, can, with some training, provide direct patient care.

Under the pharmaceutical care model, the pharmacist reviews the patient therapy for eight medication-related problems, prioritizes those problems, develops solutions, recommends a solution for each problem, and watches the patient's progress. The challenge has been how to free up and train staff pharmacists to join clinical pharmacy specialists in providing pharmaceutical care for patients. A paper on how to do this successfully has been published.[21] Some of the cited keys to success were: (a) having and training a good group of pharmacy technicians, (b) training all pharmacists to provide pharmaceutical care, (c) redesigning the work, (d) the use of automation, and (e) analyzing patient outcomes.

Focusing on Patients Needing the Most Help

Philosophically, all patients deserve pharmaceutical care. Pharmacists should review the drug therapy of every patient. However, until there are enough pharmacy technicians, enough pharmacy automation, and enough pharmacists to do this, criteria are needed to select which patients will receive pharmaceutical care. Under the clinical pharmacy model, patients were usually selected based on the clinical pharmacy specialist's judgment. This resulted in mixed results and a haphazard approach to care.

In many hospitals today, pharmacists are members of *patient-focused teams* — teams of clinical practitioners from medicine, nursing, pharmacy, and other health disciplines that focus on special populations of patients for improving the patient's outcomes, health status, satisfaction, quality of life, and cost of care.

Instead of patient-focused teams, certain categories of patients can be selected for the pharmacist to monitor, but this should be coordinated to meet the needs of the hospital, as chosen by the P&T committee and based on the most common or most significant medication-related problems in the hospital. The P&T committee may have information through its drug-use evaluation (DUE) program that certain categories of drugs are not being used ideally. Thus, these drugs are the ones pharmacists need to monitor until there is improvement. Some hospital P&T committees may want to focus on treatment failures, patients with reduced renal function, patients 65 years of age or older, or patients with more than a certain number of drugs being prescribed at one time.

Avoiding Medication Misadventures

Although it is important for pharmacists to be a part of making sure that patients receive the most appropriate drug, it is also important that they focus on preventing or minimizing the adverse effects of drugs, that is, *drug misadventures*. Drug or medication misadventures are defined as significant negative effects of drugs.[22,23] Medication misadventures reveal themselves in the form of adverse drug reactions, medication errors, drug interactions, and allergic drug reactions. Definitions and explanations of these mechanisms of medication misadventures are provided in Chapter 4, The Drug-Use Process, and the extent and cost of medication misadventures is provided in Chapter 7, Pharmaceutical Care.

Medication Errors

When a medication error occurs in the hospital, an *incident report* is completed by the person who discovers the error, which contains all the facts about the error without placing blame. All incident reports go to the risk manager. If the incident report involves medication, a copy should also go to the person in charge of quality assurance in the pharmacy.

In most hospitals, medication incident reports are investigated further, and a summary report is produced by the pharmacy for review by the P&T committee. It is important that this summary report include: (a) clinical significance — how it affected the patient, (b) whether the event could have been prevented, and (c) how it could have been prevented.

JCAHO now requires health organizations to take added steps if the event is a *sentinel event*. A sentinel event is an adverse event that ends in death or is a *near miss event*, which is an event that could have ended in a tragic outcome. For sentinel events, the health care organization must show that they have performed a *root cause analysis* (RCA) of the event. Once the root cause analysis has been completed, the health care organization must document what changes have been made to prevent a similar instance in the future.

If the adverse event was serious (ends in death); was life-threatening (real risk of dying); resulted in hospitalization (first or prolonged), disability (significant, persistent, or permanent), or a congenital anomaly; or needed intervention to prevent permanent harm or damage, the FDA would like to have the event reported. These reports are voluntary, but important, and can be filed by anyone (including patients) to the FDA's MedWatch Program.

Many medication errors are preventable, and many are preventable by pharmacists. Common causes of medication errors include: (a) use of abbreviations, (b) not reading labels, (c) sound-alike drug names, (d) look-alike names, and (e) sloppy handwriting. The pharmacy department drafts and monitors medication policies and procedures that improve drug safety in the hospital for the P&T committee. One example of an important drug safety policy concerns abbreviations. There are now well over 16,000 medical abbreviations, acronyms, and symbols, and 24,000 possible meanings.[24]

Leape and colleagues at a large urban teaching hospital showed that the presence of a pharmacist on rounds as a full member of the patient care team in a medical ICU could substantially lower the rate of prescribing errors.[25] Besides preventing medication errors, pharmacists can also reduce other adverse drug events (ADEs) such as drug interactions, adverse drug reactions, and allergic drug reactions.

Education and Training

Another important part of hospital pharmacy practice is education and training. Every pharmacist is taught that part of being a pharmacist is teaching others about pharmacy, drugs, drug therapy, and, in general, health:

Pharmacy: The pharmacist can help educate and train pharmacy students, pharmacy interns, pharmacy residents, and other pharmacists. There is special joy in helping others learn about pharmacy, and it is a way of paying back the profession. After all, if you are a seasoned pharmacist, someone helped you to learn when you were a student, intern, resident, or young pharmacist.

Medicine: Pharmacists also help train medical students, medical interns and residents, and attending physicians. Almost any physician can tell you a story about how a pharmacist taught him or her something about a drug or drug therapy.

Nursing: Many pharmacists train nursing students on the practical aspects of drugs, how to administer drugs, and how to monitor the drug's effects. Some pharmacists also teach some of the coursework (such as pharmacology) in nursing schools.

Patients: Of course, all pharmacists are involved in helping patients learn about their medication. It is also important to teach patients about pharmacy and about being a pharmacist.

PHARMACY STAFF

Hospital pharmacies are organized in different ways. A typical organizational chart in a moderate size hospital is shown in Figure 9.2. Most hospital pharmacies have managers, supervisors, pharmacists, pharmacy technicians, and other supportive personnel such as clerks and secretaries.

Pharmacy and Drug Information Service

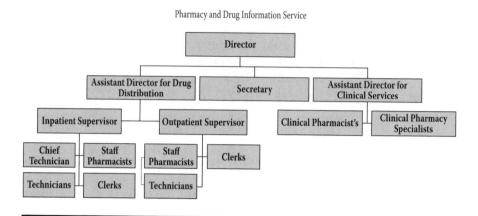

Figure 9.2   Typical organization of a moderate-size hospital pharmacy department.

PHARMACISTS

Pharmacy Managers

The managers include the Director of Pharmacy, also called the Chief of Pharmacy in government hospitals, and assistant directors. The supervisors report to the assistant directors, who report to the director. In large pharmacy departments, there may also be an Associate Director of Pharmacy position between the assistant directors and the director. Some pharmacy managers have added education and training beyond a degree in pharmacy. Many have completed a hospital or administrative pharmacy residency, and some have also completed a master's degree in business administration (M.B.A.) or in hospital or health care administration.

The Director of Pharmacy is accountable to hospital administration for the department. The director also sets the vision and direction for the department — where the department should be at a time in the future. The director is also responsible for the morale and teamwork within the department.

The pharmacy managers do the planning and help move the pharmacy program forward. They also are the ones who often work outside the department with other departments on behalf of the pharmacy. In short, they try to achieve the vision set forth by the director.

Pharmacy Supervisors

The pharmacy supervisors supervise the pharmacists and the pharmacy technicians or chief pharmacy technician. Pharmacy supervisors see that the work gets done, and they are responsible for the quality of work.

Supervisors must be able to handle people well and be able to motivate and counsel pharmacists and pharmacy technicians. Supervisors hire personnel, recommend raises and terminations, schedule employees, and interact with the supervisors of other departments.

Pharmacists

There are two categories of pharmacists who are not managers or supervisors: staff pharmacists and clinical pharmacists, although the lines between these are starting to blur because of pharmaceutical care.

Many staff pharmacists hold a B.S. degree in pharmacy, and some have a Pharm.D. degree. Despite the difference in education, if the work is the same, so is the pay. A survey reported that hospital pharmacists spend 32% of their day supervising the preparation and distribution of drugs, 23% on dispensing functions, and 18% on clinical functions.[26] Forty-five percent of the pharmacists indicated that they were performing more clinical functions compared to the previous year.

There may be two types of clinical pharmacists in the hospital: a *clinical pharmacy generalist* and a *clinical pharmacy specialist*. The clinical pharmacy generalist or clinical pharmacist probably will have a Pharm.D. degree and will have completed a pharmacy residency. These pharmacists follow patients' therapy and progress using the principles of pharmaceutical care. The clinical pharmacy specialist will usually have a Pharm.D. degree and will have completed a residency in a specialty area (e.g., critical care, ambulatory care, cardiology) and will follow special populations of patients or those patients with complex medication-related problems.

In many hospitals today, there are career ladder advancement programs that place pharmacists on a continuum — new graduate pharmacist, staff pharmacist, clinical pharmacist, and clinical pharmacy specialist.[27] In some hospitals, these positions are listed as pharmacist I, II, III, and IV. Each level has different job functions, responsibilities, and pay. Pharmacists can advance from one level to the next with more training, experience, and good job evaluations.

Most hospital pharmacists are happy with their jobs, and many would not work elsewhere. However, the rising workload has some pharmacists doing more drug distribution than clinical work. In fact, about two-thirds of pharmacists responding to a recent survey feel their workload could contribute to medication mishaps.[28] Many hospitals simply do not have the staffing to allow pharmacists to engage in clinical duties.[29]

What hospital pharmacists say they need to be able to practice clinically is: (a) more administrative support (34%), (b) more automation (26%), (c) additional pharmacy staff (17%), (d) longer hours (10%), (e) receipt of the Pharm.D. degree (7%), and (f) *outsourcing* (2%), which is contracting to prepare drugs and IVs outside of the hospital.[28] Some hospitals are losing pharmacists because of the slow pace of change, transition to pharmaceutical care is slower than they wish.[30] In addition, there can be a sizable gap in salary between what pharmacists are paid in hospitals versus what they get paid in chain store pharmacies.

Pharmacy Supportive Personnel

Pharmacy supportive personnel include pharmacy technicians, pharmacy clerks or aides, and secretaries.

> *Pharmacy Technicians:* Hospital pharmacies could not get along without pharmacy technicians. Employing good pharmacy technicians is the backbone of any pharmacy service. Pharmacists could not get the work done without them, and they allow the pharmacist to be able to practice clinically. See Chapter 5, Pharmacy Supportive Personnel. Just like with pharmacists, many hospitals have career ladder advancement programs for pharmacy technicians. An example of a continuum for the career ladder is technician trainee, technician I, technician II, and chief technician. The advancement through the ladder is based on more training, certification, experience, and job evaluation.
>
> *Pharmacy Clerks or Aides:* Pharmacy clerks or aides usually have no formal training in pharmacy and often learn on-the-job. Pharmacy clerks do routine functions in the pharmacy and do not prepare medication. Typical functions of a pharmacy clerk are to unpack medication orders, restock shelves, perform routine clerical functions, and deliver medication.
>
> *Pharmacy Secretaries:* Every hospital pharmacy needs a good secretary or two. Pharmacy secretaries need special skills in understanding drug names and pharmacy terminology. They also need to understand pharmacy's role in the hospital and know how to interact effectively with other departments in the hospital.

ACCREDITATION

The JCAHO has been accrediting hospitals for more than 50 years. Its accreditation is a nationwide seal of approval that indicates that a hospital meets high performance standards. Pharmacy services in hospitals must meet JCAHO standards for the pharmacy service, some medical staff standards involving the formulary, P&T committees, and policies and procedures involving the drug use process.

Additionally, the pharmacy must help the hospital meet the JCAHO's national patient safety goals that relate to medication and the medication use system (MUS) (seehttp://www.jointcommission.org/PatientSafety/ National-PatientSafetyGoals/), such as having a list of do-not-use abbreviations and ensuring the continuity of care when patients move from one setting to another (e.g., from home to the hospital, and from the hospital to a nursing home). This latter requirement means there must be a process of checking to make sure no medications the patient is using are missed or the dose, dosage schedule, or route of administration are changed without authorization of the prescriber.

CHECKING ON PROGRESS

Almost every year, the ASHP performs national surveys to check on the status and progress of pharmacy in hospital settings.[8,14,15,31–33] The general areas covered in these reports include prescribing and transcribing, dispensing and administration, and monitoring and patient education.

JOB SATISFACTION

Most pharmacists working in hospitals like what they are doing. A survey showed that job satisfaction among pharmacists working in one large medical center correlated highly with both intrinsic (motivators) and extrinsic (hygienes) factors.[34]

FUTURE OF HOSPITAL PHARMACY

As time goes by, the clinical duties of the pharmacist working in the hospital will increase. What will quicken this growth is the use of more board-certified pharmacy technicians, a drastic change in how drug distribution is organized, and much more automation. It will also take the realization by hospital administrators and the medical staff of how much pharmacists can improve the quality of care and reduce the morbidity and mortality from drugs.

In 2003, the ASHP launched a landmark initiative to significantly improve the practice of pharmacy in health systems. This initiative began with a member-developed vision statement that conceptualizes how pharmacy practice in hospitals and other components of health systems should look in the future. The project, which includes 6 key goals and 31 objectives and is to be achieved by the year 2015, evolved from the "ASHP Vision Statement for Pharmacy Practice in Hospitals and Health Systems." The principal themes in the statement are that "health-system pharmacists will help make medication use more effective, scientific, and safe and will contribute meaningfully to public health in their communities."[35,36]

SUMMARY

Hospital pharmacists pride themselves on controlling the drug-use process in hospitals. Hospital pharmacists have continuously implemented new policies and procedures and technology to speed the distribution of drugs and make the drug use process safer. In the future, hospital pharmacists will focus more on improving the clinical, humanistic, and economic outcomes of patients from drug therapy. Pharmacists in hospitals will be recognized for helping develop drug therapy that is more rational, more evidence-based, ideal, and delivered with care.

DISCUSSION QUESTIONS AND EXERCISES

1. Make an appointment to tour a pharmacy in a medium (100 to 300 beds) or large (more than 300 beds) hospital.
2. While you are there interview a:
   a. Staff hospital pharmacist
   b. Clinical pharmacist
   c. Pharmacist doing a pharmacy practice or specialized residency
3. How does hospital pharmacy differ from community pharmacy in:
   a. Types of patients
   b. Types of medication
   c. Amount of patient contact
   d. Interaction with other health care personnel like doctors and nurses
   e. The knowledge the pharmacist needs to practice competently
4. Based on what you know and have read thus far, what do you feel are the pros and cons of being a pharmacist in a hospital?

CHALLENGES

1. Hospital pharmacies specialize in compounding individualized sterile preparations for patients. In doing so, pharmacists must be well trained, use sterile technique, and follow USP procedures. For extra credit, and with the permission of your professor, read USP's general Chapter 797 and prepare a concise summary report on what hospital pharmacies must do to be compliant with USP standards when compounding sterile preparations.

2. Many hospital pharmacists are still tied to a drug preparation and distribution system but would like to deliver pharmaceutical care most of their day. For extra credit, and with the permission of your professor, prepare a brief report on your perfect job as a clinically oriented hospital pharmacist. What mechanisms would allow you time to spend with patients? What assurances are in place to make sure drug preparation and distribution would be error free? Describe your perfect day.

WEB SITES OF INTEREST

American Hospital Association: http://www.aha.org/aha/index.jsp
Am Society of Health-Systems Pharmacists: http://www.ashp.org/
Hospital accreditation: http://www.jointcommission.org/
JCAHO Standards for Hospitals: http://www.jcrinc.com/subscribers/perspectives.asp? durki=6065&site=10&return=2815

REFERENCES

1. Kennedy, LA. Hospital and health care institutions. In *Pharmacy and the U.S. Health Care System*. Fincham, JE, and Wertheimer, AI, eds. Pharmaceutical Products Press, Binghamton, NY, 1998, chap. 10.
2. Fast facts on U.S. hospitals from *AHA Hospital Statistics*. American Hospital Association, Chicago, 2004. Available at http://www.aha.org/aha/resource_center/fastfacts/fast_facts_US_hospitals.html. Accessed April 25, 2006.
3. *Statistical Abstracts of the United States: The National Data Book*. Health and Nutrition, U.S. Census Bureau, U.S. Department of Commerce, Washington, DC, 2006.
4. Miller, A. Promina, employer group agree to patient safety plan. *Atlanta Journal Constitution*. December 21, 2000, p. E-1.
5. Chrymko, MC, and Kelly, WN. Are there really pharmacists in hospitals? *Am J Hosp Pharm*.1989;46:2000–2001.
6. Brodie, DC. Drug-use control: keystone to pharmaceutical service. *Drug Intell*. 1967;1(Feb):63–65.
7. Buchanan, C. A brief history of unit-dose drug distribution. *J Pharm Technol*. 1985;1:127–129.
8. Reeder, CE, Dickson, M, Kozma, CM, and Santell, JP. ASHP national survey of pharmacy practice in acute acre settings — 1996. *Am J Health-Syst Pharm*. 1997;54:653–669.
9. Rucker, TD. A public-policy strategy for drug formularies: preparation or procrastination? *Am J Health-Syst Pharm*. 1999; 56:2338–2342.
10. Rucker, TD, and Schiff, G. Drug formularies: myths-in-formation. *Med Care*. 1990;28:928–942.
11. *Wolters Kluwer Health, Source Pharmaceutical Audit Suite, January 2005–December 2005. Dollars reflect wholesale acquisition cost (WAC).*

12. Bollish, SJ, Kelly, WN, Miller, DE, and Timmons, RG. Establishing an aminoglycoside pharmacokinetics monitoring service in a community hospital. *Am J Hosp Pharm.* 1981;38:73–76.

13. Kelly, WN, Gibson, G, and Miller, DE. Obtaining reimbursement for clinical pharmacokinetic monitoring. *Am J Hosp Pharm.* 1982;39:1662–1665.

14. Ringold, DJ, Santell, JP, Schneider, PJ, and Arenberg, S. ASHP national survey of pharmacy practice in acute care settings: prescribing and transcribing — 1998. *Am J Health-Syst Pharm.* 1999;56:142–157.

15. Pedersen, C, Schneider, PJ, and Scheckelhoff, DJ. ASHP national survey of pharmacy practice in hospital settings: prescribing and transcribing — 2004. *Am J Health-Syst Pharm.* 2005;62:378–390.

16. Alsuwaidan, A, Malone, DC, Billups, SJ, and Carter, BL. Characteristics of ambulatory care clinics and pharmacists in Veterans Affairs medical centers. *Am J Health-Syst Pharm.* 1998;55:68–72.

17. Cahill, RJ. Pharmacist prescribing in a community hospital. *Pharm Pract Manag Q.* 1995;15:43–45.

18. Raehl, CL, Bond, CM, and Pitterle, ME. Clinical pharmacy services in hospitals educating pharmacy students. *Pharmacotherapy.* 1998;18:1093–1102.

19. Raehl, CL, and Bond, CA. 1998 National Clinical Pharmacy Services study. *Pharmacotherapy.* 2000;20:436–460.

20. Bond, CA, Raehl, CL, and Franke, T. Clinical pharmacy services, pharmacist staffing, and drug costs in the United States hospitals. *Pharmacotherapy.* 1999;19:1354–1362.

21. Hooks, MA, and Maddox, RR. Implementation of pharmaceutical care process for professional transformation. *South J Health Syst Pharm.* 1998;3:6–12.

22. Manasse, HR. Medication use in an imperfect world: drug misadventuring as an issue of public policy. Part 1. *Am J Hosp Pharm.* 1989;46:929–944.

23. Manasse, HR. Medication use in an imperfect world: drug misadventuring as an issue of public policy. Part 2. *Am J Hosp Pharm.* 1989;46:1141–1152.

24. Davis, NM. *Medical Abbreviations: 24,000 Conveniences at the Expense of Communications and Safety,* 11th ed. Neil M. Davis Associates, Huntingdon Valley, PA, 2001.

25. Leape, LL, Cullen, DJ, Clapp, MD, et. al. Pharmacist participation on physician rounds and adverse drug events in the intensive care unit. *JAMA.* 1999;282:267–270.

26. Gannon, K. How hospital R.Ph.s spend their workday. *Drug Top.* 1999;143(Jun 21):56.

27. Meyer, JD, Chrymko, MM, and Kelly, WN. Clinical career ladders: Hamot Medical Center. *Am J Hosp Pharm.* 1989;46:2268–2271.

28. Fleming, H. No rest for the weary. *Drug Top.* 1999;143:50–56.

29. Magill-Lewis, J. Reverse trend. *Drug Top.* 2000;144:44.

30. Gebhart, F. Work in progress. *Drug Top.* 1998;142:40, 43.

31. Pedersen, CA, Schneider, PJ, and Santell, JP. ASHP national survey of pharmacy practice in hospital settings: prescribing and transcribing — 2001. *Am J Health-Syst Pharm.* 2001;58:2251–2266.

32. Pedersen, CA, Schneider, PJ, and Scheckelhoff, DJ. ASHP national survey of pharmacy practice in hospital settings: dispensing and administration — 2002. *Am J Health-Syst Pharm.* 2003;60:52–68.

33. Pedersen, CA, Schneider, PJ, and Scheckelhoff, DJ. ASHP national survey of pharmacy practice in hospital settings: monitoring and patient education. *Am J Health-Syst Pharm.* 2004;61:457–471.

34. Sansgiry, S, and Ngo, C. Factors affecting job satisfaction among hospital pharmacists. *Hosp Pharm.* 2003;38(11):1037–1046.

35. ASHP. What is 2015. Available at http://www.ashp.org/2015/2015.cfm? cfid=12314756&CFToken=24200196. Accessed April 28, 2006.

36. Zellmer, WA. Vision for pharmacy practice in hospitals and health systems. *Am J Health-Syst Pharm.* 2001;58:1505.

10

MANAGED CARE PHARMACY

In the early to mid 1980s, acute hospital (inpatient) care started shifting to ambulatory (outpatient) care, largely for cost reasons. With this shift came the practice of discharging patients from the hospital sooner and the rise of home health care. In the mid 1980s and early 1990s, health care costs, especially hospital costs, rose at unprecedented rates in the United States. Despite the rising cost of health care, the quality of health was less than in many other developed countries spending less money on health care.

Pressure mounted to solve this problem, and after a major effort to legislate health care financing and delivery solutions, the marketplace moved toward its own solution — managed care. With it came new ways of delivering care for patients and new roles for health care providers, including the pharmacist.

This chapter will introduce the reader to managed care and the impact of managed care on pharmacy. It will address the various roles and functions pharmacists play in managed care and how those roles and functions differ from practicing in other practice sites. The chapter will end with a discussion of the ethics of practicing pharmacy in managed care.

LEARNING OBJECTIVES

After reading this chapter, you should be able to:

- Explain the term *managed care*
- Explain how managed care evolved
- Explain how managed care works
- Name and explain the four basic types of HMOs
- Define the terms *HEDIS* and *NCQA*

- Explain the impact of managed care
- Discuss the impact of managed care on pharmacy practice
- Explain what a P&T committee does
- Explain the following terms:
  - P&T Committee
  - Formulary
  - Quality assurance
  - DUR, DUE, and PBM
- Explain the role of the pharmacist in managing managed care patients
- Discuss some potential ethical dilemmas

WHAT IS MANAGED CARE?

It is difficult to pin down a date when managed care started. The HMO Act of 1973 encouraged employers to offer their employees managed care over traditional health care. This act spearheaded a dramatic rise of health maintenance organizations (HMOs), especially on the West Coast of the United States. HMOs slowly sprang up in other areas of the country, most notably in Minnesota. In the 1980s, HMOs gained market share (i.e., enrolled more members).

The health care financing crisis in the early 1990s resulted in a significant, yet failed, effort of President Clinton and Congress to pass legislation that would cover more health care costs for more people. At that time, about 30% of people in the United States were without health care coverage.

Since this failed attempt to fix the health care system, the marketplace has taken over and the country has quickly moved toward HMOs and the managed care HMOs provide. In fact, the growth away from traditional health care financing toward managed costs has been explosive. Today, managed care affects over 175 million Americans, or about 59% of the population.[1] Table 10.1 shows the penetration of managed care in the United States.

Managed care is in a constant state of flux, redefining itself almost every day. Although managed care assumes many forms and is constantly changing its goals, scope, and charges, it can be defined in general terms. "Managed care is fundamentally a healthcare delivery that attempts to control cost (financial risk) of healthcare service and delivery, as well as the quality, access, and availability of that care."[2]

In practical terms, managed care means care and cost managed by those who pay for it, chiefly the employer, but it is also paid by insurers, health plans, and the government. Before this, the access to care was not managed, and the cost, availability, and delivery of care was controlled

Table 10.1   Managed Care Penetration in the United Sates, 2005

Segment	Total U.S. (No.)	Percent U.S.	Managed Care	Managed Care (%)
Medicare	42.0	14.0%	6.0	14.3%
Medicaid	44.3	14.9%	26.9	60.7%
Commercial	165.8	55.6%	142.8	86.1%
Uninsured	45.8	15.4%	0.0	0.0%
Total	298.0	100.0%	175.7	59.0%

Note: numbers are in millions.

Source: MCOL. *Managed Care Fact Sheet.* 2006.

by those who provided it; that is, physicians, other health care providers, and health care facilities. Because of this shift in power, the transition to managed care has been uneven.

Before HMOs and managed care, most of health care was provided on a *fee-for-service* basis. The patient paid the *health care provider*: the physician, pharmacist, or hospital. If there was a health care benefit, the patient's employer paid some or all of the cost either through a contracted third-party such as an insurance company or by direct payment (self-insured). Some health providers, as a service to their patients, would bill the insurance company or employer directly so the patient would not have any *out-of-pocket* expense. As health providers' costs rose, they charged more for their services. Thus, market forces controlled health care costs.

Although fee-for-service was neat and tidy, it excluded those who could not afford care or were not covered by an employer's health care plan. Although the government failed to complete health care reform in the earlsy 1990s, it acted as a catalyst to the market and fueled the growth of managed care nationwide.[3] Many legislators and employers saw managed care as a means of cutting costs while providing quality of care. However, consumers, although wanting lower costs, did not want to give up their access to care, nor did they want to make other sacrifices that would be needed to lower costs. In general, most Americans were happy with their health care.

To lower costs, managed care, through its HMOs and PPOs (preferred provider organizations), needed to make drastic changes in how health care was financed and provided. The financing was changed to *capitation* — a contracted cost between an employer or the government with a *managed care organization* (MCO) to insure a covered individual for a period of time, usually 1 year. In a sense, managed care is prepaid health care. *MCO* is a general term used for health plans that provide health care in return for preset monthly payments and coordinate care through a defined network of *primary care physicians* (family practitioners, internists, pediatricians, and hospitals). MCOs are organizations that offer a HMO, PPO, or provider-sponsored organization (PSO) plan, or any combination of these.[4] MCOs are owned by national managed care organizations, hospitals, physician groups, Blue Cross and Blue Shield, and private investors.

For the MCO to keep its costs as low as possible, it contracts with providers (hospitals, physicians, and community pharmacies) for payment rates that are usually below average. However, since patients must stay within the system, providers can count on seeing patients covered by the MCO.

Employees usually pay a premium to their employer to pay for some of the cost of their health care, and this premium changes from year to year. Under some plans, there is still some cost to be paid by the covered individual in the form of a *deductible*, which is the amount the individual pays before the annual managed care payment goes into effect, and in *copayments*, which is a percentage of the charge paid by the individual. For example, the individual may have to pay the first $300 of health care costs before any costs are paid by the MCO. After the deductible is paid, the individual may have to pay a copayment of 20% of the charge.

Many employers like managed care, because they know exactly what their health care costs are going to be for the next year and can budget accordingly. In addition, the financial risk is by the MCO, not the employer.

The MCO receives a set amount of money per covered individual for the year to provide health care no matter how sick that individual is or will become. If the individual remains healthy, the MCO profits. If the individual has a disastrous illness, the MCO might lose money, but just on that individual. The MCO does careful actuarial studies on the individuals to be covered to decide what it will charge the employer. Most MCOs are for-profit companies that must make money to satisfy their stockholders; thus, they are careful in predicting their costs and profits.

The delivery of care through an MCO is provided differently than in traditional care. The MCO delivers its medical care by creating *provider panels*, which are groups of caregivers allowed to provide service for managed care members. They are the *gatekeepers*, who control or regulate access and care and discover medical need and fiscal integrity.[2] To better control the cost of care, MCOs prescribe certain benefits and limits.

There are three basic types of managed care health insurance plans: (a) HMOs, (b) PPOs, and (c) point of service (POS) plans.

Table 10.2 Growth Trends in HMOs and HMO Enrollment, 1994 to 2004[a]

Plan	Number of Operating HMOs	Enrollment (1000)
1994	556	55,006
1995[b]	669	67,575
1996[b]	749	77,339
1997[b]	757	89,031
1998[b]	902	98,309
1999	820	104,569
2000	625	99,285
2001[b]	542	91,077
2002	504	86,455
2003	481	82,500
2004	465	78,581

[a] Operating plans only. HMOs not licensed by state agencies are excluded from all totals.
[b] Enrollment data include HMO members in Puerto Rico and other U.S. territories.

Source: Managed Care Digest, Series 2005. Aventis Pharmaceuticals, Bridgewater, NJ. http://www.managedcaredigest.com/ShowReportAction.do.

HEALTH MAINTENANCE ORGANIZATIONS

HMOs offer comprehensive health services to its members for a fixed monthly fee by employing or contracting with health providers to provide care. HMOs want their members only to see physicians and other providers in the HMO's provider network. A primary care physician coordinates needed care. The patient needs a referral from the primary physician to see a medicine specialist.

The growth in managed care, once explosive, is now dropping.[5] In 1998, there were 902 HMOs. In July 2004 there were 465. Table 10.2 shows the number of HMOs and enrollments from 1994 to 2004.

There are four basic types of HMOs:

Staff Model: The physicians and health care workers of the HMO are salaried employees of the HMO and provide care only to the HMO's enrollees, usually in clinics owned by the HMO. The contract between the HMO and physicians is an exclusive one because physicians cannot participate in the HMO unless they become HMO employees. Although this model provides the most control and the least cost, it puts heavy controls on patient choice. An example of this type of HMO is Kaiser Permanente.

Group Model: In this model, the HMO contracts with one large physician group to provide care. Although the HMO and physician group work together, they are independently owned.

IPA Model: In this model, the HMO contracts with individual or different groups of independent physicians (known as IPAs). The IPAs provide care for HMOs enrollees (and other patients as well) in their private offices.

Network Model: The HMO contracts with several large IPAs, not individual or small group practices, who care for HMO and non-HMO patients. In a network model, the provider is not the employee of the health plan. Consequently, what a network model can require of its providers is different. An example of this HMO model is Aetna.

The IPA model is the most popular, having 40.7 millions enrollees in 2004,[5] followed by the network model (21.1 million enrollees), the group model (15 million enrollees), and the staff model (1.9 million enrollees).

The advantages of HMOs are:[6]

- Low out-of-pocket costs
- Focus on wellness and preventative care
- Typically no lifetime maximum payout

The disadvantages of HMOs are:[6]

- Tight controls can make it difficult to get specialized care
- Care from non-HMO providers is generally not covered

PREFERRED PROVIDER ORGANIZATIONS

PPOs are networks of providers (hospitals, physicians, and pharmacies) that provide health care to the employees of a company or organization for a negotiated fee-for-service. PPO members pay higher copayments and deductibles when they receive care outside the PPO network. PPOs are often marketed to employers as a variation of traditional health insurance plans. The main difference between a PPO and a HMO is that the PPO incurs no risk. The financial risk remains with the employer.

The number of PPOs grew from about 824 in 1990 to 1127 in 1998.[5] Enrollment grew from 38.1 million to 98.3 million during this same time period. In 2005, there were 175.7 million enrollees in PPOs versus 67.7 million in HMOs.[1]

The advantages of PPOs are:[6]

■ Free choice of health care provider
■ Generally limited out-of-pocket costs

The disadvantages of PPOs are:[6]

■ Less coverage for treatment provided by non-PPO physicians
■ More paperwork and expenses than HMOs

POINT OF SERVICE PLANS

The POS plan is an increasingly popular plan that allows patients to select providers at the time a service is needed rather than when they join the plan.[7] Members may choose to receive services either from participating HMO providers or from providers outside the HMO's network. Patients pay less for in-network care. For out-of-network care, members usually pay deductibles for some of the cost of care.

The advantages of POS plans are:[6]

■ Maximum freedom
■ Minimal copayment
■ No decuctible
■ No "gatekeeper" for nonnetwork care
■ Limited out-of-pocket expenses

The disadvantages of POS plans are:[6]

■ Substantial copayment for nonnetwork care
■ Deductible for nonnetwork care
■ Tight controls on specialized care

STANDARDS

Shortly after MCOs started flourishing, several employers and some MCOs in the northeastern United States began discussing the possibility of developing a set of measurements that employers and patients could use to compare managed care plans. Today, the *Health Employer Data and Information Set* (HEDIS) is a set of managed care performance standards that can be used to compared managed care plans and to conduct health outcomes research.

The HEDIS performance standards cover such items as clinical quality, access to care, patient satisfaction, membership characteristics, use, and organizational and financial information. For 2001, 50% of 650 MCOs met HEDIS guidelines.[8] In 2004, compliance with five selected measures for commercial MCOs ranged from 30.7% (comprehensive diabetes care) to 96.2% (beta-blocker treatment after heart attack).

The guidelines are provided by the National Committee on Quality Assurance (NCQA). Large employers need HEDIS information from MCOs as a condition of contracting. Comparisons of MCOs are available from the NCQA, and these are updated each year from new HEDIS reports.

ACCREDITATION

MCOs often seek to have their managed care plans accredited by the NCQA, showing by *report cards* that they meet agreed upon standards of quality. Accreditation is voluntary but is often used as a marketing tool.

IMPACT OF MANAGED CARE

Good Things

After over 25 years of managed care, what has been its impact? In short, managed care has delivered on its promise to reduce health care costs. Double-digit increases in employer annual health care costs that peaked in 1988 at 18.6% fell to 8% in 1993.[9] In 1995, the average employer cost for HMOs declined by 3.8%.[10] As shown in Table 10.3, managed care was the most likely reason why annual increases in medical expenditures fell below the rise in the gross domestic product between 1990 and 1999. However, this trend failed to sustain itself after 1999.[11]

Criticisms of Managed Care

Despite its impact on reducing the rising cost of care, HMOs have their failings. The first and continuing struggle has been with choice. Most patients prefer to receive health care from someone they choose. Under managed care, more choice means more cost.

Another problem confronted by HMOs is newspaper stories about patients being denied care, about patients not being treated properly, and about patients being discharged from the hospital too early, especially mothers who have just delivered a baby.[3]

Another criticism of HMOs is that they do not serve rural areas. In addition, the savings they have achieved have been made by cutting administrative costs; denying extended hospital stays, specialized

Table 10.3 Annual Increase (%) in Medical Care Expenditures Compared to the Annual Increase in the Gross Domestic Product in the United States, 1990 to 2004

Year	Gross Domestic Product	Medical Care Expenditures
1990	1.9	11.0
1997	4.5	2.8
1998	4.2	3.2
1999	4.5	3.5
2000	3.7	4.1
2001	0.8	4.6
2002	1.9	4.7
2003	3.0	4.0
2004	4.4	4.4

Source: U.S. Census Bureau. *Statistical Abstracts of the United States: 2006.*

procedures, and technology; and slashing payments to hospitals and physicians.[12] Much of these are one-time cost savings. Meanwhile, HMO premiums have been flat. The impact on the use of health services has been small.

There is a struggle between those who want managed care and those who do not. Those who want it are employers who pay for some of the health care of their employees, the managed care industry and its stockholders, and intermediaries such as insurance companies and pharmacy benefits managers (PBMs) and their stockholders.[2] Those who do not want managed care are mostly providers, especially physicians, hospitals, and pharmacists, who are concerned about the quality of care and whose fees are being negotiated downward.

In the middle of all of this is the patient, who is not sure managed care is a blessing or a curse. Patients often worry about managed care (about access problems, lack of choice, and about the quality of care). They also read stories that say managed care is the only way to keep health care costs under control. There is little wonder that there is now a book on managed care written for patients entitled *Doctor Generic Will See You Now.* This book offers 33 rules for surviving managed care.[13] Rule one — Don't let an HMO give you nickel-and-dime care for your million-dollar body.

PHARMACY BENEFIT MANAGERS

Pharmacy benefit managers (PBMs) are companies that administer drug benefit programs for employers and health insurance carriers. Examples include Caremark, Medco, and Express Scripts. PBMs contract with MCOs, unions, Medicaid and Medicare managed care plans, and federal, state, and local governments to provide managed prescription benefits. PBMs design prescription plans, have networks of contracted pharmacies to fill prescriptions, and process pharmacy claims for their customers. In recent years, PBMs have boosted their appeal by offering such services as mail-order pharmacies, which refill drugs at cut-rate prices. Today PBMs manage about 75% of the $235 billion spent on prescription drugs every year.

The drug formulary structure developed by the PBM for its customers (employers and HMOs), or by HMOs using a PBM dictates, the ability to achieve savings. The drug formulary can be:[14]

Closed or partially closed: Requires justification for drugs not on the formulary.

Open preferred: Encourages the use of certain drugs through incentives.

Open-passive: Includes drugs that are not generally promoted to be used.

No formulary with prior authorization: Certain drugs need prior approval before they can be used.

No formulary with drug utilization review: No formulary, but drug use is monitored by retrospective reviews (after the drug has been prescribed).

Other cost-saving techniques PBMs use include generic substitution, therapeutic interchange, and thee- or four-tiered copayment structures. Tier 1 is usually payment for generic drugs; tier 2 is usually payment for brand name drugs with a generic equivalent or preferred brand name drugs; tier 3 is usually payment for brand name drugs that have generic or therapeutic equivalents or nonpreferred brand name drugs; and tier 4 is usually nonformulary drugs. The amount of copayment the patient pays goes up with each tier.

In 2004, 100% of HMOs were using a formulary.[5] Table 10.4 shows the percentage of HMOs using open versus closed formularies and the number of tiers in 2004.

PBMs like to make incentives for people to use mail-order pharmacies, rather than their local pharmacist. This is because some PBM's own their own mail-order pharmacies. The incentives include being able to obtain a 90-day supply of medication from the mail-order pharmacy (one copay), but only being allowed a 30-day supply (and three copays over 3 months

Table 10.4 Percentage of HMOs Using Open and Closed Formularies[a] by Copay Tier Design

One Tier		Two Tier		Three Tier		Four Tier		Five Tier	
Open	Closed	Open	Closed	Open	Closed	Open	Closed	Open	Closed
33.6%	66.4%	54.6%	45.4%	81.9%	18.1%	89.4%	10.6%	42.2%	57.8%

[a] Open formulary: a drug is usually covered by the HMO, even if it is not on the formulary. Closed formulary: a drug not on the formulary is generally not covered, unless it goes through a prior authorization.

Source: Managed Care Digest, Series 2005. Aventis Pharmaceuticals, Bridgewater, NJ. http://www.managedcaredigest.com/ShowReportAction.do.

to get a 90-day supply) of medication if the prescription is filled at a retail pharmacy.

IMPACT OF MANAGED CARE ON PHARMACY

The initial impact of managed care on pharmacy practice was to reduce pharmacy cost. The annual pharmacy cost per HMO member of $186.32 in 2000 has been rising and is a major concern to the managed care industry.[5] Little attention has been paid to the safety and quality of drug therapy. The major impact on community pharmacy practice has been a further disruption in the long-standing pharmacist–patient relationship by making low-cost, restrictive networks composed largely of discount and chain store providers.[14] The managed care era has also provoked feelings of dismay, frustration, mistrust, and anger by community pharmacists toward many PBMs. The history in the eyes of many community pharmacists has been that many PBMs have had cavalier attitudes and offer meager fees for dispensing a prescription for a managed care patient.

Impact on Community Pharmacy

In the case of community services, the pharmacist traditionally collects a given charge from the patient (or insurance agent) for each prescription supplied. Under the managed care concept, patients are entitled to obtain an unlimited number of prescriptions without charge (except as specified by the contract), because the pharmacist will receive a fixed sum (say $300) per year regardless of the level of patient utilization. The net result for the prescription department is that annual income now depends not on the number of prescriptions dispensed, but on the number of patients accepted from a particular insurance firm.

Implementation of the managed care concept creates a number of problems for providers, especially when applied to the ambulatory sector. Prescription department income may originate from multiple sources: (a) cash and carry customers, (b) fee for service insurance programs, and (c) managed care insurance plans where reimbursement is based on the number of individuals and not unique services furnished. Indeed, some pharmacies have accepted participation agreements with more than 50 third-party programs. However, each source may have a different formula for determining provider compensation, and few, if any, may approximate the actual cost of running the prescription department.

PBMs act as subcontractors for broader-based health insurance carriers that stress the capitation method of reimbursement. In accepting this role, PBMs often revert to paying pharmacies on a fee-for-service basis per prescription rather than on how many patients have been assigned to each pharmacy.

In order to make a prudent business judgment concerning an appropriate charge for prescriptions, the manager of the department should first know the expenses related to this function and, preferably, how such costs vary according to type of insurance coverage represented by manager's mix of customers. Yet, even among the chain store organization with a sophisticated accounting staff, many lack reliable accounting data pertaining to the operations of the prescription department per se. In short, it may be very difficult to determine whether prescription department operations are subsidized by or are subsidizing sales from another department. The complex task of departmental accounting can be even more problematic, since pharmacists often help customers outside their department (such as selecting an over-the-counter [OTC] preparations).

Further, a discrepancy could arise, as third parties of all types pay little attention to pharmacy costs, because their actuaries estimate expenses for the average patient per month and then set compensation rates designed to entice the pharmacy to enroll as a participating vendor. Thus, the particular level of reimbursement put forward by each insurance plan can be more or less than the actual cost of running the prescription department. Given this situation of receiving less than full costs from an insurance program, pharmacies must make up the difference from one or more plans that exceed this economic base, from cash and carry customers, and from the sale of nonpharmaceutical products or go out of business. Indeed, some community pharmacies contend that third-party pressures have caused their demise.

Thus, one must conclude that prescription department revenue may be dependent upon both internal and external pressures. The former is illustrated by subjective cost accounting methods, the proportion of customers with various types of insurance protection, and the nature of policies and rules utilized by these third-party organizations. However, economic results are also likely to be distorted by more external forces as well. Among others, we would have to nominate the absence of a comprehensive, national patient medical record system and the proliferation of multiple insurance schemes. Yet, if the negative consequences associated with reimbursement from competing organizations are to be minimized, some scholars contend that our country also needs to pursue a single-payer formula based upon more objective means for determining provider compensation for all patients rather than selected segments.

Given the less than optimal combination of reimbursement methods used today to reward pharmacists, one might expect that major efforts may occur from time to time to find better ways of paying pharmacists.

Impact on Pharmacy in Organized Health Care Settings

The impact of managed care on pharmacists practicing in organized health care settings such as hospitals has been pressure to reduce drug inventory costs, the cost of drugs, and personnel.

The good part is that managed care has recognized the talents of pharmacists: mostly in managing a pharmacy and helping reduce the cost of drug therapy for patients. Recognition that the pharmacist can also improve the quality of drug therapy and patient outcomes is coming more slowly.

The major ways pharmacists help managed care are prudently buying drugs, running drug formularies, conducting drug-use reviews, developing generic drug reimbursement policies, and pharmacy network contracting. However, there are various other ways pharmacists help managed care.[15]

Pharmacy and Therapeutics Committee and the MCO Formulary

The pharmacist working in managed care can make important contributions to the *pharmacy and therapeutics (P&T) committee,* which is the committee that reviews drugs for the formulary. A *formulary* is a list of pharmaceuticals that have been approved for use by the managed care plan. It is the cornerstone of the drug benefit. Formularies have been used a long time to improve the quality of drug prescribing. The first hospital formulary in the United States was the *Lititz Pharmacopeia* (1778), which was used in military hospitals during the Revolutionary War.

Formularies and P&T committees are critical to managed care, unfortunately, more from the viewpoint of cost than safety and efficacy. This is why it is important for the pharmacist to be there to champion *quality drug therapy.*

Decisions by the P&T committee about drugs should be based on efficacy, safety, and cost. Some of the considerations in reviewing a drug for formulary status include effectiveness, U.S. Food and Drug Administration (FDA)-approved indications, side effects, physician follow-up needs, effect on emergency room visits and hospitalization, laboratory costs, cost of drugs, and outcome studies.[16]

The drug receives one of six formulary labels by the HMO's P&T committee after it is reviewed:

Preferred: The drug the organization would like used.

Approved: It is acceptable, but not preferred that this drug be used.

Restricted: The drug can only be used in certain patients and in certain situations.

No reimbursement: No reimbursement means no approval.

Prior authorization: The pharmacist must receive approval to dispense the drug.

Not listed: Not approved.

One of the problems managed care is having, and one that is inherent in the formulary process, is physician compliance.[17] Physicians like to prescribe what they feel is best for the patient. If the formulary is *closed*, physicians must prescribe within the formulary, and MCOs make it difficult for them to do otherwise. Some physicians feel formularies intrude on the private practice of medicine or their right as the patient's physician. That is true when the only two people in the equation are the physician and the patient and the patient is private pay and the only one who pays. If a third party is paying some or all of the bill, the physician's authority in selecting what is best might be compromised by the payer's concern for cost.

When a physician works for or is contracted to provide services for an MCO, the physician agrees to abide by the formulary. However, that does not always mean they agree with it. Most physicians realize that some of their peers and pharmacists are members of the P&T committee, and the committee uses the medical and pharmacy literature to decide about the formulary status of drugs. However, a few will sometimes disagree with the decisions of the P&T committee and say something like "That's not true in my patients" or "That drug is not in my patient's best interest." This makes things difficult, and it is often the pharmacist who makes it better.

There are now formulary managers (some pharmacists and some not) in managed care who perform formulary police work to see who is not complying with the formulary. Sophisticated computer software is being used to match diagnoses and drugs to catch and educate *outlier physicians* about their prescribing patterns.

Others functions that emanate from this include providing educational materials about drugs, monitoring drug use, developing prescribing guidelines, and interacting with the quality assurance activities of the organization, all roles pharmacists can provide.[18]

MEDICATION THERAPY MANAGEMENT

On January 1, 2006, the government started paying for the prescriptions of Medicare beneficiaries. This *Part D Medicare* benefit could be offered by managed care plans as a stand-alone benefit (prescription drug program [PDP]) or as part of a comprehensive medical benefit. Part D Medicare regulations require plans to have a *medication therapy management program* (MTMP) for "targeted beneficiaries" (those who have multiple chronic diseases, are taking multiple Part D medications, and are likely to incur annual costs exceeding a level predetermined by the Center for Medicine and Medicaid Services [CMS]). The rule states that pharmacists may be reimbursed from the plan for providing these services. This is a wonderful opportunity for pharmacy.

QUALITY ASSESSMENT AND ASSURANCE

Quality assessment and assurance in pharmacy is accomplished using a process called a *drug utilization review* (DUR), which is an authorized, structured, and continuous program that reviews, analyzes, and interprets patterns of medication use against criteria representing how the drug should be used.[19]

DUR is becoming more and more important in managed care. Although drug therapy only represents about 8.3¢ of every health care dollar and pales in comparison to the cost of hospital care (38.4¢) and physician services (18.9¢), the amount for prescription drugs is rising at a steeper rate than the other costs.[17] The *complete DUR* is "the system by which quality drug therapy is defined, measured, and eventually achieved."[20]

The Joint Commission Accreditation of Healthcare Organizations (JCAHO) developed a standard that the medical staff of a health care organization should evaluate how drugs are used, and the Director of Pharmacy or someone of the director's choice should help with this review.

Today, PBM companies make DUR a part of the contract between themselves and an MCO or employer. How motivated PBMs are to measure quality over utilization, and thus increased cost, can be debated.

The DUR process has several steps: (a) selecting a target, (b) developing measurement criteria, and (c) monitoring drug use.

Selecting a Target

There must be a reason to perform DUR, as DUR can be expensive without a payoff. The P&T committee is in the best position to target specific areas of concern based on efficacy, misuse, overuse, safety, or cost. The measurement can concern treating a disease, the use of a drug or a drug class, or who and how the drug is prescribed.

From a clinician's viewpoint, the emphasis should be on quality — measuring actual drug therapy versus ideal drug therapy. However, from the viewpoint of finance, the question is, "Are we using the lowest cost therapy?" The compromise position is, "Are we achieving the desired outcome at the lowest price?"

Developing Measurement Criteria

The criteria must be based on the opinion of experts and well-controlled studies from the medical and pharmacy literature. The criteria should be objective and *evidence based*. The pharmacy is usually responsible for developing the DUR criteria.

Monitoring Drug Use

Pharmacists are also the ones who usually perform the DUR. There are three ways to do this:

Retrospective DUR is performed by reviewing patient records after the patient has been discharged from a health care facility or after the patient has been on the drug for some time. The advantage of retrospective review is that it is inexpensive, not as time consuming, and is less expensive than the other ways of doing DUR.

Concurrent DUR is performed shortly after the drug has been prescribed and the patient is still taking the drug. This is the easiest way for pharmacists to perform DUR and one where they can have the greatest impact. Recommendations can be made while collecting information for the DUR, and these will improve therapy or make it safer. This may be the most expensive way to do DUR, but it is one that collects the needed information and improves therapy in the process.

Prospective DUR is performed before the drug is prescribed. Electronic order screens match diagnoses and patient problems with preferred formulary drugs. These screens come into view as the physician is ordering the medication. Dose and cost information are also supplied when needed. This may be the most effective way of improving drug therapy and achieving the lowest cost; however, this is yet to be proven.

Comparing the Actual Drug Use versus the Ideal

The next step in the DUR process is to compare the actual drug use versus the ideal by analyzing trends and assessing the quality of drug therapy being delivered. This is also a function of managed care pharmacists.

Reporting Results

The next step in the DUR process is to develop a concise, well-written report of the DUR results with recommendations. This will go to the P&T committee for its review and action. The report should be clear, concise, and easy to read and use tables and graphs as much as possible. Some items often found in a DUR report are wrong use, overuse, underuse, inappropriate duration of therapy, inappropriate monitoring of the drug, therapeutic overlap, incorrect dosage, drug interactions, drug–disease contraindications, and use of an inferior agent.

Communicating Results

Once the P&T committee reviews the results, it may ask the pharmacy to provide the results of the DUR and the recommendations to the medical staff. This can be done in various ways. One is to hold a conference. Another way is to provide the medical staff with something in writing. However, neither of these mechanisms has been found to be effective. The most effective way is to show individual physicians their prescribing pattern compared to the rest of the medical staff and to the ideal. This is more effective.

Adjusting Criteria and Performing the Review Over

After communicating the results of a DUR to the medical staff and letting some time go by, the P&T committee may want to adjust the criteria as needed and perform another audit or it might select a new potential problem to review.

In recent years, the term *drug-use evaluation* (DUE) has replaced the more traditional term *DUR*. It is unclear if there is a true difference in these two terms. One definition of DUE is "a method of enhancing the appropriate, safe, and effective use of drugs by developing indicators, collecting and evaluating patient data, identifying potential problems, and implementing corrective action to improve drug use."[17] Common indicators for DUE have been overuse and underuse of a particular drug. At best, DUE uses objective outcome measures such as an improved range of motion, improved sleep, and less pain.

EDUCATION OF PROVIDERS AND MEMBERS

It is important for MCOs to educate and work with their members (patients) and their providers (primarily physicians, pharmacists, and hospitals) so it can be more successful. What the MCO needs is compliance with its preferred procedures such as the use of generic drugs and compliance with the formulary. It also needs happy members and providers. Happy providers make for happy members.

Member Education

The MCO wants happy members so it can keep them as clients. Managed care pharmacists can do quite a lot to help patients make the best use of their medication and improve member satisfaction with the prescription benefit. The main way of doing this is to spend time with the patient. It is important for the patients to know what medication they are taking, why they are taking it, how to take it properly, what to be careful about, and what may happen if it is not taken. This will improve compliance and health outcomes.

Provider Education

Provider education is mostly for physicians and pharmacists. Information on what education is needed comes from computer program information tracking the drug-use process and from DUEs. Some MCOs build performance profiles of each provider physician and each provider pharmacy. These performance profiles, sometimes called *report cards*, are mailed to the provider or the provider is visited by a health care professional. In a physician visit, the visitor may be a managed care pharmacist. These visits are sometimes called *academic detailing* or *counter-detailing*.

Academic or counter-detailing is based on unbiased, *evidence-based medicine*, as opposed to the detailing provided to physicians and pharmacists by sale representatives of pharmaceutical companies. The person doing the academic detailing shares the performance of the provider with the provider along with comparable information. The actual performance can be compared with the provider's peers or against certain *benchmark measures*, which is the ideal or a standard.

Some items often selected for DUEs are the use of generic drugs, compliance with the formulary, responses to computer alerts, and use of therapeutic interchange, which is approval to substitute one brand of drug for another. MCOs use this information to select which physicians to counter-detail. PBMs use this information to counter-detail network pharmacies and to select which pharmacies will remain in the network.

Physicians and pharmacies selected for counter-detailing are sometimes called *outliers*, as their performance profiles are outside the needed range.

Ambulatory Clinics

Ambulatory care is defined as health services provided on an outpatient basis or to refer to patients not confined overnight in a health facility. Ambulatory care is provided within a physician's office or a medical clinic. There has been a dramatic shift from inpatient to outpatient care since 1980.

If the ambulatory care is provided in a clinic, managed care pharmacists can help improve patients' clinical and economic outcomes of patients. The model for providing pharmaceutical care to ambulatory patients can be found in the ambulatory clinics of the Veterans Affairs (VA) Medical Centers.[21] Here, qualified pharmacists manage the therapy of primary care patients with chronic diseases.

Managed care has started using pharmacists in the same manner as the VA. Thus, there is a bright future for any pharmacist with additional training in ambulatory care such as an ambulatory care residency program.

HEALTH OUTCOMES

In the past, the quality of care was measured by how well the process of care was delivered. The assumption was that if the process is correct, so will be the outcome. A good example of this practice in pharmacy is measuring serum drug levels. Many clinical pharmacists spend a lot of time making sure the serum levels of a drug are in the therapeutic range. They track how often physicians take their advice to make a dosing change and if the following serum drug level is within the therapeutic, subtherapeutic, or toxic range. The thinking is that the more often the drug is in the therapeutic range, the better the outcome. However, this is a big assumption.

Today, the thinking has shifted to measuring patient outcome, and if it is poor, checking the process to see what may be wrong. An *outcome* (short for health outcome) is the result of a process of prevention, detection, or treatment. The shift in emphasis from inpatient to outpatient care reaps big dividends, especially in managed care, where successful health outcomes can be used as a marketing tool.

Outcome activities in managed care are concentrated in three areas: outcomes research, outcomes measurement, and outcomes management:[22]

> *Outcomes research* assesses the effectiveness of a given drug, medical procedure, or technology on health or its cost. The scientific finding is used as the basis of practice guidelines.

Outcomes measurement evaluates how well a given medical intervention (a drug or procedure) is meeting the expectation of the drug company, the managed care plan, or the patient.

Outcomes management sets about trying to improve health care by implementing the findings of the outcomes research and measurement, usually in the form of a *continuous quality improvement* process.

Health outcomes include clinical outcomes, humanistic outcomes, and economic outcomes:

Clinical outcomes involve measurable changes in disease. An example would be migraine headaches. What is happening to the number and intensity of the headaches? Are they getting better? Staying the same? Are they getting worst?

Humanistic outcomes involve behavior, perceptions about functioning, and the quality of care. Examples are school and work attendance, being able to walk farther, and feelings about health care providers.

Economic outcomes involve the cost of care. The question is, Did the intervention or drug improve the cost of care? To discover this, sophisticated techniques are needed. These techniques have spawned a new pharmacy discipline called *pharmacoeconomics.*

Pharmacoeconomic Studies

Pharmacoeconomic studies assess the overall value of drugs in preventing and treating disease. When performing or reading about a pharmacoeconomic outcome study, some important items need to be defined.

First, is the cost the actual cost of care or is it charges (revenue)? Second, if it is cost, how was the cost derived — from invoices or gathered using a ratio of charges to cost? Third, if it is cost, is it only the cost of the drug or does it involve total cost, which would include a share for salaries, benefits, supplies, and overhead (the cost of heat, lights, electricity)? Fourth, whose cost is it? The patient's? The managed care's or hospital facility's? The insurance company's?

It is also important to realize that drug therapy can decrease the overall cost of care. An example would be treating peptic ulcer disease. Before the H2 antagonists, such as cimetidine (e.g., Tagamet) it was expensive to diagnose and treat peptic ulcers. Sometimes the patient had to go through expensive testing and was ineffectively treated. Therapeutic failures would result in more physician visits, occasional visits to the emergency room and hospitalization, and lost time at work.

Today, the H2 antagonists and the finding that most peptic ulcer disease is caused by a bacterium, *Helicobacter pylori*, have revolutionized treating peptic ulcer disease. These drugs dramatically reduced the overall cost of this disease, but the cost of treating the disease costs more than the old treatment.

For some reason, many financial managers inside traditional hospitals, and even some in managed care facilities, do not appreciate this distinction — the drug therapy costs more, but the cost of the disease is less. Perhaps it is because so many of these managers have M.B.A. degrees and no health care backgrounds. This lack of understanding by the "financial types" inside health care facilities frustrates many physicians and most directors of pharmacy. The directors of pharmacy, in recent years, have experienced relentless pressure to keep drug costs down, and yet, what other major mechanisms are there to bring down the overall cost of a disease? There are few others.

A lot of information exists on pharmacoeconomics and how to perform pharmaceoeconomic studies.[23–29] Many pharmaceutical companies are partnering with MCOs to perform pharmacoeconomic research. The drug companies are willing to spend large sums of money to prove their drugs are valuable in the prevention or treatment of disease. The managed care company has the patients and patient database to perform the studies, and they benefit by learning what will bring down the cost of care. However, few MCOs have the kind of clinical database needed to perform efficient and high-quality outcome studies. In addition, only a few drug companies and MCOs possess the talent to perform these studies well. Fortunately, there are good health outcomes researchers in academia (pharmacy, medicine, and public health schools) and in the private sector.

The four basic types of pharmacoeconomic studies are cost minimization analysis, cost-benefit analysis, cost-effectiveness analysis, and cost utility analysis:[30]

> *Cost minimization analysis* (CMA) is used to compare treatments that have clinically identical effectiveness or outcomes to see which is less expensive.
>
> *Cost-benefit analysis* (CBA) measures all costs and benefits of interventions in dollars to determine the difference in cost and outcome.
>
> *Cost-effectiveness analysis* (CEA) compares two or more interventions for the total resources used and the health outcomes achieved.
>
> *Cost utility analysis* (CUA) is a CEA that evaluates costs and consequences of an intervention for the patient's quality of life (QOL), the ability to pay the costs, or preference for one form of treatment over another.

For these studies, there is general agreement that no claim can be made unless it is based on two well-controlled studies that show the same result. Of course, the more studies that show the same result, the easier it is to make the claim.

Patient Satisfaction

Measuring a patient's satisfaction with care is new in health care, and it has come, in part, with the *total quality improvement* (TQM) effort in health care.

The NCQA has been measuring satisfaction with managed care plans for some time. Members are asked, "How would you rate your health plan now?" Members rate their plans on a scale of 0 to 10, with 10 being the best. Those rating the plan 8, 9, or 10 represented 57% of the members in 1998 and 56.7%.[31] The NCQA also says, "We want to know your rating of all your health care in the last 12 months from all physicians and other health care providers. How would you rate all your health care?" The scale is the same (0 to 10 with 10 being the highest). Those rating all of their health care 8, 9, or 10 represented 70.3%. The comparison and conclusion based on these data are left to the reader.

Quality of Life

Everyone has a different *quality of life* (QOL), and it is reasonable to expect that everyone measures their QOL differently. Thus, measuring the QOL would be impossible. But what is possible is measuring people's perceptions of their QOL. In health care, the million dollar question is: What health care interventions improve QOL? One major intervention is drug therapy. Thus, the patient's perception of the QOL before and after starting a new drug can be used to measure the drug's perceived effectiveness in that patient. There are general QOL measurement instruments available such as the (SF-36, Short SF-12) and disease-specific QOL measurement instruments such as the St. George QOL Instrument for Respiratory Disease.

Managed care formularies and managed care pharmacists can have a significant impact on a patient's QOL. As Rucker and Schiff have suggested, formularies should maximize the cost effectiveness and help improve the quality of care.[32] Thus, what is in or not in the formulary can significantly add or subtract from the health plan members' QOL.

What pharmacists do also impacts the health plan member's QOL both indirectly and directly. Pharmacists in managed care often work "behind the scenes" to improve the quality of drug therapy. Writing safe medication policies and procedures and working on the formulary are examples. The direct impact of what the pharmacist does to improve a patient's QOL can be seen when observing a pharmacist reviewing a patient's drug therapy, identifying medication-related problems, and doing things to resolve these problems. It is also obvious when a pharmacist is observed effectively counseling patients about their medication.

Focusing on patient outcome rather than the process of delivering care is new to pharmacy. Managed care has led the way, but is still not where it needs to be.[33] Each practicing pharmacist, regardless of the practice setting, needs to focus on the health outcome important to each patient he or she provides care for. Does the patient want better sleep? Is the patient trying to return to work? Does the patient want to walk farther? Through properly selected medication, taken in the correct dose, and taken as ordered, some of these things can be possible. It is up to the pharmacist to try to make this happen.

DELIVERING PHARMACEUTICAL SERVICE AND CARE

Information Systems

No doubt having an automated pharmacy data and information system plays a role in providing quality care. The impact is yet to be measured. However, knowing what drugs are being prescribed for what types of patients is critical for correcting medication orders and for the DUE process. Unfortunately, most hospital, managed care, and pharmacy computer systems have been designed solely for administrative and billing purposes. Few computer systems have been designed for safety and the provision of care and assessing the quality of care.

Another major problem with information systems in health care is the difficulty (and seeming lack of priority) of integration of the various computer systems found within one health care system. Total hospital information systems are rarely designed with pharmacy in mind, whereas stand-alone pharmacy computer systems, although more useful, usually have not been integrated with the rest of the hospital as well as they should be.

Prescription Networks

For a managed care plan's members to have access to the medication prescribed for them, MCOs contract with community and mail-order pharmacies. Pharmacists working in managed care are often asked to help develop criteria on which pharmacies to select. If the prescription benefit is controlled by the payer (the employer), the employer may select a PBM to manage the prescription benefit, and it is the PBM that selects the pharmacies.

The pharmacy profession seeks fairness when MCOs and PBMs select pharmacies to be part of their prescription network. Pharmacy's viewpoint is that all pharmacies should be allowed to participate. However, MCOs and PBMs prefer pharmacies that will comply with their wishes about formulary compliance and generic and therapeutic substitution. In addition, MCOs and PBMs want pharmacies that will accept what most community pharmacists feel is a less than satisfactory dispensing fee for their services. Thus, the relationship between community pharmacists and MCOs and PBMs has been strained.

Much to the dismay of community pharmacists, MCOs and PBMs have been turning more and more to mail-order pharmacies (MOPs) as another way for plan members to obtain their medication. MCOs, PBMs, and patients like the price savings achieved by using MOPs; however, patients sometimes do not like to wait for their medication, and some worry about having their medication lost in the mail. Community pharmacists point out the lack of personal attention and the inability to ask questions and be counseled about the medication. MOPs answer to this critique is to provide well-written information leaflets with the medication.

Prescription Benefit Design

The design of the prescription drug benefit is complex and it would be good if the MCOs and employers who contract with MCOs would have pharmacists help them design this important benefit. However, this is seldom the case. The prescription drug benefit is often loaded with deductibles, copayments, the formulary, and sometimes *prior approval* requirements (approval before the drug can be dispensed).

The prescription benefit in managed care has spawned a whole new entity, the PBM company, which helps design and administer the prescription drug benefit for the MCO and employer. PBMs (e.g., Advance PCS and Aetna US Healthcare Pharmacy Management) are intermediaries between the MCO and the community and mail-order pharmacies. They are also the ones that will decide which drug will be paid for and how often and decide on prior approval.

The main job of the PBM is to reduce the cost of pharmaceuticals — end of story. PBMs now connect most U.S. pharmacies by computer network with the MCO rules on dispensing and educational information directed toward least-cost prescribing and dispensing. Some PBMs are independent, whereas others are subsidiaries of pharmaceutical companies or insurance companies.

Partnerships

The pharmaceutical industry has learned how to use the managed care concept to meet its business objectives. Thus, the drug companies have taken their emphasis away from traditional health delivery and are devoting more and more resources and their sales forces to managed care. Many pharmacists are being employed in pharmaceutical sales, and some pharmacists with expertise in certain diseases are being hired as medical service representatives (MSRs) to provide clinical information on the company's products to physicians and pharmacists who provide services to MCOs.

Drug companies have been forming partnerships with managed care because they see the possibility that managed care will become the dominant market for their products and have the ability to shift the market for products. Thus, the pharmaceutical industry has been financing many of the pharmacoeconomic studies performed in managed care. Because they pay for the studies, the results are kept within the company and the MCO, unless of course the results are favorable, in which event the study may be submitted for publication.

Continuity of Care

Managed care has brought into clearer focus the problems of patients moving between providers, which often results in overlaps and gaps in care. This problem is known as the *continuity of care.* Care is currently not seamless between providers. This is largely a problem of not having a national health care database shared by all providers and of not having a one-payer system for health care.

There are many challenges to integrating care for patients.[34] The greatest challenge for pharmacy is twofold. The first is the pharmacy not having access to information on the patient other than pharmacy information. Unless special efforts are made and unusual circumstances prevail, most pharmacists have little to no clinical information on a patient for whom they are about to dispense a drug.

This problem occurs in the hospital, for example, when the pharmacy is unable easily to access the latest laboratory results on a patient's renal function and the pharmacist is about to dispense a drug that can potentially harm the kidney.

This problem of the pharmacist being unconnected to patient information is most prominent in community pharmacy. The only patient information comes from the prescription, which often contains barely enough information to even dispense the medication. The prescription will have the name but probably not the address or age of the patient.

It will not have anything about any chronic diseases or conditions the patient has.

Often the pharmacist will not know for which condition the drug is being prescribed, as many drugs have multiple indications. For example, the drug propranolol (e.g., Inderal) can be used for high blood pressure, angina, conduction problems in the heart, migraine headaches, and tremors. The only way for the community pharmacist to know is to ask the patient, which can be embarrassing, as the patient thinks the pharmacist should know.

The ideal would be for pharmacists to communicate between practice sites.[35] For example, when a patient is discharged from the hospital, the hospital pharmacist could write a summary note on the patient and include his or her pharmaceutical care plan. The community pharmacist filling the patient's discharge prescription could see what the hospital pharmacist says about the patient. The home health care nurse visiting the patient can access the patient's pharmacy information by logging onto the system with a laptop computer. The issue of patient confidentiality needs to be worked out, but this problem is not as big as some make it out to be.

Disease State Management

Disease state management (DSM), or *disease management* (DM), is a patient-focused, comprehensive approach to reducing treatment variability of a specific disease to improve patient outcomes.[36] This idea is similar to pharmacy's idea of pharmaceutical care, but broader, in that it educates patients about their diseases and tries to have the patients become full partners in their own care.[37,38]

What is interesting about DSM is that pharmacists can fully participate and even get paid to do it. Community pharmacists, especially those in chain pharmacies, are working with patients, and some are charging and receiving reimbursement for their services (see Chapter 7, Pharmaceutical Care). Reimbursement has been received for pharmacists working with patients with diabetes, asthma, and other chronic diseases. In doing this, it is important for the pharmacist to document what has been done and any improvement in outcome.

How managed care has impacted pharmacy varies by site. For pharmacists working in hospitals, there has been only a small impact, unless the hospital has its own managed care plan. Some of the newer concepts such as including a pharmacoeconomic assessment when assessing a drug for the formulary and focusing on patient outcome rather than the process, have made their way into some hospitals. However, it can be argued that it is managed care that has made times hard for hospitals financially, and these hard times have had an immense impact on hospital pharmacists.

The impact on community pharmacy practice has been dramatic and frustrating. Managed care and PBMs have successfully negotiated unusually low dispensing fees with community pharmacies based on promising volume. Thus, community pharmacies are filling more and more prescriptions at lower fees, hoping to make a decent profit on volume. However, this is causing stress and potentially unsafe conditions because of the volume of prescriptions being filled. The bureaucratic process imposed by PBMs to fill a prescription is increasing, and this is increasing patient wait times and frustration. However, there is little the community pharmacist can do to change this. It is difficult to hire more help and use automation when the dispensing fee is so low.

One positive impact managed care has had on pharmacy is a new place for pharmacists to work.[39] Managed care has been employing many pharmacists for their expertise as medication experts. Managed care likes using pharmacists with training (a residency) in ambulatory care to help physicians prescribe medication according to the needs of the MCO.

Another positive impact of managed care on pharmacy has been the development of a national pharmacy organization, *The Academy of Managed Care Pharmacy* (AMCP), and its publication, the *Journal of Managed Care Pharmacy*.

Reducing Medication Errors

It has been proposed that managed care pharmacists devote more time to trying to reduce medication errors.[40] Proposed mechanisms include patient and practitioner education, and tools to improve patient compliance with taking their medication as prescribed.

BEING A PHARMACIST IN MANAGED CARE

Many of the procedures in managed care have been taken from hospitals and revised for the needs of managed care, as focused on ambulatory patients. Thus, hospital pharmacists make the transition to managed care the best.

It is helpful if the pharmacist understands the distinction between population-based issues and individual patient care, which is at the heart of understanding managed care and the role of the pharmacist in this sector of health care.

There are three expectations of pharmacists in managed care.[41] Pharmacists must shift their emphasis away from the drug product and toward the patient, deliver high-quality care that is responsive to patients' needs and be attentive to cost, and develop new skills, competencies, and attitudes toward their work. To prosper in managed care, pharmacists must be good managers and have strong clinical skills for evaluating and counseling various patients of all ages with different diseases.[18] The AMCP has published a well-written guide on the principles and practices of managed care pharmacy to help pharmacists in managed care.[42]

ETHICS

One final word on the important topic of ethics: being a pharmacist in managed care is not always easy. Managed care has brought the business of health care crashing into the practitioner's arena of clinical medicine. Physicians and pharmacists practicing in the managed care environment struggle with what is best for the patient clinically, and now they must consider what it will cost. When cost is a variable in the decision-making process, the quality of care can be compromised. Physicians and pharmacists take oaths to do what is best for the patient. Balancing quality and cost makes fulfilling these oaths more difficult and at times puts the pharmacist into a difficult ethical problem.[43–44] Pharmacists working within a managed care system must be the patient's support and protector when it comes to the appropriate use of medication.

SUMMARY

Like it or not, managed care is here to stay and it will probably get bigger as time goes by. Employers, MCOs, PBMs, and insurance companies think highly of managed care. The employers save money, the rest make money. Those paid by managed care (providers such as hospitals, physicians, and pharmacists) do not feel the same way about it for two reasons — concern about compromising patient care and low fees. Meanwhile, caught in the middle are the patients, who are confused as ever about managed care. They too are concerned about the quality of care and the freedom to choose their health providers. At the same time, they want to save money.

It is difficult to foretell how pharmacy practice may be impacted by managed care forces, or vice versa. One major reason is that the provision of pharmaceutical care represents some 10% of the larger health care delivery system, where Americans spent more than $1.7 trillion in 2003. Another is that the system in general, as many experts claim and patients have learned, often is dysfunctional. These limitations are manifest in numerous ways, such as the inability of patients to acquire or maintain adequate insurance coverage, increased reliance on patient cost-sharing, and even denial of benefits.

Prudent students should expect that changes in the administrative aspects of pharmacy will characterize their lifetime of work. Further, one must take into account the additional dynamics of scientific discovery and technological innovation pertaining to drug therapy. Thus, the conclusion seems inescapable that pharmacy careers will be dominated by forces significantly differently from those operative now.

Pharmacists must practice with competence and confidence and always care for patients and be their advocates no matter how the health care system operates or is financed. Using the principles of pharmaceutical care and pharmacy ethics will help pharmacists more effectively practice in this environment.

DISCUSSION QUESTIONS AND EXERCISES

1. You are the owner of an independent pharmacy and are offered the opportunity to provide pharmacy services for the 5000 employees and family members of a local company. There will only be 10 pharmacies eligible to provide services. However, you must drop your dispensing fee to the company's PBM from $7.00 to $6.00. Should you do this?

2. A pharmacy owner of a community pharmacy would like to contract with HMOs and be paid to help managed patients' chronic disease states such as asthma and diabetes. Do you think community pharmacists are in a good position to do this? Why or why not?

3. You are secretary of your HMO's pharmacy and therapeutics committee. A physician has requested a drug for formulary status, but your research reveals that the drug is inferior to the drug currently on the formulary. The physician says, "We need to put this drug on the formulary, because the drug company funds my research for a lot of money." How do you feel about this? What would you do?

4. Based on what you know and have read thus far, do you think drug formularies:
   a. Improve drug therapy? Why or why not?
   b. Make drug therapy safer? Why or why not?
   c. Reduce the cost of therapy? Why or why not?

5. Discuss the potential ethical dilemmas pharmacists might experience while being a managed care pharmacist. How do you feel about this?

6. A pharmaceutical company has offered to drop the price of its antihypertensive medication and make it less expensive than the other three drugs in this class of drugs. The other three drugs have the same safety profile — two are slightly more effective and one is moderately more effective than the drug being offered for less money. The HMO has accepted the drug company's offer to use

the less expensive drug. If you were a pharmacist working for this HMO, how would you feel about this? What could you do about it?

7. Make an appointment to visit an MCO and to interview a pharmacist.
8. What do you see, based on what you know and what you have read thus far, as the pros and cons of being a managed care pharmacist?

CHALLENGES

1. Some people think managed care is a mixed blessing. For extra credit, and with the permission of your professor, prepare a concise report discussing the pros and cons of managed care from the patient's, physician's, and pharmacist's (community and MCO) points of view.
2. 2. Part of the Part D Medicare regulations call for plans for medication therapy management programs. For extra credit, and with the permission of your professor, investigate and document how one of these programs works.

WEB SITES OF INTEREST

American Academy of Managed Care Pharmacy: http://www.amcp.org/
American Journal of Managed Care: http://www.ajmc.com/
Managed Care Digest: http://www.managedcaredigest.com/index.jsp
National Committee on Quality Assurance: http://www.ncqa.org/

REFERENCES

1. MCOL. Managed care fact sheet. 2006. Available at http://www.mcareol.com/factshts/factnati.htm. Accessed April 28, 2006.
2. Robbins, DA. *Managed Care on Trial: Recapturing Trust, Integrity, and Accountability in Healthcare.* McGraw-Hill, New York, 1998.
3. Kaldy, J. Looking back: failed health care reform put managed care on the map. *J Managed Care Pharm.* 1997;3:159–163.
4. Knight, W. *Managed Care.* Aspen, Gaithersburg, MD, 1998.
5. eManaged Care Trends Digest 2005. Aventis Pharmaceuticals, Bridgewater, NJ, 1990–2001. Available at http://www.managedcaredigest.com/ShowReportAction.do. Accessed April 28, 2006.
6. Anonymus. Health insurance: HMOs, PPOs, and POS plans. Available at http://www.agencyinfo.net/iv/medical/types/hmo-ppo-pos.htm. Accessed April 28, 2006.
7. Motheral, BR, and Schafermeyer, KW. Managed care. In *Introduction to Health Care Delivery: A Primer for Pharmacists.* McCarthy, RL, and Schafermeyer, KW, eds. Aspen, Gaithersburg, MD, 2001, chap. 21.

8. NCQA. The State of Health Care Quality — 2005: Industry Trends and Analysis. Available at http://www.ncqa.org/Docs/SOHCQ_2005.pdf. Accessed May 20, 2006.

9. *Foster Higgins National Survey of Employer-Sponsored Health Plans.* New York, Foster Higgins. 1996.

10. Geisel, J. Health plan costs remaining stable — managed care key to control. *Bus Insurance.* 1996;1(5):1.

11. U.S. Census Bureau. *Statistical Abstracts of the United States: 2006.* Tables 128 and 653.

12. Wilson, CN. The case against managed care. Part 2. *Hosp Pharm.* 1998;33:614–628.

13. London, O. *Dr. Generic Will See You Now: 33 Rules for Surviving Managed Care.* Ten Speed Press, Berkeley, CA, 1996.

14. Richardson, J. PBMs: the basics and an industry overview. June 26, 2003. Available at http://www.ftc.gov/ogc/healthcarehearings/docs/030626richardson.pdf. Accessed April 28, 2006.

15. Cardinale, V. Managed care: different career opportunity. *Drug Top.* 1991;135(Aug suppl):12–13.

16. Rich, S. Managed competition and formulary decisions. In *Managed ,Competition and Pharmaceutical Care.* Pathak, DS, and Escovitz, A, eds. Pharmaceutical Products Press, New York, 1996, p. 101–108.

17. Sax, MJ, and Emigh, R. Managed care formularies in the United States. *J Managed Care Pharm.* 1999;5:289–295.

18. Graham, P, and Schlaifer, M. Managed care. *Tex Pharm.* 1998;117:15.

19. Edgren, B. DUR and DUE in managed competition. In *Managed Competition and Pharmaceutical Care,* Pathak, DS, and Escovitz, A, eds. Pharmaceutical Products Press, New York, 1996, p. 117–127.

20. Stolar, MH. Drug use review: operational definitions. *Am J Hosp Pharm.* 1978;35:76–78.

21. Alsuwaidan, A, Malone, DC, Billups, SJ, and Carter, BL. Characteristics of ambulatory care clinics and pharmacists in Veterans Affairs medical centers. *Am J Health-Syst Pharm.* 1998;55:68–72.

22. Frankel, RB. Outcomes management and cost considerations: the role of pharmacists. In *Managed Competition and Pharmaceutical Care,* Pathak, DS, and Escovitz, A, eds. Pharmaceutical Products Press, New York, 1996, p. 109–116.

23. Basskin, LE. *Practical Pharmacoeconomics: How to Design, Perform and Analyze Outcomes Research.* Advanstar Communications, Cleveland, 1998.

24. Bootman, JL, Townsend, RJ, and McGhan, WF. *Principles of Pharmacoeconomics.* Harvey Whitney Books, Cincinnati, OH, 1991.

25. Edwards, R, Wiholm, BE, and Martinez, C. Concepts in risk-benefit assessment. *Drug Saf.* 1996;15(1):1–7.

26. Summers, KH, Hylan, TR, and Edgell, ET. The use of economic models in managed care pharmacy decisions. *J Managed Care Pharm.* 1998;4:42–50.

27. Bootman, JL, and Harrison, DL. Pharmacoeconomics and therapeutic drug monitoring. *Pharm World Sci.* 1997;19:178–181.

28. Sanchez, LA. Pharmacoeconomic principles and methods: including pharmacoeconomics into hospital pharmacy practice. *Hosp Pharm.* 1994;29:1035–1040.

29. Sanchez, LA. Evaluating the quality of published pharmacoeconomic evaluations. *Hosp Pharm.* 1995;30:146–152.

30. Brixner, DI, Szeinbach, SH, Ryu, S, and Shah, H. Pharmacoeconomic research and applications in managed care. In *Managed Care Pharmacy Practice,* Navarro, RP, ed. Aspen, Gaithersburg, MD, 1999, chap. 17.

31. 2000 State of Managed Care Report. The National Council on Quality Assurance (NCQA). Available at www.ncqa.org. Accessed February 28, 2001.

32. Rucker, TD, and Schiff, G. Drug formularies: myths-in-formation. *Med Care.* 1990;28:928–942.

33. Parker, DA. Advancing outcomes research in managed care pharmacy: a call to action. *J Managed Care Pharm.* 1998;4:257–267.

34. Vogenberg, FR. Trends in managed care pharmacy benefits. *Hosp Pharm.* 1999;34:1263–1267.

35. Navarro, RP, Christensen, D, and Leider, H. Disease management programs. In *Managed Care Pharmacy Practice,* Navarro, RP, ed. Aspen, Gaithersburg, MD, 1999, chap. 16.

36. Ponte, CD. Managed care and the pharmacy profession revisited. *J Managed Care Pharm.* 1999;5:78.

37. Munroe, WP, and Dalmady-Israel, C. Community pharmacist's role in disease management and managed care. *Int Pharm J.* 1998;12(Suppl):S3–S4.

38. Desselle, S, and Hunter, TS. The evolution of pharmaceutical care into managed care environments. *J Managed Care Pharm.* 1998;4:55–58, 61–62.

39. Schafermeyer, KW. The impact of managed care on pharmacy practice. *Pharm Pract Manage Q.* 2000;19:99–116.

40. Grissiner, MC, Globus, NJ, and Fricker, MP. The role of managed care pharmacy in reducing medication errors. *J Managed Care Pharmacy.* 2003;9(1):62–65.

41. Trinca, CE. Pharmacist career path opportunities in managed care. In *Managed Care Pharmacy Practice.* Aspen, Gaithersburg, MD, 1999, chap. 21.

42. Ito, SM, and Blackburn, S., eds. *A Pharmacist's Guide to Principles and Practices of Managed Care Pharmacy.* Foundation for Managed Care Pharmacy, Alexandria, VA, 1995.

43. Aroskar, MA. Ethical aspects of pharmacy practice in managed care. In *Managed Care Pharmacy Practice,* Navarro, RP, ed. Aspen, Gaithersburg, MD, 1999, chap. 22.

44. Robbins, DA. *Integrating Managed Care and Ethics: Transforming Challenges into Positive Outcomes.* McGraw-Hill, New York, 1998.

11

HOME HEALTH CARE PHARMACY

Today, patients often receive care and treatment at home rather than in an organized health care setting. This is called home health care. Home health care provides the patient with familiar surroundings and an environment where the patient is surrounded by family and saves money.

Most home health care patients are still moderately ill and need the attention of health professionals who help them with their care. They often need medication that is potent and should be carefully prepared by a pharmacist using special techniques.

This chapter is about home health care and the role of the pharmacist in the care of patients at home. It begins with the development of home health care and discuss what home health is and how it is provided. Common pharmacy services provided to home health patients will also be covered. The chapter ends with a discussion of what it is like to be a pharmacist in home health care practice.

LEARNING OBJECTIVES

After participating in this learning session, you should be able to:

- Define home care
- State why home care has become important
- Explain the role of the home care pharmacist
- Discuss the home care market
- Explain how a typical home care agency is set up
- Explain how home care is provided
- Explain the types of services home care pharmacies provide

- Explain what it is like to practice home care pharmacy
- Discuss the rewards of home care pharmacy

BACKGROUND

Home health care, sometimes called home health or home care, is defined by the U.S. Department of Health and Human Services (HHS) as "that component of a continuum of comprehensive health care whereby health services are provided to individuals and families in their place of residence for the purpose of promoting, maintaining, and restoring health or of maximizing the level of independence, while minimizing illness."[1] In July 2000, The American Society of Health-System Pharmacists (ASHP) issued its guidelines for the pharmacist's role in home care and defined home care as "the provision of specialized, complex pharmaceutical products and clinical assessment and monitoring of patients in their homes."[2] There has been concern that the ASHP has defined home care too narrowly.[1,3] Home care involves medical, nursing, and social services, as well as therapeutic treatment. In addition, home care is practiced in settings such as hospices and long-term care facilities.

Patients used to stay in the hospital longer than they do now. It was not unusual for a patient suffering a heart attack, a myocardial infarction, to be in the hospital for several weeks. New mothers used to stay in the hospital for 5 to 7 days after delivery. Today, a patient experiencing a myocardial infarction (without complications) will usually stay in the hospital less than a week, whereas a new mother may stay only a day or two after delivery. The average *length of stay* (LOS) in hospitals in the United States dropped from 7.8 days in 1970 to 4.8 days in 2003.[4]

The primary reason for this drop in LOS is cost. Hospital reimbursement has dropped because of a capitation (a fixed rate of reimbursement based on diagnosis) system of reimbursement for many patients (e.g., Medicare) and the negotiating power of managed care (see Chapter 10, Managed Care).

The main concern about sending patients home from the hospital earlier is whether patients are clinically and physically ready to be sent home. One way to help ensure that patients will have continuing care through their recuperation is for them to receive home health care. In addition, some patients, rather than having to go a hospital, can be cared for in their home.

Home health patients often need complex IV medications that were previously only provided in hospitals. Pharmacists have been employed in home health care agencies to prepare drug infusions, which are drugs slowly administered into a vein, for home health patients.

STATISTICS

In 1986, there were 5,250 home care agencies in the United States.[5] In 1998, there were more than twice this number (11,400). Since 1998, the number has been dropping. According to the U.S. Census Bureau, the ownership of home care agencies in 1996 was 54.3% proprietary (private, for-profit), 34.3% voluntary (not-for-profit), and 11.4% government and other.[6,7]

During 1996, home care agencies cared for 8.2 million patients.[6] Of this total, 59,400 patients received *hospice* care either in their homes or at hospices. A hospice is more like home than an institution, providing supportive care for terminally ill patients. As shown in Figure 11.1, the number of home care patients per 1,000 population is dropping. In 2000 there were 1.5 million home care patients. Of this total, 105,500 were hospice patients.[7] Home health agencies' average weekly visits also dropped, from 521 in 1999 to 479 in 2003.[8] Since 1996, the average length of home health service declined from 97.9 days to 69.5 days in 2000.[9]

The decline in home care patients and length of service is explained by the Balanced Budget Act of 1997, which curbed the increased spending on home health care. This act mandated the creation of prospective payment services whereby Medicare payments for home health services moved away from a cost-based payment system to fixed, predetermined rates.

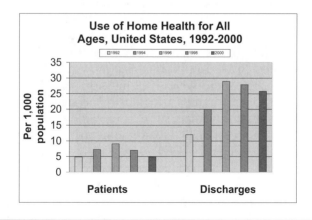

Figure 11.1 Use of home health care by population of all ages: United States, 1992–2000. *(Source: Bernstein, AB, Hing, E, Moss, AJ, et al. Health Care in America: Trends in Utilization. Hyattsville, MD: National Center for Health Statistics. 2003.)*

HOME CARE AGENCIES

Home health care agencies provide services to ill, disabled, and infirm people in their homes. The agency may be located within another health facility, but must be licensed by the state, accredited by a national body (usually JCAHO), and certified by Medicaid and Medicare. Home care agencies must provide nursing care and at least one therapeutic service to patients, and services must be provided under the direction of a physician.[8]

Home health care involves providing nursing care, equipment, and treatment for the patient. Nursing care must be provided by or under the direction of a registered nurse. Home care agencies are designated as either "Part A" or "Part B" agencies, or both. These designations come from Medicare, where nursing services are provided under Part A Medicare and equipment and treatment are provided under Part B Medicare.

Pharmacy services, treatment, and equipment, are provided to patients through Part B home care agencies. Pharmacies provide infusion services and home medical equipment (HME). Pharmacy services for home care can be provided by a hospital-based home care agency, a free-standing home care agency, or a specially equipped community pharmacy.[10] The infusion part of the business is the most profitable.

Home Infusions

The home infusion business has experienced phenomenal growth. Between 1982 and 1986, home infusion grew by a compounded annual growth of 64%.[11] However, this figure dropped to 24% during 1986 to 1993, largely because of the impact of managed care. The growth rate in 2006 was estimated to be 10 to 12%.[12] It is now a $12 to 15 billion per year industry. In 2006, there were 4500 infusion sites.[13]

Something new in the home care industry are stand-alone *ambulatory infusion centers* (AICs). AICs specialize in providing infusion therapy and nursing care to noninstitutionalized, nonhomebound patients in a center that provides high-quality, low-cost care. Patients come to the AIC for part of a day, then return home after they receive their care, or they come to the center to pick up their home infusions or supplies. This idea is thought to be more efficient and takes less home care staffing to manage.

An emerging market for nonhospital infusion services is long-term care. There are roughly 16,000 long-term care facilities in the United States providing care for 1.5 million patients.[14] (see Chapter 12, Long-Term Care Pharmacy).

PROVIDING HOME CARE

Much has been made of integration in health care, although the idea is simple. Free-standing home care agencies offer a single product line such as private duty nursing or HME, or infusion therapy. There are also home care agencies that provide more than one product, with the most common being nursing care and infusion therapy. However, only a *health care system* can provide integrated care — emergency care, chronic care, ambulatory care, home care, and long-term care.

Receiving home care from a health care system offers several advantages. First, patients' records are more easily available to all health care providers, and there is less duplication of services provided. The continuity of care is also better, and the care is more efficient and less time consuming for the patient.

Patient Eligibility

To be eligible to be reimbursed for home care, Medicare, Medicaid, and most insurance companies require the patient to be homebound, meaning the patient has physical or medical conditions that limit his or her ability to leave home. Second, the patient must require skilled, intermittent care to treat the qualifying condition. Third, the referring physician must approve the plan of treatment in writing and state that the patient is homebound and needs skilled nursing care.[15]

The 2003 David Jayne Medicare Homebound Modernization Act expanded eligibility from strictly residents confined at home to any individual who: (a) has been certified by a physician as having a permanent and severe condition that will not improve and that requires the individual to receive assistance from another individual with at least three out of five activities of daily living for the rest of the individual's life and (b) requires one or more described home health services to achieve a functional condition giving the individual the ability to leave the home.

Standard Treatment

A standard protocol for treating home care patients includes an initial visit, continuing nursing visits, home health aid visits (for non–nursing chores), physical therapy, HME, and perhaps drug infusions and treatment.[16]

Home Care Patients

Most patients receiving home care are elderly, and many are undernourished. A study revealed that of the 241 home care patients (60 years or age or older) studied, the mean number of medical conditions was 4.9, the average number of prescription medications was 7.2 (range 0 to 26), and the average number of over-the-counter medications was 1.8 (range 0 to 11).[17] In addition, most patients were at high nutritional risk.

Accreditation

The JCAHO accredits home care agencies. Under JCAHO, pharmacy services providing home infusion have their own set of standards. The standards for providing pharmacy services for home care patients are more progressive than the standards for hospital pharmacies and expect the pharmacist to provide pharmaceutical care.

The JCAHO standards are a basic road map to ensure patient safety and positive patient outcomes. Most home care pharmacy services have written policies on how to provide quality care. It is recommended that these policies be patterned after the JCAHO standards and that these standards be incorporated into the daily practice of the pharmacists providing service to home care patients.[18] In this way, the pharmacy is always ready for a JCAHO visit.

The JCAHO has consolidated accreditation of long-term care pharmacy services and free-standing (pharmacy-based) ambulatory infusion services with its home care pharmacy accreditation program.[19]

HOME HEALTH CARE PHARMACY SERVICES

Great satisfaction can come from providing pharmacy services for home care patients.[20] The pharmacist plays a vital role for these patients, as most patients need complex intravenous pharmaceuticals that must be carefully compounded. Home services can be provided from a hospital pharmacy, a free-standing infusion service, or a community pharmacy, all of which need to be specially equipped.

Total Parenteral and Enteral Nutrition

It is critical that the pharmacists and pharmacy technicians are well trained as to how to prepare these life-maintaining specialty solutions, the most complex of which is called *total parenteral nutrition* (TPN). TPN is an intravenous solution containing all the needed nutrition (proteins, carbohydrates, fats, vitamins, and minerals) to sustain life. From the standpoint of calories, it is like putting a complete meal in an IV container. Patients need this when they cannot eat and are unable to absorb nutrients from their gastrointestinal (GI) tract.

A TPN solution needs to be carefully prepared to ensure accurate content and in such a way as to remain sterile (germ free), because it is infused into the patient's vein. Important guidelines on implementing safe practices for parenteral nutrition formulations have been published by the American Society for Parenteral and Enteral Nutrition (ASPEN).[21]

Enteral nutrition is a term used to describe complete and specialty nutrient mixtures that can be prepared and administered orally or nasally through a feeding tube in patients who have a gastrointestinal tract that can absorb the nutrients. These mixtures do not have to be prepared using *aseptic technique* — preparing a sterile product.

Pharmaceutical Care

Largely because of the JCAHO standards, home health care pharmacists do not have a choice about clinical practice and practicing pharmaceutical care. The JCAHO standards demand that the pharmacist know the laboratory results for each patient, and that the pharmacist practice with the entire team caring for the patient. It also means identifying, classifying, and resolving home care patients drug-related problems (DRPs).[22] In one study, 80 patients were referred to pharmacists from agency personnel, and pharmacists discovered 271 DRPs in this group of patients.[23] Every patient referred had at least one DRP, and 32% of DRPs were identified by a visit to the patient's home. Nearly 65% of pharmacist recommendations were implemented.

Pain Management and Hospice Care

Some home health care agencies and hospices provide compassionate care and pharmacy services to terminally ill patients. In a hospice program, the dying patient has rights that are respected.[24] These rights include:

- The right to enjoy the best quality of life possible
- The right to die with dignity, as patient perceives dignity
- The right to participate in their own care, their remaining life span, dying, and the event of death
- The right to remain a viable family member in the environment of choice

Some pharmacists work with other health care providers (physicians and nurses) to provide pain management and other therapies for terminal patients. This practice is called *collaborative drug therapy management*

(CDTM).[25] Pain control for the patient with cancer in the home care setting can be challenging and rewarding for the pharmacist.[26]

Home Medical Equipment

Home care pharmacies often provide *home medical equipment* (HME) for patients. HME has replaced the older term *durable medical equipment* (DME). Examples of HME include aids to daily living, hospital equipment for the home, ostomy aids and supplies, incontinent supplies, self-monitoring equipment, ambulatory aids such as walkers and wheelchairs, dressings, and prostheses. The HME pharmacy business can be quite rewarding if done properly.[27]

Total Quality Management

During the late 1980s and early 1990s, a wave of enthusiasm swept the health care environment, especially in hospitals, for *total quality management* (TQM). A major principle of TQM is, "We will do the right thing the first time, and every time." Home care services have been an excellent place to implement TQM. If things are not done correctly, the patient is vulnerable to harm, because health care providers are not available all the time and the patients are moderately ill.[28]

Opportunities

The scope of home infusion therapy prepared by pharmacists will continue to expand. This expansion will be based on changing patient needs and increased comfort levels among physicians.[29] This trend will be fueled by the increasing number of elderly patients, but its success will be determined by satisfactory refund by third-party payers and managed care.

THE PHARMACIST'S ROLE IN HOME HEALTH CARE

The role of the pharmacist in home health care is important. The ASHP has developed guidelines to help pharmacists practicing in home health care.[30] These guidelines cover 15 responsibilities pharmacists have when practicing in the home care environment. Guidelines have also been published for pharmacists providing home care services from a community pharmacy.[31]

Pharmacist Functions

The services provided to home health care patients include preparing infusion products and providing medications and HME. It also includes providing pharmaceutical care (PC). In the home care pharmacy, pharmacists are required (by JCAHO) to maintain medication profiles, written care plans, and communication notes.[32] The care plan should identify actual or potential patient problems or needs. The pharmacist also documents the patient's goals of therapy and the progress toward those goals. The JCAHO also expects home health care pharmacists to identify, resolve, and prevent medication-related problems. A useful community pharmacy model on how to provide PC in home health care patients has been developed.[33]

Many opportunities exist for pharmacists to practice clinically in the home care environment. In a recent study, pharmacists working with a home care agency found that many home care patients were elderly, took many medications, and were at risk for DRPs and suboptimal therapy.[34] Another recent study found that adverse drug events (ADEs) were common during the month following hospital discharge.[35] The ADEs were more common in women and often resulted in medication changes.

Pharmacy technicians are the key to freeing up the home care pharmacist to work directly with patients.[36] Pharmacy technicians can also become experts in preparing the various infusion preparations needed by home care patients.

Competency in Home Care

Pharmacists working in home care need to be expert in infusion therapy, understand the home care patient, and have good PC skills. A competency assessment for the home care pharmacist has been developed.[37] The instrument tests the following skills: communication, completion of initial pharmacy assessment and reassessment, obtaining a medication profile, medical history taking, nutritional screening, assessment of laboratory data, development of a patient care plan, and checking the pharmaceutical preparation.

CAREER OPPORTUNITIES

Employment opportunities in home care include positions with hospital-based programs, private home care companies, and some community pharmacies that specialize in providing medication and infusion services for patients. Home care offers pharmacists three types of positions: management, clinical practice, and pharmacy operations. In smaller operations, pharmacists may perform a combination of these duties. During a typical day in a home care operation, a pharmacist might perform some or all of the following functions:[38]

Formulate and recommend treatment regimens:

- Interview patients, obtain medication histories, assess allergies, and determine disease status
- Provide education, conduct training, and counsel patients
- Check the preparation of infusion products and infusion devices
- Supervise pharmacy technicians
- Make treatment recommendations and check patient progress
- Help patients with questions, infusion problems, and device needs
- Review and assess compliance with therapy, quality of care, and therapeutic outcomes
- Document the pharmaceutical care delivered

REWARDS AND SATISFACTION

No reference could be found on the rewards and satisfaction of pharmacists working in home care. However, observation and personal testimonies suggest that practicing home care pharmacy is rewarding. Satisfaction comes from working with ill patients, many of whom are elderly, to preserve or improve their health and quality of life. Home care pharmacy requires pharmacists to practice pharmaceutical care. Home patients have many special needs, including parenteral antibiotics, chemotherapy, pain management, and caregivers who are understanding. Pharmacists can become experts in many of these therapies.

Success Stories

An interesting story in *Drug Topics* entitled "Six who Made it Big in Home Care" may be of interest to the reader.[39] In this article, six community pharmacists tell what it takes to succeed in the home care business. The title of each vignette reveals the story of home care delivered from a community pharmacy:

- "How I Discovered a Sleeper in Ostomy Supplies" by Frank L. Smith
- "Building a Lasting Business in Medical Durable Medical Equipment," by Stanley D. Siskind
- "How I Turned $1,400 in Diabetes Items into $22,000," by Marty Rubin
- "How I Found the Sweet Smell of Success in Oxygen Equipment," by Roy M. Shuman
- "How I Built Up My Breast Prosthesis Business," by Paul W. Hal
- "How I Entered the Field of High-Tech Products," by Barry D. Derman

SUMMARY

Home care has grown because of increased cost pressures in hospitals and shifting emphasis by managed care and payers to send patients home from the hospital earlier. In addition, patients like being at home in familiar surroundings with family. Because these patients are usually moderately ill, they need professional care. Part of that care is treatment with specially compounded medications that need to be carefully prepared under the watchful eye of a pharmacist. In addition, the home care pharmacist has become part of a technical and clinical team of health professionals who provide specialized care for the home care patient. This involvement can be satisfying for a patient-oriented pharmacist.

DISCUSSION QUESTIONS AND EXERCISES

1. Home care pharmacies prepare intravenous additive infusions for patients. What is an IV infusion?
2. Home care pharmacies also prepare total parenteral nutrition (TPN) infusions for patients. How does TPN differ from other intravenous additive infusions?
3. Intravenous infusions must be aseptically prepared. What constitutes aseptic preparation?
4. Are there certain IV additive infusions that should not be prepared by pharmacy technicians? By certified pharmacy technicians?
5. All intravenous products prepared by pharmacy technicians must be checked by a pharmacist — the ingredients, the amount of the ingredients, and the label. If a pharmacist was not present when the IV product was prepared, how will the pharmacist know how much of each ingredient was used?
6. Pharmacists have two primary roles when working in home care — oversight of the drug preparation and dispensing process and monitoring patients for appropriate drug therapy. Which role would you prefer and why?
7. Home care pharmacy practice may include pain management and hospice care. Is this something that interests you? Why or why not?
8. Make an appointment to tour a home care pharmacy and interview a home care pharmacist.
9. What do you feel are the pros and cons of being a home care pharmacist?
10. Based on what you know and have read so far, is working as a home care pharmacist something you would like to do? Why or why not?

CHALLENGES

1. The role of home care pharmacists is much more clinical than that of pharmacists in most other settings. For extra credit, and with the permission of your professor, prepare a concise report comparing and contrasting the roles of the average pharmacist in home care and the average pharmacist in hospitals. Explain differences and advance arguments and mechanisms on how the clinical role of the hospital pharmacist might look more like the role of pharmacists in home care.

2. The public's perception of pharmacy is formed largely from what it sees in community pharmacies. That perception reveals trust, but also technical expertise, rather than clinical expertise like that seen in home care pharmacy. For extra credit, and with the permission of your professor, prepare a concise report comparing and contrasting the roles of the average pharmacist in home care and the average pharmacist in community pharmacy. Explain differences and advance arguments and mechanisms on how the clinical role of the community pharmacist might be made to look more like the role of pharmacist in home care.

WEB SITES OF INTEREST

National Association for Home Care & Hospice: http://www.nahc.org/
National Home Infusion Association: http://www.nhianet.org
American Society for Parenteral and Enteral Nutrition: http://www.nutritioncare.org/
JCAHO Home Health Standards: http://www.jcrinc.com/subscribers/perspectives.asp?durki=6064&site=10&return=2815

REFERENCES

1. Macklin, R, Defining home care. *Am J Health Syst-Pharm.* 2001;58:422.
2. American Society of Health-System Pharmacists. ASHP guidelines on the pharmacist's role in home care. *Am J Health Syst-Pharm.* 2000;57:1252–1257.
3. Filibeck, DJ. Defining home care. *Am J Health Syst-Pharm.* 2001;58:422–423.
4. *Hospital Statistics, 2000 Edition.* American Hospital Association, Chicago, 2000.
5. *Managed Care Digest Series 2000.* Aventis Pharmaceuticals, Kansas City, MO, 2000.
6. U.S. Census Bureau. *Statistical Abstract of the United States: 1999,* 119th ed. Government Printing Office, Washington, DC, 1999.
7. U.S. Census Bureau. *Statistical Abstracts of the United States:2004–2005.* Government Printing Office, Washington, DC, 2005.

8. Verispan. Home Health Agencies. Available at http://www.firstmark.com/pdf_files/MarketSegments_rep.pdf. Accessed April 30, 2006.

9. Bernstein, AB, Hing, E, Moss, AJ, et al. *Health Care in America: Trends in Utilization.* Hyattsville, MD: National Center for Health Statistics, 2003. Available at http://www.cdc.gov/nchs/data/misc/healthcare.pdf. Accessed April 29, 2006.

10. Bailey, R. Home health care industry continues growth, independent pharmacies are ideal outlets. *Commun Pharm.* 1997;89(6):38–41.

11. Monk-Tutor, MR. The U.S. home infusion market. *Am J Health-Syst Pharm.* 1998;55:2019–2025.

12. Critical Care Systems. Frequently asked questions about home infusion therapy. Available at http://www.criticalcaresystems.com/insideccs/faq.html. Accessed April 29, 2006.

13. National Home Infusion Association. Frequently asked questions about infusion therapy. Available at http://www.nhianet.org/faqs.htm. Accessed April 29, 2006.

14. National Center for Health Statistics. Centers for Disease Control and Prevention. 2005. Available at http://www.cdc.gov/nchs/hus.htm#updated. Accessed April 30, 2006.

15. Christiansen, K. A paradigm shift for the home care provider. In *Home Care and Managed Care: Strategies for the Future,* Linne, EB, ed. American Hospital Association, Chicago, 1995, chap. 2.

16. Frank, RA, and Callahan, HE. Marketing and financial management strategies for managed home care. In *Home Care and Managed Care: Strategies for the Future,* Linne, EB, ed. American Hospital Association, Chicago, 1995, chap. 3.

17. Gunning, K, Saffel-Shrier, and Shane-McWhorter, L. Medication use and nutritional status in elderly patients receiving home care. *Consult Pharm.* 1998;13:897–911.

18. Chamallas, SN, and Cote, LK. Preparing for a Joint Commission survey: a pharmacist's perspective. *Am J Health-Syst Pharm.* 2000;57:275–277.

19. American Society of Health-System Pharmacy. Joint Commission folds other pharmacy services into home care program. *Am J Health-Syst Pharm.* 2000;57:1646.

20. Melikian, DM. Establishing a home infusion pharmacy service. In *Home Health Care Practice,* 2nd ed., Catania, PN, and Rosner, MM, eds. Health Markets Research, Palo Alto, CA, 1994, chap. 18.

21. Kumpf, VJ. Implementation of safe practices for parenteral nutrition formulations. *Am J Health-Syst Pharm.* 1999;56:815–817.

22. Audette, CM, Triller, DM, Hamilton, R, and Briceland, LL. Classifying drug-related problems in home care. *Am J Health-Syst Pharm.* 2002;59:2407–2409.

23. Triller, D, Clause, SL, Briceland, LL, and Hamilton, RA. Resolution of drug-related problems in home care patients through a pharmacy referral service. *Am J Health-Syst Pharm.* 2003;60:905–910.

24. McPherson, ML. Hospice pharmacy practice. In *Home Health Care Practice,* 2nd ed., Catania, PN, and Rosner, MM, eds. Health Markets Research, Palo Alto, CA, 1995, chap. 8.

25. Barry, CP, and Fuller, TS. Home and hospice care. *Hosp Pharm.* 1998;33:797–799, 818.

26. Falkenstrom, MK. Pain management of the patient with cancer in the homecare setting. *J Intraven Nurs.* 1998;21:327–334.

27. Walley, GJ. There's home health care gold in your pharmacy: making the most of HME opportunity. *Commun Pharm.* 1999;91(5):19–21.

28. Davis, ER. *Total Quality Management for Home Care.* Aspen, Gaithersburg, MD, 1994.

29. Hawkins, PR. Home infusion challenges and opportunities. *Hosp Pharm Rep.* 1999;13:42–51.

30. American Society of Health-System Pharmacists. ASHP guidelines on the pharmacist's role in home care. *Am J Health-Syst Pharm.* 2000;57:1252–1257.

31. Morlock, C. Pharmacist involvement in home care practice. *US Pharm.* 1997;22(suppl 1):4, 6–8, 10.

32. Lima, HA. Pharmaceutical care in the home infusion health care setting. *Pharm Pract News.* 1999;26:33–36.

33. Brown, NJ. A model for improving medication use in home health care patients. *J Am Pharm Assoc.* 1998;38:696–702.

34. Triller, DM, Hamilton, RA, Briceland, LL, et al. Home care pharmacy: extending clinical pharmacy services beyond infusion therapy. *Am J Health-Syst Pharm.* 2000;57:1326–1331.

35. Gray, SL, Mahoney, JE, and Blough, DK. Adverse drug events in elderly patients receiving home health services following hospital discharge. *Ann Pharmacother.* 1999;33:1147–1153.

36. Simmons, SD. Technicians instrumental in home, long-term care pharmacies. *Mich Pharm.* 1996;34:35–37.

37. Gallagher, M. Home care pharmacist competency assessment program. *Am J Health-Syst Pharm.* 1999;56:1549–1553.

38. Harris, WL. Career opportunities in home health care. *Am J Hosp Pharm.* 1990;47:1267.

39. Chi, J. Six who made it big in home health care. *Drug Top.* 1985;129:32–34, 38–40.

12

LONG-TERM CARE PHARMACY

Long-term care "covers a diverse array of services provided over a sustained period of time to people of all ages with chronic conditions and functional limitations."[1] The needs of long-term care patients range from needing help in performing daily activities to needing total care. Many providers in various settings such as people's homes, assisted living facilities, and nursing homes take care of these needs.

Long-term care pharmacy has become a specialty area of practice. A pharmacist with a special interest in caring for long-term care patients has the title *consultant pharmacist*. There is much to the practice of consultant pharmacy, and this area of practice can be exciting and rewarding.

This chapter will explore long-term care and the role pharmacists play in this important area of health care. It will begin by describing long-term care patients and their medication-related problems. Next, the chapter will describe the various types of long-term care environments and the standards for long-term care. The central focus of the chapter will be on the role of consultant pharmacists in long-term care. The chapter will end with a description of the satisfaction and rewards of having a career in long-term care.

LEARNING OBJECTIVES

Following this learning session, you should be able to:

- Define the term *long-term care*
- Explain the goals of long-term care
- Discuss how the population is aging
- Explain some of the therapeutic issues of long-term patients
- Discuss the different types of long-term care facilities
- Explain what consultant pharmacy practice is like

- Discuss some services provided by consultant pharmacists
- Discuss the kind of growth expected in:
  - Long-term care
  - Consultant pharmacy practice
- Discuss the satisfaction level of consultant pharmacists

THE AGING POPULATION

As described in defining long-term care, patients of any age may need long-term care. Patients experiencing the disabling effects of chronic disease and those experiencing the long-term disabling effects of accidents may need long-term care whether at home or in an *extended care facility* such as a nursing home. However, most long-term care patients are elderly (65 years of age or older).

The Elderly

The growth in the number of elderly in the United States is increasing at an historical rate. In 2006, there were 38 million seniors. That number will rise to 75 million by 2030. According to the American Society of Consultant Pharmacists, "Every day in the United States, another 6,000 people reach the age of 65.[2]

Goals of Long-Term Care

The goals of long-term care involve the restoration or maintenance of health and function. Care is centered on allowing maximum patient autonomy and minimizing complications and dependency. The type and extent of care depend on the patient's health status, support, and the potential for recovery.

Diseases

The elderly, as a group, experience chronic diseases as they get older. Figure 12.1 shows the disease prevalence of the 65 years and older population.[3] These diseases are consistent with aging, but they can be managed with good diagnosis, treatment, and monitoring. Pharmacists can help make sure long-term care patients are treated properly.

Drug Therapy in the Elderly

Medication needs to be carefully prescribed in the elderly because of the large variation in how patients respond to therapy. The sources of this

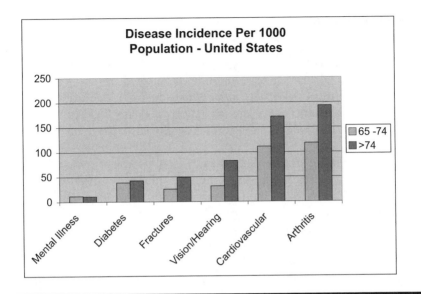

Figure 12.1 Disease prevalence in the elderly. (*Source:* The Centers for Disease Control and Prevention. *The National Center for Health Statistics. 65+ in the United States: 2005.* Atlanta, GA, 2005.)

variation include the presence of multiple chronic diseases, or *comorbidity*, physiological changes that go with aging, and the wide properties of drugs used to treat diseases of the elderly.[4] For some reason, there can also be an enhanced drug effect in older people.

Comorbidity

The presence of more than one disease can complicate diagnosis and treatment. Nearly 40% of the elderly have arthritis plus another serious health condition.[5] One study showed that people over 55 years had an average of 2.68 chronic conditions.[6] Sorting out what is going on in the patient can be difficult, and individualizing therapy is a necessity.

When comorbidity is present, there is also the possibility of *drug–disease interaction*, which occurs when a drug used for one condition worsens another condition.[5] An example of this is when beta-blockers (such as propranalol) are used to treat a heart condition in a patient who also has respiratory problems. Although the drug will help the heart condition, it may reduce breathing in a patient already experiencing breathing problems. In addition, the presence of certain diseases together may dramatically reduce the effectiveness of some drugs. As the number of coexisting diseases increases, the predictability of how a drug will work decreases.

Physiological Changes

It is well documented that the elderly vary in how their bodies handle drugs more than younger people. Age-related physiological change affects how drugs are absorbed, distributed, metabolized, and excreted from the body. Each of these four *pharmacokinetic* features can affect the active drug in the blood and at the site of action. Too much drug can cause an overdose, and too little drug could cause the disease or condition to be under-treated.

Drug absorption can be altered in the aging patient owing to reduced gastric acidity, increased gastric emptying time, and reduced intestinal blood flow. Thus, the rate and extent of drug absorption can be altered.

Some drugs distribute to lean body tissue, whereas others distribute to fat. As a person ages, there is less lean body mass and more fatty tissue. There is also less total body water and less serum albumin. Using normal adult doses, without consideration of the lean body mass and total body water, can commonly result in too much or, less commonly, in too little drug being distributed to the site of action.

Most drugs are lipid soluble (dissolve in fat) drugs that are absorbed in the small intestine and pass through lipid membranes to the site of action. The drug then leaves the site and is available for *metabolism*, usually being transformed from a lipid-soluble drug to a water-soluble drug, which it needs to be in order to be *excreted* into the urine by the kidney. Metabolism is dependent on blood flow (reduced in older patients) through the liver (size also reduced) and the presence of certain liver enzymes. As people age, both of these functions can be altered, resulting in the drug being metabolized either too quickly or too slowly. If the drug is still being administered at the same rate, it can build up in the bloodstream and cause toxicity or be reduced and be less effective.

Most drugs are eliminated from the body by the kidney. Reduced renal (kidney) function and blood flow occurs with age, and this reduction is predictable. In elderly patients, kidney function may be reduced by as much as 50% by age 75 years.[5]

Enhanced Effects

When compared with younger people, the elderly are more likely to experience an enhanced, atypical response to their medication.[5] For some reason, with age, organ systems can become more sensitive to the effects of certain drugs. This is especially true for drugs affecting the central nervous system such as narcotic analgesics and tranquilizers.

Medication-Related Problems

Because of comorbidities, physiological changes, and enhanced drug effects, the elderly experience more *medication-related problems* (see Chapter 7, Pharmaceutical Care) than those in other age groups.[7] Investigators have described the prevalence, types, and effects of adverse drug events (ADEs) in patients 65 years old or older taking multiple (five or more) medications.[8] Thirty-five percent of patients reported having at least one ADE within the previous year. Various medications were involved, but the ADEs were mostly associated with cardiovascular (33%) and central nervous system agents (29%).

Surprisingly, almost all the ADEs were classified as predictable (type A) adverse events, which means they could have been prevented. Pharmacists, using the pharmaceutical care model, should be able to prevent many of these medication-related problems.

Poly-Pharmacy

Poly-pharmacy is the act or practice of prescribing too many medicines or is a prescription made up of many medicines or ingredients. Twice as many medications are prescribed to patients over 65 years of age compared with younger patients.[9] The older population uses approximately 30% of all prescription medications, along with an unknown percentage of non-prescription medications.

A study showed that one-third of seniors take medications prescribed by two or more physicians.[10] More than one quarter (28%) have been to at least three physicians in the past six months. One third of older adults take eight or more medications.

LONG-TERM CARE FACILITIES

There are several types of long-term care (LTC) facilities.

Nursing Homes

The best-known type of LTC facility is the nursing home, which largely came about from the Social Security Act of 1935. In nursing homes, patients (resident is the preferred term) cannot do one or more of the normal activities of daily living: ambulating, eating, bathing, dressing, or toileting.[11]

Nursing homes provide intense services and have various health care workers including physicians, nurses, dieticians, physical therapists, respiratory therapists, social workers, and consultant pharmacists.

Low-income residents are eligible for Medicaid, and this helps pay the nursing home expenses.

Assisted Living

There are two less intense levels of community-based LTC, generally called *assisted living*.

> *Independent Living:* The first level of community-based LTC is a relatively new idea called *independent living*. These facilities allow residents to do as much as possible for themselves, yet provide support and back-up. Such facilities often provide assistance in taking medication, housekeeping, eating, and doing laundry. They also have attractive cultural and recreational facilities. The cost is borne by the resident or is provided through estate planning.
>
> *Intermediate Care:* An emerging level of LTC between independent living and nursing homes is called *intermediate care*. This level of care is less intense than nursing home care but more intense than assisted living. More services are offered than in assisted living, and the care allows the resident to remain as independent as possible before progressing to nursing home care. For example, impairment may occur in one or more basic measures of function.

Continuing Care Retirement Community

The *continuing care retirement community* (CCRC) provides individuals a continuum of care that is needed as they move through the last part of their life. A CCRC usually provides for all levels of care, from independent living through nursing home care. Some CCRCs also provide acute, Alzheimer's, and hospice care.

Statistics

In 2003, there were 16,323 LTC facilities, a slight decline from 2000.[12,13] The decline is most likely attributed to the increased focus of nursing homes on patients with greater disability and postacute care needs and a preference for alternatives to nursing home care.

In 2003, there were 1.5 million nursing home residents.[13] The occupancy rate was 82.6%. Most (about 75%) nursing home residents were female. Fourteen percent of the residents were age 65 to 74 years, 36% were age 75 to 85 years, and 50% were 85 years old or older.

Quality of Care

Local, state, and national policy makers have questioned the quality of LTC. The public, including the families of residents of LTC facilities, especially nursing homes, have also questioned the quality. Concerns about the quality of care and treatment of residents persist despite some improvements in these facilities in recent years.

In 2001, the Institute of Medicine (IOM), with the support of the Robert Wood Johnson Foundation, launched a study on "Improving Quality in Long-Term Care."[1] This study is a follow-up to one completed in 1986. In general, the IOM found that the quality of care in nursing homes had improved since 1987. They also found that the quality of life for nursing home residents had shown some improvement, but to a lesser extent.

The IOM offered 14 recommendations in the following areas:

- Access to appropriate services (1)
- Quality assurance through appropriate oversight (5)
- Strengthening the work force (5)
- Building organizational capacity (1)
- Reimbursement issues (2)

State standards exist for assisted living facilities; however, the IOM reported that these standards are variable. For nursing homes, there are both federal and state regulations to protect the quality of care. To monitor and assess compliance with these regulations, state agencies perform on-site surveys. After surveying a facility, state surveyors decide whether the facility has met or not met each standard.

Unfortunately, the quality of care in nursing homes has not improved much since the IOM report. For example, one study found that for-profit nursing homes are 46.5% more likely than nonprofit nursing homes to be cited for poor quality.[14] Almost two-thirds of nursing homes are for-profit. Poor-quality-of-care nursing homes have resulted in at least one national citizens' coalition for nursing home reform.[15]

The American Geriatrics Society has a position statement on measuring the quality of care for nursing home residents.[16] Additionally, the quality of care in the nation's nursing homes may get a boost from a recent quality improvement initiative from the Centers for Medicare and Medicaid Services (CMS).[17]

Financing Long-Term Care

Long-term care does not come cheap — the estimated annual costs are from $70,000 to $100,000.[18] "Even so, 95% of us lack insurance to protect ourselves from the potentially catastrophic financial demands of such vital services." An article titled "Financing Health Care for an Aging Population" stated that the United States has a broken financing system that so far is unable to cope with an aging population.[19] Although seniors acquired help by the complex Medicare prescription benefit in 2006, no solution is on the radar screen for helping to finance long-term care.

CONSULTANT PHARMACY PRACTICE

Pharmacists specializing in LTC pharmacy are called *consultant pharmacists* "because the relationship between the facility or agency and the pharmacist is contractual (rather than that of employee–employer) in about 95% of situations."[11] A new term for pharmacists with specialized knowledge in geriatrics, geriatric pharmacotherapy, and the unique needs of the senior population is *"senior care pharmacist."*[20]

Settings

According to Posey,[11] consultant pharmacists work in various settings:

- An independent or chain store pharmacy that provides limited long-term services
- Stand-alone long-term care pharmacies
- Pharmacies that provide no drugs but consult on the proper procedures and therapies in the facility
- Pharmacies located in nursing homes

Federal Laws

Federal law mandates consultant pharmacy services to nursing homes. Nursing homes, to qualify for Medicaid, must have the drugs of all residents reviewed by a pharmacist at least once a month. Today, this is the only clinical pharmacy service recognized by federal law.

Managed Care

More and more managed care plans are starting to look at long-term benefit plans for their enrollees. It is important that these plans include a long-term pharmacy benefit plan. There are various arrangements (from fee-for-service to full capitation) under which consultant pharmacists can provide services to patients using a managed care plan (see Chapter 10, Managed Care Pharmacy).

Standards of Practice

The American Society of Consultant Pharmacists (ASCP) has developed progressive standards, many of which call for incorporating pharmaceutical care into the daily routine of each practicing consultant pharmacist. These standards of practice have helped standardize and improve pharmacy services to extended care facilities and have raised the pharmacist's clinical practice.

Accreditation

Accreditation of LTC pharmacy comes from the Joint Commission on Accreditation of Healthcare Organizations (JCAHO). This accreditation process started around 1996, and the standards are progressive, especially concerning the pharmacist's clinical practice. Consultant pharmacists have done a wonderful job in meeting the standards and in being accredited.[21]

Services

Services pharmacists provide to LTC facilities can be divided into provider services and consultant services. These services can be combined or provided individually.

Provider Services

Provider services are supplied at various levels depending on the needs of the LTC facility. The most basic service is dispensing medications to the residents of the facility.

Many of the services listed in Table 12.1 can be provided using automation.[22] The ASCP and several other professional pharmacy organizations commissioned the Automation in Pharmacy Initiative, a white paper on automation in pharmacy.[23] This paper puts forth the important issues in automating the distributive functions and highlights the importance of automation in quality assurance. Some recommended areas on which to focus include:[24]

- Order entry
- Downtime and system failures
- Filling and refilling medication containers
- Storage
- Education and training
- Machine errors

Table 12.1   Selected Provider Pharmacy Functions

Drug Distribution
Drug delivery (routine and emergency)
Drug packaging and labeling
Medication reordering
Auditing for controlled medications
Emergency medication supply
Monitoring of proper storage of medication
Forms and Reports
Patient profile
Medication administration
Patient cardex
Physician order forms
Automatic stop orders
Treatment records
Patient care plans
Drug utilization review
Billing statements
Other
Policy and procedure development
Drug information
Durable medical equipment
Medical/surgical supplies
Enteral products
Intravenous services

Source: From Simonson, W, and Feinberg, JL. *Consultant Pharmacy Practice.* American Society of Consultant Pharmacists and Roche Laboratories, Nutley, NJ, 1991. With permission.

- Labeling
- Servicing equipment
- Medication error detection

The importance of automation to pharmacy has many benefits: (a) improved efficiency, (b) improved accuracy, (c) reduction of medication errors, (d) automated charting of medication, (e) automated billing of medication, and (f) freeing up of the pharmacist to provide more patient-focused care.[25]

Table 12.2 Selected Consultant Pharmacist Activities

Development of innovative medication distribution systems
Drug-regimen review (DRR)
Drug use review (DUR)
Drug use evaluation (DUE)
Quality assurance
Infection control
Formulary development
Nutritional support services
Policy and procedure development
Committee participation
Therapeutic drug monitoring
Facility staff education and training
Medication pass review
Participation in state survey process
Geriatric research

Source: From Simonson, W, and Feinberg, JL. *Consultant Pharmacy Practice.* American Society of Consultant Pharmacists and Roche Laboratories, Nutley, NJ, 1991. With permission.

Consultant Services

Consultant pharmacy services range from the federally mandated drug regimen review (DRR) to doing geriatric research. Some of the many consultant pharmacy services are listed in Table 12.2. "The extent of involvement and variety of services offered depends on the consultant pharmacist's interest, motivation, formal training or experience, work environment, and reimbursement for services."[22]

The three methods of reviewing drug therapy for quality are *drug regimen review* (DRR), *drug-use review* (DUR), and *drug-use evaluation* (DUE).

Drug Regimen Review

At the heart of consultant pharmacy services is DRR.[26] A consultant pharmacist must review a resident's medications at least every 30 days. Doing this improves therapy, reduces medication-related morbidity and mortality, and reduces cost, achieving quality drug therapy.

The best way to undertake DRR and to achieve quality drug therapy is to have a well-functioning interdisciplinary team with each team member focusing on the same goal. The effect of such a team was measured.[27] The team was composed of a geriatric physician, geriatrics medical fellow, nurse practitioner, medical resident, clinical pharmacist, geriatric pharmacy resident, social worker, rehabilitation therapist, dentist, and nursing staff. Although the change in the number of drugs did not change over a 4-month period, there was a significant decrease in the number of unnecessary medications (1.57 ± 1.47 to 0.34 ± 0.65; $P < 0.001$).

DRR is performed *concurrently*, which means while the patient is taking the medication. Thus, recommendations to change therapy can have an immediate effect on the quality of drug therapy. For this review, the pharmacist reviews the resident's medical history, prognosis, treatments, orders, laboratory tests, medication history, and care plan.[28] The pharmacist then focuses on the treatment goals set up for the patient by an interdisciplinary team of which the pharmacist is a member.

The pharmacist's attention is then turned to the appropriateness of therapy and uses identifying medication-related problems, as developed under the pharmaceutical care model of delivery care (see Chapter 7, Pharmaceutical Care).

Commercially available software is helpful to pharmacists in performing DRR. The software helps capture the data, tracking various kinds of medication, producing reports, making recommendations, and capturing recommendation outcomes.[29]

Consultant pharmacists look for specific problems when doing DRR. For example, there is a national or regional average for the number of prescriptions the average elderly person has each month. Patients who take more than the average number of prescriptions may be taking unnecessary therapy. National and regional figures are also available for the number of medication administration errors found monthly by other consultant pharmacists. Such *benchmarks* can be useful.

Some other useful signs to be looking for are: (a) multiple orders for the same drug for the same patient; (b) drugs administered after *stop orders* (automatic stops on medication); (c) PRN (medication ordered as needed) drugs administered each day for more than 30 days; (d) drug interactions; (e) wrong dosage of laxatives, tranquilizers, analgesics, antipsychotics, or antidepressants; and (f) failure to order diagnostic tests during chronic therapy.[30]

Since consultant pharmacists have been performing DRR for a long time, an expert panel was recently assembled to identify elderly patients at risk for medication-related problems. The expert panel agreed on various medications or medication classes (Table 12.3) that call for scrutiny in the elderly.[31]

Another finding is that LTC residents are sometimes undertreated for conditions such as pain, depression, and osteoporosis. Various software programs incorporate disease state management programs to help consultant pharmacists identify problems and improve patient outcomes.

Table 12.3 Inappropriate Medication and Medication Classes for Use in the Elderly

Antihistamines
Blood products/modifiers/volume expanders
Platelet aggregation inhibitors
Cardiovasculars
Antihypertensives
Peripheral vasodilators
Antiarrhythmics
Central nervous system agents
Narcotics
Sedatives and hypnotic agents
Antidepressants
Gastric medications
Antiemetics
Anticholinergic/antispasmodics
Antidiarrheals
Genitourinary medications
Antispasmodics
Hormones/synthetic/modifiers
Hypoglycemic agents
Musculoskeletal medications
Nonsalicylate nonsteroidal anti-inflammatory drugs
Skeletal muscle relaxants

Source: Modified from Hanlon, JT, Shimp, LA, and Semla, TP. *Ann Pharmacother.* 2000;34:360–365. With permission.

Another important function of consultant pharmacists during the DRR process is to identify, resolve, and prevent ADEs. A recent study determined that nursing home residents experience 1.89 ADEs every 100 months, and 0.65 potential ADEs (those that may have caused harm but did not do so because of chance or because they were detected) every 100 months.[32] Of the ADEs, one was fatal, 6% were life-threatening or serious, and 56% were significant.

Overall, 515 of the ADEs were preventable: 72% of the fatal, life-threatening, or serious events and 34% of the significant ADEs. Errors resulting in preventable ADEs occurred most often at the stages of prescribing and ordering. Psychoactive medications (antipsychotics, antidepressants, and sedatives and hypnotics) and anticoagulants were the most common drugs associated with preventable ADEs.

Some common ADEs in the elderly may tip off the consultant pharmacist that the resident is experiencing trouble with his or her medication. These include confusion, depression, lack of appetite, weakness, drowsiness, ataxia, forgetfulness, tremor, constipation, dizziness, diarrhea, or urinary retention.[22]

According to the ASCP, drugs that often cause ADEs in elderly patients include nonsteroidal anti-inflammatory drugs (NSAIDs), diuretics, beta-blockers, digoxin, antihypertensives, sedative and hypnotics, tranquilizers, anticholinergics, antipsychotics, and antidiabetic drugs.[22]

Drug-Use Review

DRR is performed on one patient at a time, and the consultant pharmacist's recommendations are provided to the patient's physician. DUR is the process of reviewing drug therapy on a broader basis, that is, on a drug used in many patients or by many physicians. DURs supply trend information. Once a drug is selected for review, criteria on how the drug should ideally be used are developed. Pharmacists usually perform this function. The review can take place *retrospectively* by reviewing the records of patients who have received the drug in the past or *concurrently* — on patients still taking the drug. A table of results of how the drug is being used in the facility versus the ideal way the drug should be used is developed for review by the pharmacy and therapeutics (P&T) committee or presented to the physicians at an education meeting or through a newsletter.

Drug-Use Evaluation

DUE is a process of reviewing drug therapy that is even broader than DUR. In DUE, a disease is selected to see how it is being treated; thus, the process will review the use of many drugs.

The importance of DRR, DUR, and DUE is that medication-related problems are identified and solutions put in place to help the patient (DRR) or many patients (DUR and DUE). Consultant pharmacists are to be congratulated on the fine job they are doing. A study showed that consultant pharmacists were able to reduce or stop the use of 43% of unacceptable medications.[33]

Another study of 3464 interventions made by consultant pharmacists found that 85.7% of the interventions requested a response by the physician (14.3% were informational). Of the interventions seeking a response, physicians accepted the advice of the pharmacist 68% of the time.[34] The most common interventions were for unnecessary medication, laboratory monitoring, and more laboratory checking.

Consultant pharmacists provide value to LTC facilities and their residents. A study discovered most LTC facilities pay $3.28 for each resident each month for consultant pharmacist services (range was $3.14 to $4.04).[35] The savings generated by discontinuation of unnecessary drugs as recommended by the pharmacist more than pays for these services.

One of the methods pharmacists have developed to reduce unnecessary medication is the use of the *stop order*, which is not an order at all but rather a policy developed by the P&T committee to stop the use of certain drugs after a certain time unless the physician reorders the medication. The beauty of a stop order policy is that it reminds physicians to routinely review the active orders for a patient. The downside is that certain important medications may be stopped when the physician does not want them stopped; that is why physicians are given several warnings by the pharmacy before the medication is stopped. However, in LTC facilities, physicians may only see their patients once a month and miss the stop order warning. This is where the consultant pharmacist's DRR should help.

An example of a LTC stop order policy looks like this: antibiotics (7 days), antiemetics (4 days), antihistamines (7 days), cold preparations (5 days), all other medication (30 days).

Drug Safety

Since the IOM's report, *To Err is Human* in 1999, there has been a stepped up effort by consultant pharmacists to improve medication safety. The ASCP has published a list of the top ten drug interactions in long-term care.[36] The ten drug interactions are:

1. Warfarin — NSAIDs
2. Warfarin — sulfa drugs
3. Warfarin — macrolides
4. Warfarin — quinolones
5. Warfarin — phenytoin
6. ACE inhibitors — potassium supplements
7. ACE inhibitors — spironolactone
8. Digoxin — amiodarone
9. Digoxin — verapamil
10. Theophylline — quinolones

Note: The NSAID class does not include COX-2 inhibitors. Quinolones that interact include ciprofloxacin, enoxacin, norfloxacin, and ofloxacin.

GROWTH IN LONG-TERM CARE

The elderly population is growing dramatically. It is estimated that the greatest impact will be felt between 2010 and 2030 when those on the leading edge of the baby boom generation begin to reach age 65 years.[37] Patients in nursing homes are expected to get there quicker and be sicker. This is already starting to happen. Because of declining reimbursement for hospitals, patients are being discharged sooner. In about 1966, the average nursing patient took 3 to 10 medications a day, or an average of 3.8 drugs.[38] In 1996, the nursing home patient took an average of 6.3 medications a day.

GROWTH IN CONSULTANT PHARMACY PRACTICE

George F. Archambault, who first coined the phrase "consultant pharmacist" in the 1950s, probably never imagined the growth of consultant pharmacy practice during the past 50 years. This growth has occurred because of the growing number of elderly, whose numbers are projected to exceed 70 million by 2030.[37] The growth in consultant pharmacy practice also has to do with the dedication and enthusiasm of many hard-working consultant pharmacists and their professional organization, the ASCP.

REWARDS AND SATISFACTION

Despite LTC being regulated, consultant pharmacists have focused on the right things and have documented their successes. Consultant pharmacists have been able to combine the clinical aspects of hospital pharmacy practice with the business challenges of community pharmacy.[11] They like working with physicians and other health care professionals, feel like they have a direct impact on patient well-being, have autonomy, and like the rewards.[38]

Consultant pharmacists also like the variety in their daily routine: monitoring the dispensing process, counseling physicians, performing pharmacokinetics, reviewing therapy, counseling patients, and committee work.[39]

The less appealing aspects of consultant pharmacy are conflicts with management and other health care professionals, dealing with those who do not adapt to change, and the travel associated with monthly DRRs.[11,39]

FUTURE OF CONSULTANT PHARMACY PRACTICE

Recent changes in the nursing home survey process have started to focus on quality. Surveyors use 24 quality indicators when selecting a sample of residents to review. The quality indicators help consultant pharmacists provide better services to patients.[37] Also, the arrival of the Medicare nursing facility prospective payment system created a financial reason for all decisions. Thus, consultant pharmacists must now consider cost during their DRRs.[37] The cost of drug therapy now includes the cost of therapeutic failures and medication-related problems, not just the cost of the medication, distribution, and use. There will also be more of a focus on reviewing the use of psychotropics, not just in nursing homes but also in assisted living facilities, and on patient outcomes.[39]

SUMMARY

The U.S. population is getting older. By 2030, there will be 70 million Americans 65 years old or older. With this growth has been the growth in LTC and consultant pharmacy practice. Consultant pharmacists are a dedicated and motivated group of health care professionals who are focusing on what is important — quality drug therapy and improved health outcomes in LTC residents. Their job combines clinical and business skills and offers various functions throughout the workday. They also are on the leading edge of pharmaceutical care, and they have provided leadership to the profession of pharmacy in thinking about automation.

DISCUSSION QUESTIONS AND EXERCISES

1. How do you feel about working with elderly patients?
2. It is federally mandated that the medication regimen of all patients in nursing homes in the United States be reviewed by a pharmacist every 30 days and recommendations made to the prescribing physician. Is this something that interests you? Why or why not?
3. During drug regimen review (DRR), you (the pharmacist) discover a drug being prescribed for a patient that, according to FDA labeling, is absolutely contraindicated in the patient and thus poses a potential danger to the patient.
   a. What would you do?
   b. What would you do if the prescribing physician still wants to use the drug?
4. You note that you and other LTC pharmacists provide many DRR recommendations to one physician versus other physicians, and that this physician rarely accepts the pharmacist's recommendations.
   a. Should you do anything about this?
   b. If yes, what would you do?

5. Patients in LTC facilities often receive too many central nervous system (CNS) depressants or experience exaggerated effects from these agents. What are the signs and symptoms of too much CNS depression?
6. Make an appointment to interview a long-term care pharmacist.
7. What do you see as the pros and cons of being a long-term care pharmacist?
8. Based on what you know and what you have read thus far, is long-term care pharmacy something you are interested in doing? Why or why not?

CHALLENGES

1. The prevalence of polypharmacy is higher among those 65 years of age or older. For extra credit and with the permission of your professor, research and prepare a concise report titled "The Problems and Solutions to Poly-Pharmacy in the U.S."
2. The Medicare Modernization Act, which authorized Medicare's payment for Part D prescription expenses, affects many long-term care residents. For extra credit, and with the permission of your professor, research and prepare a concise report titled "The Affect of the Part D Medicare Benefits on Long-Term Care Residents."

WEB SITES OF INTEREST

American Society of Consultants Pharmacists: http://www.ascp.com

Aging population: http://www.census.gov/prod/1/pop/p23-190/p23-190.html

American Geriatrics Society: http://www.americangeriatrics.org/

Getting started in consultant pharmacy: http://ascp.com/com/start/

REFERENCES

1. Institute of Medicine. *Improving the Quality of Long-Term Care*. National Academy Press, Washington, DC, 2001.
2. American Society of Consultant Pharmacists. ASCP fact sheet. Available at http://www.ascp.com/about/ascpfactsheet.cfm. Accessed May 4, 2006.
3. The Centers for Disease Control and Prevention. *The National Center for Health Statistics. 65+ in the United States: 2005*. Author, Atlanta, GA, 2005.
4. Williams, ME. *The American Geriatric Society's Complete Guide to Aging and Health*. Harmony Books. New York, 1995.
5. Nash, DB, Koenig, JB, and Chatterton, ML. *Why the Elderly Need Individualized Pharmaceutical Care*. Thomas Jefferson University, Philadelphia, 2000.

6. Verbrugge, LM, Lepkowski, JM, and Imanaka, Y. Comorbidity and its impact on disability. *Milbank Q.* 1989;67:450–484.

7. Hanlon, JT, Shimp, LA, and Semla, TP. Recent advances in geriatrics: drug-related problems in the elderly. *Ann Pharmacother.* 2000;34:360–365.

8. Hanlon, JT, Schmader, KE, Koronkowski, MJ, et al. Adverse drug events in high risk older outpatients. *J Am Geriatr Soc.* 1997;45:945–948.

9. Corcoran, ME. Polypharmacy in the older patient with cancer. Available at http://www.moffitt.usf.edu/pubs/ccj/v4n5/article5.html. Accessed May 4, 2006.

10. ASHP. New study reveals one-third of seniors take medications prescribed by two or more doctors. Available at http://www.ashp.org/public/news/breaking/shoearticle.cfm?id=2528. Accessed May 4, 2006.

11. Posey, LM. *Pharmacy Cadence.* PAS Pharmacy/Association Services, Athens, GA, 1992.

12. U.S. Census Bureau. *Statistical Abstract of the United States: 1999,* 119th ed. Government Printing Office, Washington, DC, 1999.

13. Bernstein, AB, Hing, E, Moss, AJ, et al. *Health Care in America: Trends in Utilization,* Hyattsville, MD: National Center for Health Statistics, 2003.

14. University of California at San Francisco. For-profit nursing homes more likely than non-profits to be cited for poor quality. Available at http://www.chc.ucsf.edu/archives/forprofitnursinghomes.htm. Accessed May 2, 2006.

15. National Citizens' Coalition for Nursing Home Reform. Available at http://www.nccnhr.org/default.cfm. Accessed May 2, 2006.

16. American Geriatrics Society (AGS) Position Statement. Available at http://www.americangeriatrics.org/products/positionpapers/unintended_conseq.shtml. Accessed May 2, 2006.

17. Centers for Medicare and Medicaid. Nursing home quality initiatives: overview. Available at http://www.cms.hhs.gov/NursingHomeQualityInits/. Accessed May 2, 2006.

18. Durenberger, D. The Commonwealth Fund. The U.S. long-term care system: ripe for reform. Available at http://www.cmwf.org/publications/publications_show.htm?doc_id=331496. Accessed May 2, 2006.

19. Derr, JF. The Commonwealth Fund. Financing health care for an aging population. Available at http://www.cmwf.org/publications/publications_show.htm?doc_id=331494.

20. American Society of Consultant Pharmacists. What is a senior care pharmacist? Available at http://www.ascp.com/consumers/what/index.cfm. Accessed May 4, 2006.

21. Williams, L. Accreditation tune-up: the top ten JCAHO survey pitfalls — and how to avoid them. *Consult Pharm.* 1999;14:259–271.

22. Simonson, W, and Feinberg, JL. *Consultant Pharmacy Practice.* American Society of Consultant Pharmacists and Roche Laboratories, Nutley, NJ, 1991.

23. Barker, KN, Felkey, BG, Flynn, EA, and Carper, JL. White paper on automation in pharmacy. *Consult Pharm.* 1998;13:256–293.

24. Josephson, DC. Automation's emerging role as a new quality assurance tool for the long-term care pharmacist. *Consult Pharm.* 1998;13:1028–1032.

25. Riley, K. The expanding role of automation in long term care pharmacy. *Consult Pharm.* 1996;11:749–762.

26. American Society of Consultant Pharmacists. Drug regimen review. Available at http://ascp.com/resources/drr/. Accessed May 4, 2006.

27. Jeffery, S, Ruby, C, Twersky, J, and Hanlon, JT. Effect of an interdisciplinary team on suboptimal prescribing in a long term care facility. *Consult Pharm.* 1999;14:1386–1391.

28. American Society of Consultant Pharmacists. Consultant pharmacist services. Available at http://www.ascp.com/member/policy/ltc/cps.shtml. Accessed April 18, 2001.

29. Meade, V. Large LTC providers set the pace. *Consult Pharm.* 1999;14:509–520.

30. Anonymous. U.S. tells how to measure consultant RPH's performance. *Am Drug.* 1981;183:106.

31. Hanlon, JT, Shimp, LA, and Semla, TP. Recent advances in geriatrics: drug-related problems in the elderly. *Ann Pharmacother.* 2000;34:360–365.

32. Gurwitz, JH, Field, TS, Avorn, J, et al. Incidence and preventability of adverse drug events in nursing homes. *Am J Med.* 2000;109:87–94.

33. Byars, JR, Gruber, J, and Harmon, JR. Results of an effort to curtail the number of "unacceptable" medications in the elderly population via drug regimen review. *Consult Pharm.* 1999;14:363–370.

34. Johnston, AM, Doane, K, Phipps, S, and Bell, A. Outcomes of pharmacists' cognitive services in the long-term care setting. *Consult Pharm.* 1996;11:41–50.

35. Malone, DC, and Gwyn, B. Consultant pharmacist services and payment in long-term care facilities. *Consult Pharm.* 1997;12:781–790.

36. American Society of Consultant Pharmacists. Patient safety. Available at http://www.ascp.com/advocacy/briefing/patientsafety.cfm. Accessed May 4, 2006.

37. Bryan, G, and Martin, CM. The changing face of long-term care. *Consult Pharm.* 2000;15:715–723.

38. Bennett, BV. Long-term care: 30 years later. *Drug Top.* 1996;140:74–75.

39. Sogol, EM. Career paths: geriatric pharmacy. *U.S. Pharm.* 1991;16:66–69.

40. Buerger, DK. Are you positioned for success on the new frontier? *Consult Pharm.* 1999;14:204–206.

13

GOVERNMENT PHARMACY

One of the advantages of being a pharmacist is the variety of places to work. One of those places is within the goverment. Unfortunately, pharmacist positions in the government do not have the visibility and recognition they deserve.

This chapter is about the opportunities pharmacists have and the kinds of work pharmacists do in government service. It will discuss the U.S. Public Health Service (PHS) and the various areas pharmacists can work within the PHS, for example, the Indian Health Service (IHS), the Food and Drug Administration (FDA), the Centers for Disease Control and Prevention (CDC), and federal prisons.

Pharmacists also work in federal hospitals such as the National Institutes of Health (NIH), the Environmental Protection Agency (EPA), the Agency for Toxic Substances and Disease Registry (ASTDR), the Agency for Health-care Research and Quality (AHRQ), and the Health Care Financing Agency (HCFA).

This chapter will also discuss how pharmacists work and provide service within the Veteran's Administration Hospitals (VA hospitals), the Drug Enforcement Agency (DEA), and the Department of Defense (DOD) — the Army, Navy, and Air Force. The chapter will end with discussion of some of the rewards and satisfactions of working for the government.

LEARNING OBJECTIVES

After participating in this learning session, you should be able to:

- Identify the eight agencies where pharmacists work in the PHS
- Explain the mission of the PHS

- Explain opportunities for pharmacists within the Department of Defense
- Explain opportunities for pharmacists within the Veterans Administration

U.S. PUBLIC HEALTH SERVICE

President John Adams set up the PHS on July 16, 1798, to provide care and relief of sick and disabled navigators.[1] Since this beginning, the PHS has protected and advanced our nation's health and has contributed to the delivery of health care worldwide.

The PHS has ten agencies: the Centers for Disease Control and Prevention (CDC), the Agency for Toxic Substances and Disease Registry (ATSDR), the National Institutes of Health (NIH), the Food and Drug Administration (FDA), the Substance Abuse and Mental Health Services Administration (SAMHSA), the Health Resources and Services Administration (HRSA), the Agency for Healthcare Research and Quality (AHRQ), the Indian Health Service (IHS), Office of Public Health and Sciences (OPHS), and the Program Support Center (PSC).[2]

The U.S. PHS is a part of the U.S. Department of Health and Human Services (HHS). There are about 6,100 commissioned corps officers and over 50,000 civil service employees in the PHS. Over 930 of these are pharmacists.[3] Today, the greatest need in government pharmacy is for clinical pharmacists to work with medically underserved populations. Most PHS pharmacists begin their careers in a clinical setting, advancing to senior clinical positions or moving to research or administration.

Centers for Disease Control and Prevention (CDC)

The CDC started in Atlanta, Georgia, in 1946. The CDC's mission is to promote health and quality of life by preventing and controlling disease, injury, and disability.[4] The CDC is the leading federal agency responsible for protecting the health of the American public by overseeing disease trends; studying disease outbreaks and health and injury risks; fostering safer, more healthful environments; and implementing illness and injury control and preventions.

The CDC employs about 8837 people. In 2006, eight commissioned pharmacy officers worked at the CDC in the drug service, the chronic disease service, vaccine safety and development, and sexually transmitted diseases. Pharmacists seeking a job at the CDC who are not commissioned officers in the PHS increase their chances of employment by having the MPH degree or an MS degree in biostatistics and epidemiology.

Food and Drug Administration (FDA)

The FDA ensures the safety of foods and cosmetics and the safety and efficacy of pharmaceuticals, biological products, and medical devices. The FDA was established in 1906, but it was not a part of the PHS until 1968. The FDA was founded in Rockville, Maryland.

In 2006, 307 (243 commissioned corp and 64 noncommissioned) of the 10,000 employees of the FDA were pharmacists. Although pharmacists work in most of the centers of the FDA, a majority of the work is completed in the Center for Drug Evaluation and Research (CDER) or the Center for Biologics Evaluation and Research (CBER).[1] Locations range from FDA headquarters in Rockville, Maryland, to locations in 150 cities nationwide.

All FDA pharmacists play a role in bringing new drugs and biologics to consumers and help regulate the manufacture and distribution of a wide variety of existing products. FDA pharmacists may work in pharmacology, toxicology, radiopharmacy, pharmacokinetics, or pharmacoepidemiology.

Examples of projects FDA pharmacists have been involved in include proposals to increase both the written and oral patient drug information, reporting adverse drug events through the FDA's MedWatch program, and surveillance of adverse effects of vaccines through the Vaccine Adverse Event Reporting System (VAERS), a joint program between the FDA and the CDC.

Indian Health Service (IHS)

The IHS is the PHS agency responsible for providing health services to approximately 1.5 million American Indians and Alaska Natives who belong to more than 557 federally recognized tribes in 35 states. Presently, the IHS and tribally managed programs operate in over 230 hospitals and ambulatory clinics. This task is complicated by the broad cultural, economic and geographic diversity of the groups served. As a result, health programs must be individually designed to address the needs of each community.

The IHS was founded in 1924 and currently has about 16,251 employees, of whom 433 are pharmacy officers and civilian pharmacists[5]: 75% of the practicing pharmacists are commissioned officers, 5% are civil servants, and 20% are direct hires by the tribes.

IHS pharmacists practice in a true pharmaceutical care environment where they fully utilize their knowledge and skills. The IHS has pioneered many progressive and innovative advances over the past 30 years. Pharmacists have access to the patient's entire health record including laboratory results, immunization status, and past medical history to assess the appropriateness of drug therapy. Problems are resolved with providers prior to dispensing medications, and all patients are counseled on their medication therapy. In many locations, pharmacists are credentialed to provide primary care and use their prescriptive authority to evaluate and manage the care of certain patients.[6]

The IHS has developed a rapid and reliable method of medication counseling for patients. The method uses a series of short questions and probes the patients for what they know about their medication (see Chapter 7, Pharmaceutical Care).

There are several examples in the literature of how IHS pharmacists provide clinical services for patients on reservations.[7,8] Articles show the rewards of working for the IHS: hands-on patient care, interdisciplinary teamwork, and a stimulating clinical experience not found elsewhere.

National Institutes of Health (NIH)

The NIH, set up in 1887, is the world's premier medical research organization. The NIH supports over 38,000 research projects nationwide in diseases including cancer, Alzheimer's, diabetes, arthritis, heart ailments, and AIDS. The NIH includes 27 separate health institutes and centers.[5] In 2006, the NIH employed 17,543 people, of which 19 were commissioned pharmacy officers.

"The Clinical Center, located in Bethesda, Maryland, a 450-bed research hospital, employs many pharmacists. Other pharmacists are employed by the National Cancer Institute (NCI), the National Institute of Neurological Disorders and Stroke, the National Institute of Allergy and Infectious Diseases, and other NIH institutes."[1] The Clinical Center pharmacy has inpatient and outpatient services, a manufacturing facility, and a full analytical section to support investigators in their research. Clinical pharmacy specialists, supported by other pharmacists, provide a full range of services, including therapeutic drug monitoring and review, protocol compliance monitoring, and institutional review board membership.

Federal Bureau of Prisons (BOP)

The BOP was established in 1930 to provide more progressive and humane care for federal inmates, to professionalize the prison service, and to ensure consistent and centralized administration of the 11 federal prisons in operation at the time.

In 2006, the BOP consisted of more than 106 institutions, 6 regional offices, a central office (headquarters), 2 staff training centers, and 28 community corrections offices. The BOP is responsible for the custody and care of approximately 185,000 federal offenders. Approximately 85% of these inmates are confined in BOP-operated correctional facilities or detention centers.[9]

The BOP protects public safety by ensuring that federal offenders serve their sentences of imprisonment in facilities that are safe, humane, cost-efficient, and appropriately secure. The BOP helps reduce the potential for future criminal activity by encouraging inmates to participate in a range of programs that have been proven to reduce recidivism. The BOP's approximately 35,000 employees ensure the security of federal prisons, provide inmates with needed programs and services, and model mainstream values. In 2006, 131 commissioned pharmacy officers worked for the BOP. An article on what it is like to be a BOP pharmacist has been written.[10]

Environmental Protection Agency (EPA)

The mission of the EPA is to protect human health and the environment. Since 1970, the EPA has been working for a cleaner, healthier environment for the American people. In 2006, the EPA employed 18,000 people across the country — at least one is a commissioned pharmacy officer. EPA staff are highly educated and technically trained. "EPA pharmacists work on various public health and sanitation programs ranging from watching viruses and bacteria in shellfish to developing detection methods for microorganisms in drinking water."[1]

Agency for Toxic Substances and Disease Registry (ATSDR)

The mission of the ATSDR is to serve the public by using the best science, taking responsive public health actions, and providing trusted health information to prevent harmful exposures and disease related to toxic substances.

The ATSDR began in 1980 in Atlanta, Georgia, is associated with the CDC, and helps prevent exposure to toxic substances from waste sites on the EPA's National Priority List. In 2006, there was one commissioned pharmacy officer working in this agency. "Pharmacists with backgrounds in pharmacology and toxicology evaluate data and information on the release of hazardous substances into the environment, develop toxicological profiles, and set up research in toxicology and health effects where needed."[1]

Agency for Healthcare Research and Quality (AHRQ)

The AHRQ, established in 1989, supports research on health care systems, health care quality and cost issues, access to health care, and effectiveness of medical treatments. The agency has 296 employees.[5] In 2006, two pharmacists (health science administrators) at AHRQ provided management for information development, helped develop grant announcements, and tracked the progress of research that the agency funds.

Centers for Medicare and Medicaid (CMS)

The CMS administers the Medicare and Medicaid programs, which provide health care to about one in every four Americans. Medicare provides health insurance for more than 42.1 million elderly and disabled Americans. Medicaid, a joint federal–state program, provides health coverage for 44.7 million low-income persons, including 21.9 million children, and nursing home coverage for low-income elderly. The CMS also administers the State Children's Health Insurance Program, which covers more than 4.2 million children.

The CMS was established as the Health Care Financing Administration in 1977. In January 2006, the CMS started a Part D prescription benefit for Medicare beneficiaries. In early 2006, the CMS employed 4943 people. Of these, 10 were commissioned pharmacy officers.

Substance Abuse and Mental Health Services Administration (SAMHSA)

The SAMHSA (a) works to improve the quality and availability of substance abuse prevention, addiction treatment, and mental health services; (b) provides funding through block grants to states to support substance abuse and mental health services, including treatment for more than 650,000 Americans with serious substance abuse problems or mental health problems; (c) helps improve substance abuse prevention and treatment services through the identification and dissemination of best practices; and (d) monitors prevalence and incidence of substance abuse. SAMHSA was established in 1982. In 2006, SAMHSA employed 558 people, 3 of whom were pharmacists working in the pharmacologic alternative service.

Other Areas

In 2006, 21 commissioned pharmacy officers worked for the Department of Homeland Security(DHS), 28 worked in the Health Resources and Services Administration (HRSA), and 19 worked in the Office of the Secretary (OS).

Commission Corps

As one of the seven uniformed services of the United States, the U.S. PHS Commissioned Corps is a specialized career system designed to attract, retain, and develop health professionals who may be assigned to federal, state, or local agencies for international organizations to accomplish its mission. The Commissioned Corps of the PHS is led by the Surgeon General and provides a wealth of opportunities for pharmacists.[11]

Most PHS pharmacists are members of the Commissioned Corps, with organization, structure, pay grades, and titles similar to the U.S. Navy.[3] Pharmacists who have a Pharm.D. degree and join the PHS are commissioned at a grade of 0–3, Senior Assistant Pharmacist, which equals the rank of lieutenant in the Navy or captain in the Army and Air Force.[11] PHS pharmacists who have a Pharm.D. degree plus a specialty certification from the Board of Pharmaceutical Specialties (BPS) are eligible for extra pay.[12]

The IHS, FDA, SAMHSA, and BOP offer extern rotations to senior pharmacy students.[13] PHS programs have a total of 52 extern agreements with 50 schools of pharmacy. Students interested in externship assignments should contact their school externship and rotation coordinator. If the school does not have an agreement with the desired program, or to try another location, have the rotation coordinator contact the appropriate program manager.

The PHS offers excellent opportunities for pharmacy students for paid employment for periods of 31 to 120 days throughout the academic year through the Junior Commissioned Officer Student Training and Extern Program (COSTEP). Junior COSTEP allows students to serve in assignments at any time during the year; however, the majority of students are hired for the summer months.

COSTEP participants earn approximately $2,100 per month, plus travel costs and other benefits. This program is highly competitive, and the number of individuals selected is based upon the needs of PHS programs. Applications for summer employment are due December 31.

In Senior COSTEP, students are assisted financially during their final year of pharmacy school in return for an agreement to work for the PHS after graduation. The student is appointed as an active-duty PHS officer during the senior year and receives monthly pay and allowances as an ensign (0-1) grade officer. The student agrees to work for the program that provided the financial support for twice the time supported following graduation. This program is very competitive. Applications for Senior COSTEP are due December 31 of the junior year.

DEPARTMENT OF DEFENSE (DOD)

Over 1500 pharmacists work for the U.S. Army, Navy, and Air Force.

U.S. Army

The Army Medical Department (AMEDD) maintains the health of the men and women assigned to the Army's fighting forces and provides health care to the family members of active duty personnel and military retirees and their families. In 2006, the AMEDD had many commissioned pharmacy officers and civilian pharmacists working in the United States, Europe, Japan, Korea, and Panama.[14] These pharmacists were supported by enlisted pharmacy technicians and civilian technicians. AMEDD trains its own pharmacy technicians with an 18-week, structured course.

Army pharmacists are an integral part of the Army health care team; they certainly do more than just handle prescriptions. Ambulatory care, inpatient drug distribution systems, nuclear pharmacy, oncology pharmacy, drug monitoring, and patient education services and nutrition support are just a few of the pharmacy practice activities you might be involved in. You could be assigned to a community hospital, an Army Medical Center, a troop medical clinic, or a field environment either in the United States or overseas.[14]

Pharmacy services are provided at fixed military medical treatment facilities located on large Army installations and field hospitals. Army pharmacy is similar to civilian pharmacy except that Army hospitals often include high-volume outpatient pharmacies. "Army pharmacists are being given direct patient care roles on interdisciplinary teams."[14]

All Army pharmacists must join in field exercises to be prepared to provide services under combat conditions. An advantage of being an Army pharmacist is broad opportunities to gain further education and training.

U.S. Navy

The mission of the Navy medical department is to provide prompt and effective health care to combat forces in times of conflict and to deliver cost-effective, high-quality services in peacetime.[13] The Navy's health care team delivers care to active-duty personnel, retired military individuals, and family members at three naval medical centers, 26 naval hospitals, eight medical clinics, and 153 naval branch medical clinics worldwide.[16]

Complementing the Navy's land-based medical treatment facilities are deployable units: two 1000-bed hospital ships, six fleet hospitals, three medical battalions, and medical expansion assets to convert amphibious ships into casualty receiving and treatment ships.[16]

In 2006, the Navy had many pharmacy officers on active duty and civilian pharmacists. "Navy pharmacy is a leader on the Navy health care team, and provides the professional expertise necessary for model pharmaceutical services for the fleet."[16]

Navy pharmacists are supported by 945 pharmacy technicians. The Navy has two technician training schools.[16] The curriculum is 23 weeks long. Graduates receive the Navy enlisted classification (NEC) of Navy Pharmacy Technician.

All Navy hospitals have unit dose drug distribution systems and complete IV admixture programs. Navy pharmacists use automation and a computer system that uses a universal pharmacy profile that is also used by the other military branches.

Navy pharmacists with proper education and training are encouraged to become involved in direct patient care and may be certified to perform specific direct inpatient and outpatient care. "Navy pharmacists have proven that their unique medical education provides valuable information and skills in all areas of military medicine."[16]

U.S. Air Force

The Air Force medical service has 87 medical treatment facilities — 38 are small, 27 are medium-sized, and 22 are large, such as Wilford Hall Medical Center, a 500-bed facility at Lackland Air Force Base in San Antonio, Texas. The average number of beds at an Air Force medical treatment facility is less than 30.[17] However, the outpatient pharmacies in these facilities fill 300 to 4000 prescriptions a day.

During combat, the Air Force typically deploys medical services through air-transportable clinics and hospitals, which are designed to be complete, efficient, and quickly mobile.

The Air Force pharmacy team consists of more than 1300 pharmacists and pharmacy technicians. Almost all of the 257 Air Force pharmacists are commissioned officers. Air Force pharmacists are military officers first, and they continually voice the core values of the Air Force: integrity, service before self, and excellence.[18]

The Air Force pharmacy team provides timely and cost-effective health care to over 8 million DOD beneficiaries — many of whom are elderly retirees suffering from chronic illnesses. Pharmacists in the Air Force are focusing less and less on dispensing and distributive services and more and more on patient counseling and disease state management.

There are opportunities for pharmacists to advance through educational programs and the Air Force Institute of Technology program. Advancement in experience, education, and rank often means relocation from one facility to another. The reader may be interested in reading an article entitled "How One Hospital Pharmacist's Career Took Wing in the Air Force."[18]

Pharmacy technicians, civilian and military, are taking on more responsibility in drug dispensing and distribution as pharmacists take on more clinical responsibility. Most Air Force pharmacy technicians are certified, and there is a 12-week course at the School of Healthcare Sciences at Sheppard Air Force Base, Texas.

Opportunities with the DOD

The DOD, the largest U.S. employer, offers many rewarding and challenging jobs for pharmacists and technicians, as a service member or a civilian, throughout the United States and the World.[19]

DEPARTMENT OF VETERANS AFFAIRS

The primary objective of the Veterans Affairs (VA) health administration is to provide consistent, high-quality medical care to eligible veterans as prescribed by federal law. Other objectives include educating health care professionals, performing basic and applied research, and offering emergency preparedness and backup to the nation in case of a natural disaster or national emergency.

Today's VA health care system is transforming itself from a medical center—based organization of 173 hospitals and 134 nursing homes, into 22 health care networks (VISINS) that stress primary and ambulatory care.[20] With this has come improved roles for over 4000 pharmacists. The VA has targeted various pharmacy areas for implementation or improvement. These include staff development, prescribing authority for pharmacists, automation, design changes for the pharmacies, residency programs, and a pharmacy benefit management (PBM) product line. There is also interest in doing pharmacoepidemiological and pharmacoeconomic research in the geriatric population.

The VA pharmacy program is well known for two, innovative, high-quality services: the Consolidated Mail Outpatient Pharmacy System and the ambulatory pharmaceutical care program in which ambulatory care pharmacists have the ability to manage and prescribe medication for patients.

Four VA pharmacy programs were highlighted for their clinical services in an article in the *Journal of the American Pharmaceutical Association*.[21]

Consolidated Mail Outpatient Pharmacy System

The Consolidated Mail Outpatient Pharmacy (CMOP) System is a regionalized state-of-the art mailout pharmacy system. In 2004, the VA's CMOP dispensed about 88 million prescriptions, representing 76% of all VA prescriptions, including 95% of refill prescriptions. The VA currently has seven CMOPs in the following locations: Leavenworth, KS; West Los Angeles, CA; Bedford, MA; Murfreesboro, TN; Hines, IL; Dallas, TX; and

North Charleston, SC (see Chapter 6, Pharmacy Technology and Automation).

Ambulatory Pharmaceutical Care

The practice of pharmaceutical care in the ambulatory care clinics of the VA may be the most advanced. A survey published found 512 ambulatory care clinics within the 50 VA medical centers (VAMCs) that responded to the survey.[22] There were 242 clinical pharmacy specialists practicing in the 50 VAMCs. Clinical pharmacists managed almost 30% of the clinics, most of which were therapeutic drug monitoring, anticoagulation, walk-in, or lipid management. In 68% of the clinics, the pharmacists had prescribing privileges. About 77% of the clinical pharmacists had the Pharm.D. degree, and most were in the clinic 5 days a week.

A recent report in the *Journal of the American Pharmaceutical Association* provided a glimpse of the pharmaceutical care being provided by pharmacists in the ambulatory care clinics of four VAMCs:[21]

Reno, Nevada: At the Reno VA, there is the feeling that the CMOP has allowed their pharmacists to do other things, such practice pharmaceutical care. Pharmacists collaborate in the therapeutic management of patients in the oncology, AIDS, *H. pylori* (ulcer), lipid, and hypertension clinics. Driving the whole process has been the electronic medical record that allows pharmacists full access to laboratory results and records of all patient encounters.

Fort Myers, Florida: Some of the pharmacists practicing at this VA say things like, "My whole focus is on making patients smarter and more informed..."; "... most of the time I am pulling patients out of the jaws of therapeutic defeat"; or, "We use current (treatment) guidelines of the National Cholesterol Education Program religiously."

Little Rock, Arkansas: A pharmacist at this VA follows some 300 psychiatric patients, most of whom have diagnoses of depression, bipolar affective disorder, schizophrenia, or posttraumatic stress disorder. The pharmacist meets with each patient for about 30 minutes and only refers the patient back to the primary care physician if the patient becomes unstable or needs assessment.

Oakland, California: In this VA, pharmacists are quantifying their clinical interventions in cost savings to the VA system. Software has been developed to track interventions, outcomes, and the cost impact. About 100 of the pharmacists' interventions were tracked for 3 months. Most of the interventions were for lack of a current indication and for drug therapy needed. The cost avoidance and savings projections amounted to $216,800.

Independent Prescribing Privileges

All the VA pharmacists working in the ambulatory care clinics work in ambulatory care teams. Each team is composed of a variety of providers that may include physicians, nurse practitioners, physician assistants, dieticians, and social workers. Patients are followed by their disease state.

Most of the VA's ambulatory care pharmacists have prescribing privileges, but they must use them under the protocol of the physician. This is called *collaborative practice*. However, a VA in West Palm Beach, Florida, may have been the first to allow their ambulatory care pharmacists to prescribe, change, or stop medications on their own authority. "Our notes are independent; our prescriptions are totally independent. The only prescribing limitations are the ones we put on ourselves."[23]

The pharmacists with independent prescribing authority must have the Pharm.D. degree and have completed a residency in general or ambulatory care pharmacy practice. Other members of the primary care team refer patients to the pharmacist.

A Focus on Patient Outcomes

The Veterans Health Study (VHS) has as its focus the development, testing, and application of patient-centered assessments for monitoring patient outcomes in ambulatory care.[24] One VA pharmacy service (Reno) has taken a lead in this area.[25] A recent publication concluded that "a system using pharmacists as independent practitioners to promote primary care has achieved high-quality and cost-effective patient care."

Pharmacist Career Ladder Program

The VA is also well known for working on career ladder programs for pharmacists. An example of such a program is at the Albuquerque VAMC, a 457-bed acute care teaching hospital with a 47-bed nursing home care unit.[26] The center's policy is to establish clinical privileges for all pharmacists with direct patient contact.

Some former barriers to this included inadequate instruction, not enough incentives, fragmentation of clinical services, and subjectivity of measuring competence. In response to this, a pharmacist credentialing committee created a career ladder with three levels of clinical privilege. The first level integrated basic clinical pharmacy knowledge with dispensing activities. The second level increased the number of clinical skills needed and allowed the pharmacist to act as a therapeutic consultant. The third level incorporated the skills necessary for specialty practice. Each level carries a modest pay increase.

Satisfaction

The satisfaction the pharmacists have with clinical privileges within the VA system can best be summarized by quotes from one of the pharmacists, Judy Siler, at the VA in Little Rock, Arkansas:[21]

> "I wish every pharmacist could have a job like mine."
>
> "This is the most fulfilling role for a pharmacist I've ever had."
>
> "I see things differently now, not just appreciate the economic aspect, but the difference that medications can make in people's lives."
>
> "I love it, the patient's love it, and the physicians and other clinicians are very supportive of my role."

FEDERAL HOSPITALS

One note before moving to other opportunities for pharmacists in the government is in order. It is about the basic pharmacy services — basic drug preparation and dispensing — within federal hospitals, which is quite outstanding. The American Society of Hospital Pharmacists (ASHP) now the American Society of Health-System Pharmacists, conducted a national survey of pharmaceutical services in federal hospitals.[27] The results were impressive, with 85% of the responding hospitals offering complete unit-dose services and 83% offering complete, comprehensive IV admixture services. Over 88% offered service to ambulatory care patients, had a computerized pharmacy system, provided drug therapy monitoring and patient education, and had a well-controlled formulary.

DRUG ENFORCEMENT ADMINISTRATION (DEA)

The mission of the DEA is to enforce the controlled substances laws and regulations of the United States. Its mission also is to bring to the criminal and civil justice systems of the United States anyone or any organization that grows, manufacturers, or distributes controlled substances through illicit traffic in the United States. It also recommends and supports non-enforcement programs aimed at reducing unlawful controlled substances on the domestic and international markets.[28]

The DEA has two types of enforcement officers — special agents and diversion investigators.[29] Special agents carry weapons, work undercover, make arrests, and conduct physical surveillance. They focus on stopping the illegal import and production of controlled substances. Diversion investigators do none of these things. They focus on regulating legitimate handlers of controlled substances and investigate violations by these handlers.

The DEA employs about a dozen pharmacists with the following job titles: Diversion Program Manager, Diversion Investigator, Staff Assistant, Pharmacologist, and Special Agent.

WORKING FOR STATE GOVERNMENT

Pharmacists also work in various positions in state government such as boards of pharmacy, departments of public health, the Department of Social Welfare, which administers the Medicaid program, and state drug enforcement agencies.

REWARDS AND SATISFACTION

There is one common theme when discussing the rewards of working for the government with pharmacists, and that is the satisfaction of helping people. Pharmacists working for the government often use terms such as interesting, *rewarding, satisfying,* and *making a difference,* when describing their jobs. The level and extent of pharmaceutical care in the federal government may be the highest anywhere in the country, and the leaders are the pharmacists working in the IHSs and the VAMCs. The other pharmacy services in the federal government, such as those at the NIH, are not far behind.[30]

SUMMARY

Working for the government is frequently an overlooked career choice for new pharmacy graduates. This is probably because there has not been enough information presented to pharmacy students. There are vast and interesting opportunities for pharmacists in the government.

The U.S. Public Health Service, the Department of Defense, and the Veterans Administration in particular have been on the leading edge of pharmaceutical care and offer those with a Pharm.D. degree and a residency opportunities that often exceed those in the private sector.

Although starting salaries for government pharmacists may not be as competitive as other opportunities, the job and retirement benefits may be superior and the job satisfaction high.

DISCUSSION QUESTIONS AND EXERCISES

1. What do you see as being unique or special about working for the government as a pharmacist?

2. Some pharmacists with Pharm.D. degrees and advanced training (a residency, certification or special course work) may prescribe medication in collaboration with physicians. Does this interest you? Why or why not?

3. Based on what you have learned thus far, do you think pharmaceutical care (see Chapter 7) in government health care facilities is more advanced, less advanced, or the same as in the private sector?

4. If you worked in a government facility as a pharmacist, would you prefer working in an acute care (inpatient) setting or ambulatory care (outpatient) setting? Why?

5. Arrange the following areas of government service in order of your interest. For example: VA>PHS>DOD>Other.
   a. Department of Defense (DOD)
   b. Veterans Administration (VA)
   c. Public Health Service (PHS)
   d. Other (DEA, Federal Hospitals, etc.)

6. Make an appointment to visit and interview a pharmacist who works for the government.

7. Based on what you know and what you have read thus far, what do you see as the pros and cons of being a government pharmacist?

8. Is working for the government as a pharmacist something you may want to do? Why or why not?

9. If you answered yes to question 8, would you like to work as a commissioned pharmacy officer or a civilian pharmacist?

10. If you answered "as a commissioned pharmacy officer," investigate the Commissioned Corps Web site at http://www.usphs.gov.

CHALLENGES

1. Pharmacy practice in the U.S. government is progressive. After thoroughly reading this chapter, prepare a concise report for extra credit, if your professor agrees, about what you think is the best opportunity for you as a government pharmacist. Your research should go beyond what is provided in this chapter. Explain why you may pursue this opportunity by discussing the positives and negatives and end your report with the statement, "Therefore, I want to ___ because ___."

2. Pharmacy practice in the U.S government is progressive, and pharmaceutical care may be advancing at a faster rate there than in the private sector. For extra credit, and with the permission of your professor, explore this observation to see if it is true, and if so, thoroughly explore and advance written arguments for why this is happening.

WEB SITES OF INTEREST

U.S. Public Health Service Commissioned Corp: http://www.usphs.gov/

Commissioned Corp — Pharmacists: http://www.usphs.gov/html/pharmacist.html

USPHS residency and student programs: http://www.hhs.gov/pharmacy/student.html

Centers for Disease Control and Prevention: http://www.cdc.gov

Food and Drug Administration: http://www.fda.gov

Indian Health Service: http://www.pharmacy.ihs.gov/

National Institutes of Health: http://www.nih.gov

NIH Clinical Center: http://clinicalcenter.nih.gov/

Federal Bureau of Prisons: http://www.bop.gov/jobs/job_descriptions/pharmacist.jsp

Environmental Protection Agency: http://www.epa.gov

Agency for Toxic Substances and Disease Registry: http://www.atsdr.cdc.gov/

Agency for Healthcare Research and Quality: http://www.ahrq.gov/

Substance Abuse and Mental Health Services Administration: http://www.samhsa.gov

Department of Defense: http://www.defenselink.mil/

U.S Army: http://www.goarmy.com/amedd/m_service/pharmacy.jsp

U.S. Navy: http://navymedicine.med.navy.mil/navypharmacy/index.cfm?docid=11752

U.S. Air Force: http://allpharmacyjobs.com/air_force_jobs.htm

Department of Veterans' Affairs: http://www.vacareers.va.gov/

Drug Enforcement Agency: http://www.dea.gov

REFERENCES

1. Paavola, FG, Dermanoski, KR, and Pittman, RE. Pharmaceutical services in the United States Public Health Service. *Am J Health-Syst Pharm.* 1997;54:766–772.
2. US Public Health Service. Agencies and programs. Available at http://www.usphs.gov/html/agencies_programs.html. Accessed May 9, 2006.
3. U.S. Public Health Service. The Mission of the Commissioned Corp. Available at http://www.usphs.gov/html/mission.html. Accessed May 10, 2006.
4. Centers for Disease Control and Prevention. About the CDC. Available at http://www.cdc.gov/about/default.htm. Accessed May 10, 2006.
5. U.S. Department of Health and Human Services. HHS: What we do. Available at http://www.hhs.gov/about/. Accessed May 10, 2006.
6. Indian Health Service. IHS pharmacy program. Available at http://www.pharmacy.ihs.gov/. Accessed May 10, 2006.
7. Jacobson, WR. Practicing pharmacy on the reservation. *Pharm Times.* 1991;57:98–102.

8. Johnson, TM. On the front lines of pharmaceutical care: lipid management at an Indian Health Service clinic. *Consult Pharm.* 1998;13:886–894.

9. Federal Bureau of Prisons. About the federal bureau of prisons. Available at http://www.bop.gov/about/index.jsp. Accessed May 10, 2006.

10. Lawson, R. Unique challenges, satisfying opportunities with the Federal Bureau of Prisons. *Consult Pharm.* 1997;12:814–815.

11. U.S. Public Health Service Commissioned Corps. The mission of the U.S. Public Health Service and the Commission Corps. Available at http://www.usphs.gov/html/mission.html. Accessed May 10, 2006.

12. Anonymous. Pharm.D. degree, specialty certification boost earnings of PHS pharmacists. *Am J Health-Syst Pharmacists.* 1997;54:1236.

13. U.S. Public Health Service Commissioned Corp. Pharmacist Professional Advisory Committee. Residency and student programs. Available at http://www.usphs.gov/html/pharmacist.html. Accessed May 10, 2006.

14. Williams, RF, Moran, EL, Bottaro, SD, et al. Pharmaceutical services in the United States Army. *Am J Health-Syst Pharm.* 1997;54:773–778.

15. Bayles, BC, Hall, GE, Hostettler, C, et al. Pharmaceutical services in the United States Navy. *Am J Health-Syst Pharm.* 1997;54:778–782.

16. Snook, DF, Whiten, RE, Holt, MR, et al. Pharmacy practice in the United States Navy. *Am J Hosp Pharm.* 1987;44:761–765.

17. Young, JH. Pharmaceutical services in the United States Air Force. *Am J Health-Syst Pharm.* 1997;54:783–786.

18. McCormick, E. How one hospital pharmacist's career took wing in the Air Force. *Pharm Times.* 1994;60(May):8HPT–10HPT.

19. U.S. Department of Defense. Recruiting information and career opportunities. Available at http://www.defenselink.mil/other_info/careers.html Accessed May 1, 2001.

20. Ogden, JE, Muniz, A, Patterson, AA, et al. Pharmaceutical services in the Department of Veterans Affairs. *Am J Health-Syst Pharm.* 1997;54:761–765.

21. Posey, LM. Expanding pharmacy's horizons: VA's pharmacotherapy innovations. *J Am Pharm Assoc.* 1997;NS37:379–382.

22. Alsuwaidan, A, Malone, DC, Billups, SJ, and Carter, BL. Characteristics of ambulatory care clinics and pharmacists in Veterans Affairs medical centers. *Am J Health-Syst Pharm.* 1998;55:68–72.

23. Ukens, C. Pharmacists independently prescribe in VA care teams. *Drug Top.* 1997;141:59.

24. Kazis, LE, Miller, RD, Skinner, KM, et al. Applications of methodologies of the Veteran's Health Study in the VA healthcare system: conclusions and summary. *J Amb Care Management.* 2006;29(2):182–188.

25. Carmichael, JM, Alvarez, A, Chaput, R, et al. Establishment and outcomes of a model primary care pharmacy service system. *Am. J. Health Syst. Pharm.*, 2004;61:472–482.

26. Swanson, KM, Hunter, WB, Trask, SJ, and Beck, SM. Pharmacist career ladder with clinical privilege categories. *Am J Hosp Pharm.* 1991;48:1956–1961.

27. Crawford, SY, and Santell, JP. ASHP national survey of pharmaceutical services in federal hospitals: 1993. *Am J Hosp Pharm.* 1994;51:2377–2393.

28. U.S. Department of Justice. DEA mission statement. Available at http://www.dea.gov/agency/mission.htm. Accessed May 1, 2001.

29. Anderson, PD. A pharmacist's career with the Drug Enforcement Administration: an interview with Louis Fisher, R.Ph., Diversion Program Manager, New England Field Division. *J Pharm Practice.* 2000;13:194–198.

30. Wrsight, LJ. United States Public Health Service bicentennial 1798–1998: a focus on oncology pharmacy practice at the National Institutes of Health. *J Oncol Pharm Pract.* 1998;4:139–142.

14

DRUG INFORMATION AND POISON CONTROL

Pharmacy emerged from its traditional dispensing and drug distribution roles in the early 1960s to fulfill a more clinical role. During this time, pharmacy also discovered that it was a knowledge-based profession. It was also discovered that pharmacy could and should move beyond its knowledge of the practice of pharmacy and its basic knowledge of drugs — there was a need to help with the rational use of drugs.

Studies revealed that drug prescribing was less than ideal. Some of the reasons for this were less emphasis on pharmacology and therapeutics in medical schools and the rapid development of new drugs. Physicians had trouble keeping up with so many new drugs and with trying to learn how these drugs fit into the overall drug therapy process. It became obvious to the profession that pharmacists could help improve therapeutics by providing unbiased, up-to-date drug information to physicians.

It was also during this time that hospital emergency rooms could no longer keep up-to-date on the ingredients in commercial products that could be harmful. The answer to this was the development of regional poison control centers. Because of the pharmacist's education and training, some pharmacists started working in these centers.

This chapter is about the provision of drug and poison information. It will cover how drug information centers and poison control centers function. Emphasis will be placed on the process of receiving and answering questions and what it is like for a pharmacist to work in these centers.

LEARNING OBJECTIVES

After participating in this learning session, you should be able to:

- ■ Discuss the difference between a drug information center and a drug information service
- ■ Identify the functions of a drug information center
- ■ Discuss the value of a drug information center
- ■ Discuss what may be different about working in a drug information service in a drug company
- ■ Explain some of the resources used in poison control centers to answer questions
- ■ Explain how a typical poison control center is staffed
- ■ Explain what it is like for pharmacist to work in a poison control center

DRUG INFORMATION

The term *drug information* has different meanings. Technically, drug information means "information about drugs that is printed in a reference or verbalized by an individual."[1] Drug information can be about the drug itself or about the use of the drug. Drug information can also refer to a place (*drug information center*) or to a person (*drug information specialist*).

Brief History

The first drug information center (DIC) was opened at the University of Kentucky Medical Center in the early 1960s.[2] The DIC was separated from the pharmacy service and was dedicated to providing drug information. The specific function was to provide comprehensive drug information to the staff physicians, dentists, and nurses and to evaluate and compare drugs. Another role of the DIC was to help educate students of the health care profession about drugs.

Shortly after the University of Kentucky started their drug information center, several DICs were started, mainly in academic health care centers. One such center deserves mention. In the late 1960s, the DIC at the University of Michigan Medical Center received a large federal grant to study the provision of drug information and to provide a network of DICs in Michigan.[3–5]

The pharmacists working in these centers quickly developed ways of classifying questions, performing systematic searches, matching resources with types of questions, and developing systems to track questions with answers. In addition, these pharmacists became knowledgeable about drugs and where to find information about drugs. Thus, in the eyes of many physicians and other pharmacists, they became true drug information specialists. As time passed, DICs expanded services to include drug use evaluation (DUE) for pharmacy and therapeutics committees and provision of continuing education about drugs through newsletters and conferences.

Drug Information Centers

During the 1970s and 1980s, DICs and drug information services (DISs) were started in many hospitals. A DIS is a distinct and promoted service of the pharmacy; however, the service does not have a separate area or a dedicated staff like a DIC. Most of the pharmacists take part in the DIS. In a DIC, drug information specialists provide the drug information.

DICs are found in academic health centers,[6] community hospitals,[7] government hospitals,[8] managed care organizations,[9] and schools of pharmacy and the pharmaceutical industry.[10] A survey in 2004 revealed 81 (down from 103 in 1999) institutional drug information centers in the United States that met the criteria of an organized DIC.[11] The survey did not include the pharmaceutical industry. Table 14.1 shows the distribution of DICs by affiliation. A reference listing DICs by state is also included.[11]

Table 14.1 Distribution of Drug Information Centers by Affiliation

Affiliations[a]	Number (%)[b]
Hospital or medical center	57 (72)
College or school of pharmacy	48 (61)
College or school of medicine	17 (22)[c]
College or school of allied health	15 (19)
Library	13 (16)
College or school of nursing	11 (14)
Poison control center	7 (9)
Other[d]	1 (1)

[a] Centers could have multiple affiliations.
[b] Rounded to the nearest whole number.
[c] Significantly different from value in 1992 ($x^2[1] = 8.01$, $P < 0.05$
[d] Area health education center.

Source: Data taken from Rosenberg, JM, Koumis T, Nathan JP, et al. Am J Health-Syst Pharm. 2004;61(19):2023–2032.

A few drug information centers are now charging a fee-for-service. One survey of drug information centers in the United States, Canada, and the United Kingdom revealed that 18% of respondents charge some type of fee-for-service.[12]

There are also online drug information sites. The number of these sites is undetermined.

Functions

The functions of most DICs are to answer drug information questions, to develop drug evaluations and comparisons for pharmacy and therapeutics committees, and to provide education about drugs.

Answering Drug Information Questions

The primary function of any DIC is to answer questions about drugs and drug therapy. These questions come from various people. Some DICs limit their service to health care professionals only, whereas others also respond to questions from the public.

Methods vary for receiving, researching, and providing answers to drug information questions. However, most DICs and pharmacists follow a basic pattern[13]:

1. *Receive and understand the question:* This seems easy, but it can be tricky. The basic steps in answering a drug information question are to:
   a. *Identify the requester:* This is critical, especially in telephone inquiries, in case the call is disconnected. It is also important to know the caller's background: Is it a physician, pharmacist, nurse, or consumer?
   b. *Identify the question type:* The question type determines where to look for answers.
   c. *Get suitable background information:* Is there a patient involved? What is the diagnosis? What other drugs is the patient taking?
   d. *Reformulate the question:* It was learned early in the development of DICs that many drug information requestors do not ask what they really want to know. The adage "ask a silly question, get a silly answer" is applicable to answering drug information questions.[14] In addition, the background information uncovered may change the nature of the question.
2. *Search for data:* A search for answers to a question is based on the question type. Is it about the dose? Is it about an adverse effect? Is it about how one drug compares with another? Certain references

are better than others for answering certain types of questions.[15,16] When searching for answers to questions, it is important to keep in mind the three general sources of information:[17]

a. *Tertiary literature:* This includes textbooks and drug compendia, which should be consulted first, as they provide rapid access to information. They also familiarize the reader searching the biomedical literature by indexing and abstracting services such as Medline, *International Pharmaceutical Abstracts* (IPA), and the Iowa Drug Information System (IDIS). These services reference secondary review articles and the primary literature.

b. *Primary literature:* This contains the research articles published in professional journals. These provide specific, detailed information that is difficult to find without using the secondary literature sources.

c. *The Internet:* This holds broad information, most of which is considered tertiary literature. However, unlike the other three sources of information, the accuracy and completeness of the information cannot be guaranteed. Anyone can put anything on the Internet, whereas the other sources of health care information must go through review by editors and peers. At best, the Internet should be considered to be a starting point for answering drug information questions. All information should be confirmed with a second source.

3. *Analyze data and develop a response:* Once the correct resources have been checked, the next step is to review the various sources found. The strengths and weaknesses of the various sources need to be considered. Reviewing the primary literature needs to be done carefully using *drug literature review* techniques taught in pharmacy school.

4. *Communicate the response:* Providing a response to a drug information question can be done orally (over the telephone or in person), in writing, or a combination of the two. Talking with the person asking is always preferred, and doing it in person is better than talking over the telephone. If suitable, providing something in writing is also preferred.

5. *Follow-up:* DICs should periodically perform random checks on the quality of their drug information service. The person asking the drug information question evaluates the quality of the response by judging the quality of the answer and the timeliness of the response.

6. *Documentation:* It is important for communication, quality assurance, and archival reasons to document information on the drug information question, requester, answer, and references used. Once a specific answer to the drug information question is formulated,

it should be documented with the references used. In 2001, 36.4% of DICs use computerized databases to help in answering and managing drug information requests.[18–20]

The issue of quality assurance in answering drug information questions has been a long-standing interest of the profession. How accurate are the answers being provided? In 1977, out of concern for the rapid growth of DICs and lack of DIC standards, Halbert et al. evaluated the performance of DICs in answering a drug information question by anonymously calling each known DIC.[21,22] The quality and timeliness of responses varied widely. Similar studies were performed in 1994 and 2000.[23,24] In 2005, a quality assurance survey of 64 Internet pharmacies found that the percentage of correct answers to five drug information questions ranged from 7% to 96%.[25]

Another important issue in answering drug information questions is ethics. Many drug information questions, especially those from consumers, raise issues of confidentiality, truth telling, respect for the law, invasion of privacy, and social responsibility. Pharmacists need to be sensitive to the ethical dilemmas often found in drug information questions.

A national survey of ethical issues presented to drug information centers was performed.[26] Six drug information questions, each posing an ethical dilemma, were presented to each DIC. Centers were asked if they would answer the question, and if they would, how. The range on the willingness to answer the questions was 23 to 96%. Answers to the questions varied, but overall, the pharmacists' responses suggested a high degree of moral and social responsibility.

Drug Evaluations

Another important function of many DICs, especially those in hospitals and managed care organizations, is to provide background on a drug requested for formulary status. This background is in the form of a comprehensive, unbiased drug evaluation. The basic content of a drug evaluation is some brief and basic information about the drug, a review of clinical studies on the drug's efficacy and safety, a comparison of the drug to the current formulary drug, a pharmacoeconomic analysis, and references.

Education

Most DICs are involved in educating health care professionals, consumers, and pharmacy students about drugs and drug therapy. Many DICs publish drug information newsletters that include information about new drugs, highlight recently published studies, compare drugs, and print some recently received drug information questions with answers. Drug information pharmacists are often asked to present similar information at various professional meetings.

Key Resources

The key resources for drug information are:

- Micromedex Healthcare Series
- *Handbook of Injectable Drugs*
- Natural Medicines Comprehensive Database
- *Hansten and Horn's Drug Interactions Analysis*
- *Management, and Martindale: The Complete Drug Reference*[11]

Drug Information in the Pharmaceutical Industry

The techniques used to answer drug information questions in a DIC within a pharmaceutical company are the same as used by DICs in other locations. What differs is the questions and who is asking.[27] DICs in the pharmaceutical industry handle more questions from the public, and most of their questions are about dosage and drug administration. They also receive requests for reprints of journal articles and for sample drugs. The most common requests handled by hospital-based DICs concern therapeutic use, drug efficacy, and adverse drug events.

Marketing

DICs continually need to market their services through newsletters, the development of a Web site, the use of phone stickers, and talking up the DIC.[28] An example of an exceptional DIC Web site is located at http://www.samford.edu/schools/pharmacy/dic/index.html.

Some drug information centers have developed fee structures to provide drug information services, chiefly answering questions, doing drug evaluations, or pharmacy and therapeutics committee support, to others outside their primary service area.[29,30] Some DICs have pooled their resources and have set up networks to provide service to a wide area. "By the way of a telecommunications platform and the Internet, the Drug Information Network aims to capture a greater share of the growing market for the information on drugs and health than could the individual centers combined."[31]

Value

DICs provide value by supplying up-to-date, unbiased, and timely drug information about drugs and drug therapy. The value is in the quality of the information and the time saved. One study determined the workload and impact of one DIC by measuring the number of practitioner hours saved (PHS) and the associated monetary value.[32] During a 3-month period, 308 responses were recorded, which represented 266 PHS. The economic impact, extrapolated over a 1-year period, was $43,950.

Drug information pharmacists provide added value when they effectively answer drug information questions involving judgment. This is because of the quality of the information provided. There are two basic types of drug information questions. The first is the library-type question. Library-type questions ask for a fact — a question is asked and an answer is delivered. For example, "What is the normal dose of oral furosemide in adults?" The answer is 40 mg. A drug information question involving judgment is different. For example, "I have a patient with Lyme disease. Do you think the new drug, panaceamycin, would be the best drug to use in this patient?" The answer is not simple and involves clinical expertise and judgment on the part of the pharmacist.

Drug Information Pharmacist

Drug information pharmacists have varied educational and training backgrounds, but most have a Pharm.D. degree and have completed a specialized residency in drug information. There are several drug information residencies in hospitals, schools of pharmacy, and the pharmaceutical industry. There are also drug information residencies that combine experience in industry and academia.[10]

Although drug information residencies are considered to be a specialized residency, and drug information pharmacists work in a specific area, the practice of drug information is not a pharmacy specialty. Drug information pharmacists are considered to be clinical pharmacists and have a strong knowledge base about drugs and drug therapy. However, they are generalists; that is, they know some information about a lot of drugs rather than knowing a lot of information about a specific pharmacotherapeutic area. An excellent commentary on drug information specialists is available.[33]

Rewards and Satisfaction

A survey of pharmacists who had completed postgraduate training in drug information expressed a high level of satisfaction with their career choice.[34] Most satisfaction was with the geographical location, opportunities for creativity and innovation, respect from the supervisor, interactions with other professionals, autonomy, benefit to society, compatibility with family commitments, opportunities for advancement, and competitive salary.

Future of Drug Information

The practice of providing drug information has been changing.[35] Drug information pharmacists are being better trained. The activities of drug information pharmacists in hospitals have broadened to include performing drug-use evaluations in health care institutions, pharmacoeconomics, and health outcomes. In addition, drug information pharmacists have embraced information technology. These changes show how drug information pharmacists and centers are adapting to the changing health care environment. Thus, the future is bright for this interesting area of pharmacy practice.[36]

POISON INFORMATION

Some readers may not realize that some pharmacists work in poison control centers. Although this is an important and narrowly defined area of practice, poison control practice is yet to be recognized by the pharmacy profession as a specialty area. Thus, pharmacists who are poison information specialists are not yet eligible for board certification by the Board of Pharmaceutical Specialties (BPS). However, they can become a certified poison information specialist by meeting criteria of the American Association of Poison Control Centers (AAPCC).

Brief History

Before 1950, there was no formal system in the United States for poison prevention or treatment. These important works were left to hospital emergency rooms. Information about the potential poisons in various commercial products was lacking, and physicians had to treat most victims of poisoning based on patient history and symptoms.

In the 1930s, pharmacist Louis Gdalman set up a poison information service at St. Luke's Hospital in Chicago, Illinois.[37] In 1950, this poison control center was described as "nothing more than a desk, chair, and telephone located in the inpatient pharmacy." In 1953, based on recommendations of the American Academy of Pediatrics, the poison center at Presbyterian–St. Luke's Hospital was formally recognized.

The number of emergency room–based poison centers rose to a high of 600 during the 1960s and 1970s.[38] The AAPCC was founded in 1958. A goal of the AAPCC was to improve the treatment and outcomes of poison patients. In 1978, the AAPCC developed criteria for certification of regional poison centers. In 1983, the AAPCC took over (from the federal government) and improved the collection and analysis of poison data. Budget cuts during the 1980s and 1990s decreased the number of poison control centers in the United States.

Poison Control Centers Today

In 2000, there were 84 poison control centers in the United States and its territories.[39] In 2002, there were 63 poison centers.[40] Of these, 52 (82.5%) were AAPCC certified. The certification standards for poison control centers are extensive and rigorous.[41] Some of the requirements for certification include the provision of free service 24 hours a day, 7 days a week, questions answered by certified poison specialists, and supervision by a board-certified medical toxicologist and clinical toxicologists. There also must be public education provided.

Poison centers provide various services: telephone management advice about poison patients, telephone follow-up, poison prevention information, professional education about the recognition and management of poisoning, data collection and analysis, and community resource functions.

Statistics

In 1998, all poison control centers answered 3.45 million calls.[39] In 2002, poison centers answered 3.64 million poison questions.[40] About 65% were human exposures, and a majority of poison exposures were in children under the age of 6 years.

Most (87%) of the poison exposures were unintentional and most (74%) were by ingestion. During 2003, there were 19,437 deaths (6.7 per 100,000) from unintentional poisoning in the United States.[42] The most frequent causes of poison death are analgesics, antidepressants, stimulants and "street" drugs, cardiovascular drugs, sedatives and hypnotics, and antipsychotic agents.[38]

Resources

Poison control center resources include computerized information systems such as Poisindex (Micromedex, Inc., Englewood, CO), which provides the identification of poisons, ingredients, dosage, symptoms, and treatment information on exposure to drugs, chemicals, and plant and animal toxins. Other resources include textbooks on pharmacology, toxicology, industrial chemicals, plants, snakes, mushrooms, and ocular and dermal toxicology.[38]

Cost Effectiveness

Poison control centers have been under great pressure to keep services and remain financially viable. Funding has always been a battle. Most funding comes from state budgets and host institutions. The federal government provides less than 5% of the funding needed to run poison control centers.

The AAPPC keeps good track of funding, and the poison control centers try to be cost effective. A study revealed that poison control centers are consistently cost effective.[43] The average cost-effectiveness ratio (cost for a successful outcome) was approximately half of that achieved without the services of a regional poison control center.[44]

Answering Poison Questions

Each poison control center has written policies and procedures on how questions are to be answered. The most important procedure is to get the telephone number of the person calling in case contact is lost. Each call is documented into an automated data collection system. Information recorded includes a history of the poisoning event including information about the substance, amount, route, time of exposure, patient age, weight, prior medical conditions, and current symptoms.

While this is being done, information on the poison is being gathered from a computerized information system. Treatment information and advice are then provided. If needed, the poison control center will call 911 or an ambulance and then an emergency department to let the staff know to expect a patient poisoned from a certain substance.

Staffing

Individuals with specialized skills and training work in poison control centers. Staffing is likely to include[38]:

- *Medical Director*, who may be trained in pediatrics or emergency medicine and is usually a board-certified medical toxicologist.
- *Managing Director*, who may be a board-certified clinical toxicologist. This individual usually is a pharmacist, nurse, or toxicologist.
- *Specialists in poison information*, the nurses, pharmacists, and physicians who answer the poison information questions. Qualifications for certification as a specialist in poison information (CSPI) have been published.[38]
- *Educators* are individuals who may or may not have a health care background. Educators provide poison prevention education in the community.

- *Consultants* in the community such as mycologists (mushroom experts), entomologists (insect experts), hepetologists (snake experts), and experts in hazardous materials, water quality, and other areas are usually available to help poison controls centers when they are needed.

Disaster Planning and Terrorism

Poison Centers are expanding their roles to include responses to disasters and terrorism. In 2004, the Pittsburgh Poison Center was deemed the best prepared poison center to respond to a terrorist strike.[45] The Utah Poison Center planned its disaster responses when Salt Lake City was preparing for the 2002 Winter Olympics.

The Poison Information Pharmacist

The AAPCC regulations state the person who answers the poison center must be a nurse or pharmacist who is a CPIS. Although this is a career option for pharmacists, most pharmacists, especially new graduates, do not consider it.[46] Pharmacy schools need to do a better job of making pharmacy students aware of this option. In 2002, there were 179 pharmacists working in 63 poison control centers. Of these, 108 had a B.S. degree, 7 had an M.A. degree, and 64 had a Pharm.D. or Ph.D. degree.[40]

Rewards and Satisfaction

Several articles have been published about poison control work as a career for pharmacists.[46–49] All of these articles provide testimonials to the high level of satisfaction pharmacists have in working in this area. One pharmacist stated in another article, "This has been, without a doubt, the most rewarding pharmacy employment experience I have had."[49] The highlights for this pharmacist were working with other credentialed health professionals and being an integral part of a lifesaving emergency service.

Although not written by a pharmacist, a reference is provided about the experiences of a new poison information specialist.[50] This interesting article provides an inside look at what takes place inside a regional poison control center and why poison information specialists enjoy their jobs so much.

Future of Poison Information

A recent paper written on the past, present, and future of poison control centers states that, although poison control centers are an essential public resource, and have been shown to be cost effective, funding support will continue to be a problem.[31] In 2004, the Institute of Medicine (IOM) recommended that the basic funding for poison control centers be federal.[51] It is hoped that the federal government will address the needs of poison control centers soon.

SUMMARY

Drug and poison information centers provide a useful, value-added service to health professionals and the public. Pharmacists play an important part in delivering these services. Pharmacists who work in drug information centers and in poison control centers provide specialized knowledge and have a high-level of satisfaction.

DISCUSSION QUESTIONS AND EXERCISES

1. What is the importance of drug information? What need does it fill?
2. Why is it important for every pharmacist to take on the role of drug information provider?
3. Select five secondary sources of drug information. Go to the library and review these resources. What are the strengths of each reference?
4. Select three electronic databases for drug information. Go to the library and learn how to use these databases. What are the strengths of each database?
5. While in the library, select one primary literature reference in medicine (e.g., *JAMA, Lancet,* or *Annals of Internal Medicine*) and one primary literature reference in pharmacy (e.g., *American Journal of Health-System Pharmacists, Pharmacotherapy,* or *Journal of the American Pharmacy Association*). What is your opinion of these sources of drug information?
6. Make an appointment to interview a pharmacist or pharmacy resident working in a drug information center.
7. What do you feel are the pros and cons of being a drug information pharmacist?
8. Based on what you know and have read thus far about being a drug information pharmacist, is this something you may want to do? Why or why not?
9. Make an appointment to interview (by telephone or in person) a poison information pharmacist.
10. What do you feel are the pros and cons of being a poison information pharmacist? Is this something you may want to do? Why or why not?

CHALLENGES

1. The number of drug information centers have been dwindling, but the quality of the drug information personnel has improved. For extra credit, and with the permission of your professor, research and write a concise report on the number of pharmacist-operated drug information centers since their beginning, track volume, note various trends, and provide theories on why the number of drug information centers are dropping. Is this a good thing or a bad thing for pharmacy?

2. There were 19,437 deaths due to unintentional poisoning in 2003. Also during this time there were 63 poison control centers (PCCs) with annual costs exceeding 107 million dollars. The Institute of Medicine has recommended that PCCs be funded with federal dollars. For extra credit, and with the permission of your professor, make an argument (in writing), based on facts, for the federal funding of PCCs based on preventing deaths from unintentional poisoning.

WEB SITES OF INTEREST

Drug Information Association: http://www.diahome.org/en/

Drug Information Journal: http://www.findarticles.com/p/articles/mi_qa3899

American Association of Poison Centers: http://www.aapcc.org/

REFERENCES

1. Amerson, AB. Introduction to drug information. In *Drug Information: A Guide for Pharmacists*, Malone, PM, Kier, KL, Mosdell, KW, and Stanovich, JE, eds. Appleton & Lange, Stanford, CT, 1996, chap. 1

2. Parker, PF. The University of Kentucky drug information center. *Am J Hosp Pharm.* 1965;22:42–47.

3. Pearson, RE, Salter, FJ, Bohl, JC, et al. Michigan regional drug information network. Part 1. Concepts. *Am J Hosp Pharm.* 1970;27:911–913.

4. Pearson, RE, Thudium, VF, and Phillips, GL. Michigan regional drug information network. Part 2. Drug therapy analysis: a model. *Am J Hosp Pharm.* 1971;28:513–515.

5. Pearson, RE. Michigan regional drug information network. Part 3. Utilization of information received from a drug information center. *Am J Hosp. Pharm.* 1972;29:229–234.

6. Matuszewski, KA. Drug information activities in academic health centers: 1996 survey. *Drug Inf J.* 1998;32:539–546.

7. DiPirro, MN, Kelly, WN, and Miller, DE. Developing a clinically oriented drug information service in a community hospital. *Hosp. Pharm.* 1975;10(10):434, 436–440.

8. Haynes, LM, Patterson, AA, and Wade, SU. Drug information resources in the Veteran Affairs health care system. *Hosp Pharm.* 1995;30:297–301.

9. McCloskey, WW, and Vogenberg, FR. Drug information resources in managed care organizations. *Am J Health-Syst Pharm.* 1998;55:2007–2009.

10. Malecha, SE, Cha, AJ, and Holt, RJ. Establishing a combined drug information residency in industry and academia. *Am J Pharm Ed.* 2000;64:177–180.

11. Rosenberg, JM, Koumis T, Nathan JP, et al. Current status of pharmacist-operated drug information centers in the United States. *Am J Health-Syst Pharm.* 2004;61(19):2023–2032.

12. Anson, MA, Moody, ML, and Stachnik, JS. Fee-for-service drug information centers. *Drug Inf J.* 2003;37(2):233–239.

13. James, K, and Millares, M. Responding to drug information inquiries: the process and resources. In *Applied Drug Information: Strategies for Information Management,* Millares, M, ed. Applied Therapeutics, Vancouver, WA, 1998, chap. 1.

14. Kirkwood, CF. Modified systematic approach to answering questions. In *Drug Information: A Guide for Pharmacists,* Malone, PM, Kier, KL, Mosdell, KW, and Stanovich, JE, eds. Appleton & Lange, Stamford, CT, 1996, chap. 2

15. Price, KO, and Goldwire, MA. Drug information resources. *Am Pharm.* 1994; NS34:30–39.

16. University of Washington Health Sciences Libraries. 1994–2006. Drug information resources: resources by topic. Available at http://www.healthlinks.washington.edu/howto/drugs/material/step3.html. Accessed May 8, 2006.

17. Mosdell, KW, and Malone, PM. Drug information resources. In *Drug Information: A Guide for Pharmacists,* Malone, PM, Kier, KL, Mosdell, KW, and Stanovich, JE, eds. Appleton & Lange, Stamford, CT, 1996, chap. 3.

18. Tsourounis, C, and Schroeder, DJ. Implementation of a computerized drug information database. *Am J Health-Syst Pharm.* 1997;54:1763–1764.

19. Gora-Harper, ML, and Smith, R. Paperless system of managing drug information requests. *Am J Health-Syst Pharm.* 1996;53:678, 683.

20. Erbele, SM, Heck, AM, and Blankenship, CS. Survey of computerized documentation system use in drug information centers. *Am J Health-Syst Pharm.* 2001;58:695–697.

21. Halbert, MR, Kelly, WN, and Miller, DE. Drug information centers: lack of generic equivalence. *Drug Intell Clin Pharm.* 1977;11:728–735.

22. Halbert, MR, Kelly, WN, and Miller, DE. Omission in drug information centers: lack of generic equivalence article (letter). *Drug Intell Clin Pharm.* 1978;12:53.

23. Beaird, SL, Coley, RM, and Blunt, JR. Assessing the accuracy of drug information responses from drug information centers. *Ann Pharmacother.* 1994;28:707–711.

24. Calis, KA, Anderson, DW, Auth, DA, et al. Quality of pharmacotherapy consultations provided by drug information centers in the United States. *Pharmacotherapy.* 2000;20:830–836.

25. Holmes, ER, Desselle, SP, Nath, DM, et al. Ask the pharmacist: an analysis of online drug information services. *Ann Pharmacotherapy.* 2005;39:662–667.

26. Kelly, WN, Krause, EC, Krowinski, WJ, et al. National survey of ethical issues presented to drug information centers. *Am J Hosp Pharm.* 1990;47:2245–2250.

27. Rumore, MM, and Rosenberg, JM. Comparison of drug information practice in hospitals and industry. *Drug Inform J.* 1989;23:273–283.

28. Ruppelt, SC, and Vann, AR. Marketing a hospital-based drug information center. *Am J Health-Syst Pharm.* 2001;58:1040.

29. Price, KO, Rosenberg, JM, and Rumore, MM. Fee-for-service and cost justification activities of pharmacist-manned drug information centers in the United States. *Drug Inform J.* 1991:25:139–153.

30. Anonymous. How one hospital is charging for drug information. *Drug Top.* 1990;134(suppl):26.

31. Thompson, CA. Drug information centers pool resources. *Am J Health-Syst Pharm.* 1997;54:1930–1931.

32. Marrone, CM, and Heck, AM. Impact of a drug information service: practitioner hours saved. *Hosp Pharm.* 2000;35:1065–1070.

33. Brand, KA, and Kraus, ML. Drug information specialists. *Am J Health-Syst Pharm.* 2006;63:712–714.

34. Beckwith, C, and Tyler, LS. Career expectations of pharmacists with postgraduate training in drug information. *Am J Hosp Pharm.* 1994;51:1197–1201.

35. Forsstrom, K. Anticipating Future Trends in the Practice of Drug Information. Residency Project Report. Mercer University School of Pharmacy, 1998. Available at Mercer University's Swilley Library, Atlanta, GA.

36. Thompson DF. A personal view of the history and future direction of drug information. *Ann Pharmacotherapy.* 2006;40:307–308.

37. Burda, AM, and Burda, NM. Taking a stand against accidental childhood poisoning: the founding of the nation's first poison control center in Chicago. *J Pharm Pract.* 2000;13:6–13.

38. Gould Soloway, RA. Poison centers: an overview of the past, present, and future. *J Pharm Pract.* 2000;13:14–26.

39. American Association of Poison Control Centers. 1999 Poison center survey. Available at http://www.aapcc.org/surveyresults99.htm. Accessed June 12, 2001.

40. American Association of Poison Control Centers. 2002 Poison center survey. Available at http://www.aapcc.org/2002_poison_center_survey_results.htm. Accessed May 6, 2006.

41. Anonymous. Criteria for certification as a regional poison center. *Vet Hum Toxicol.*1996;38:145–150.

42. Centers for Disease Control and Prevention. National Center for Injury Prevention and Control. 2003 United States unintentional poisoning deaths and rates per 100,000. Available at http://webappa.cdc.gov/cgi-bin/broker.exe. Accessed May 8, 2006.

43. Harrison, DL, Draugalis, J, Slack, MK, and Langley, PC. Cost-effectiveness of regional poison control centers. *Arch Intern Med.* 1996;156:2601–2608.

44. Thompson, CA. Pittsburgh poison center is terrorism response leader. *Am J Health-Syst Pharm.* 2004;61:2243–2244.

45. Crouch, BI. Role of poison control centers in disaster response planning. *Am J Health-Syst Pharm.* 2002;59:1159–1163.

46. Maxwell, T. How about poison control as a pharmacy career? *Drug Top.* 1990;134:21.

47. Fish, SS. Poison information specialist: a career option neglected by pharmacists. *Pharm Times.* 1988;54:105–108

48. Shaw, K. The pharmacist as poison prevention specialist. *Pharm Times.* 1998;64:51–59.

49. Woolley, V. Exploring your choice for the future: perspectives in pharmacy-poison information. *Wash Pharm.*1992;34:21.

50. Lowe, TJ. Experiences of a new poison specialist. *Vet Hum Toxicol.* 1997;39:51–52.

51. Thompson, CA. Poison control centers' basic funding should be federal, IOM says. *Am J Health-Syst Pharm.* 2004;61:1322, 1324.

15

PHARMACY ACADEMIA

At the core of pharmacy is knowledge. Various study commissions in pharmacy have confirmed this by stating that pharmacy is a knowledge-based profession. The knowledge starts with study, and study starts in pharmacy school. It continues, if one wishes, into graduate studies or a residency or fellowship training. Being a pharmacist also includes a commitment to *lifelong learning*. This means pharmacists must continually keep up with the latest developments in drug therapy, changes in pharmacy laws, and changes in the profession.

The part of pharmacy responsible for much of this training is academia — the faculty of the 89 colleges and schools of pharmacy in the United States. Academia is also a place of scholarship and the discovery of new knowledge. It is where new ideas in the science and practice of pharmacy are generated and tested. In a sense, academia is the brain trust of the profession.

This chapter is about schools and colleges of pharmacy and the role of faculty in teaching and research and the service provided by the academic pharmacy community. How schools of pharmacy are structured and accredited and how curriculums are developed and assessed will be discussed. This chapter will talk about what it takes and what it is like to be a pharmacy faculty member. A broad role of faculty will be stressed to provide the reader with an appreciation for pharmacy faculty being more than teachers. The chapter will end with some information on the rewards and satisfaction of pharmacy faculty members.

LEARNING OBJECTIVES

After participating in this learning session, you should be able to:

- Provide some brief history on academic pharmacy

- State how pharmacy schools differ
- Discuss the issue of supply and demand for pharmacists
- Explain how pharmacy faculty differ
- Explain the main responsibilities of pharmacy faculty
- Explain the scholarship of teaching
- Define the term *life-long learning*
- Explain the scholarship of research
- Explain how pharmacy faculty are evaluated
- Discuss how satisfied faculty are in workin in academia

A BRIEF HISTORY

Formal pharmacy education in the United States made slow progress before the Civil War (1861 to 1864). Much of the training of a pharmacist was apprenticeship; that is, practical training directly provided by a pharmacist to a pharmacist trainee. There was no formal pharmacy training.

There is some doubt about which college or university was the first to provide formal pharmacy coursework on a collegiate level.[1] There may have been some course work in pharmacy during Civil War times at what is now known as The Philadelphia College of Pharmacy. In 1860, the University of Michigan (Ann Arbor) offered a laboratory course in pharmacy for medical students. In 1865, Baldwin University (Berea, Ohio) became the first to offer pharmacy instruction as part of a general college program. The Medical College of South Carolina (Charleston) graduated a few men in pharmacy in 1867.

However, the course in pharmacy launched at the University of Michigan in 1868 became a separate school of pharmacy in 1876.[1] This school was noted for its pioneering and controversial approaches to pharmacy education. Dr. Albert B. Prescott, a medical doctor, abandoned the traditional requirement of pregraduation apprenticeship and developed laboratory courses in the science of pharmacy (see Figure 15.1). The pharmacy coursework at the University of Michigan was based on a curriculum that included basic sciences that demanded students' full-time attention.[1]

SCHOOLS AND COLLEGES OF PHARMACY

Universities name their individual subunits either colleges or schools. In pharmacy, there are both. Traditionally, a college of pharmacy is part of a university, whereas a school of pharmacy is part of a college. However, today, there is basically no difference between a college and a school of pharmacy.

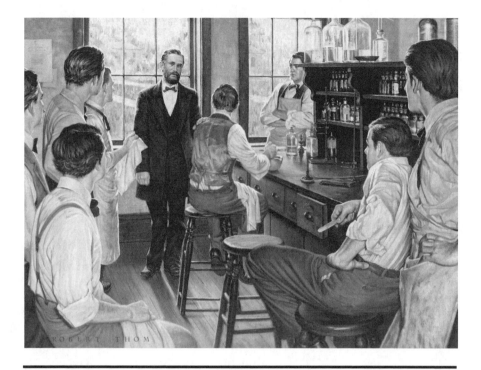

Figure 15.1   A revolution in pharmaceutical education. (From Bender, GA, and Thom, RA. *Great Moments in Pharmacy: The Stories and Paintings in the Series, a History of Pharmacy in Pictures,* by Parke Davis & Company and Northwood Institute Press, 1965. Courtesy of Pfizer, Inc.)

Statistics

The following statistics about schools and colleges of pharmacy have been supplied by the American Association of Colleges of Pharmacy (AACP).[2]

- During fall 2005, there were 89 accredited colleges and schools of pharmacy, up from 82 in 2000.
- Thirty-three were private institutions (up from 27 in 2000).
- Ninety-five colleges and schools offered the Pharm.D. degree as a first professional degree. Thirty-one colleges and schools offered the Pharm.D. degree as a post-B.S. degree in fall 2006.
- Sixty-eight colleges and schools (up 4 from 2000) offered graduate programs in the pharmaceutical sciences at the M.S. or Ph.D. level in fall 2006.

Accreditation

The American Council on Pharmaceutical Education (ACPE) accredits schools and colleges of pharmacy. A survey team from the ACPE visits each school and college of pharmacy usually every 6 years. The ACPE makes sure the colleges and schools of pharmacy are living up to the minimum standards for higher education in pharmacy.

Structure

Few schools and colleges of pharmacy are structured exactly the same; however, there is a typical model. Every college or school of pharmacy has a dean, who is the chief academic officer for the school. In this capacity, the dean is accountable for all actions of the school.

Under the dean may be associate or assistant deans, who have responsibility for specific program areas. For example, there may be an associate dean for academics, one for administration, one for enrollment, and one for student affairs (sometimes called the dean of students). These assistant and associate deans may perform full-time administrative work or may also have some teaching responsibilities.

Many schools and colleges of pharmacy divide faculty into various departments such as the Department of Pharmaceutical Science, the Department of Pharmacy Administration, and the Department of Pharmacy Practice. Sometimes the Department of Pharmacy Administration is part of one of the other two departments. A department chairperson oversees managing the department, and there may be a vice-chairperson if the department is large.

Sometimes large departments are subdivided into various specialty areas. For example, the Department of Pharmaceutical Science may be divided into divisions such as medicinal chemistry, pharmacology, and pharmaceutics. The Department of Pharmacy Practice may be divided into various clinical areas such as medicine, ambulatory care, and community pharmacy.

Other positions in academia include the director of continuing education and the director of professional affairs, both of whom may be in faculty or staff positions. Other staff positions include secretaries, work-study students, and other support staff.

PHARMACY STUDENTS

The following statistics about pharmacy students have been supplied by the AACP.[2]

- Total first professional degree enrollment was 43,884 (up 35% since 2000) in fall 2004 (43,884 in Pharm.D. degree programs and 24 in B.S. degree programs). The number of students holding a B.S. degree in pharmacy and enrolled in Pharm.D. degree programs was 3,492.
- Of the total number of students enrolled in first professional degree programs for fall 2004, 66.5% were women and 12.95% were underrepresented minority students.
- The attrition rates (those dropping out) averaged 4.68% during 2000–2004.
- Total fall 1999 full-time graduate student enrollment was 3,347 (2,566 in Ph.D. degree programs and 781 in M.S. degree programs), an increase of 20%. Just over 50.5% were females, and U.S.-educated pharmacists made up 7.2% of the total Ph.D. degree enrollment.
- In 2003–2004, 8,158 first professional degrees in pharmacy, 335 Ph.D. degrees and 651 M.S. degrees, were awarded.

SUPPLY OF PHARMACISTS

Pharmacy academia has done an excellent job of supplying pharmacists for the profession. For example, pharmacy academia, unlike some professions, has never supplied too many pharmacists. The profession can be proud that work is always available for pharmacists. Although this is good, there have been a few times when there have not been enough pharmacists, most notably in the late 1980s and currently in 2006.

There were about 196,000 pharmacists in the United States in 2000. In 2004, there were close to 230,000. The supply of pharmacists has consistently increased each year, and this growth has been faster than the growth in population. Thus, "supply factors are not the primary forces explaining today's pharmacist workforce problems."[3] As shown in Figure 15.2, the schools of pharmacy have been graduating between 7000 and 8000 new graduates each year during the 1990s. The lowest number of new graduates was 6956 in 1990 and the highest number was 8003 in 1998.

A reason for the shortage of pharmacists during this time has more to do with the increased use of medication than the supply of pharmacists. A growing number of elderly have chronic diseases (arthritis, hypertension, diabetes, asthma, hyperlipidemia, and angina), and physicians are treating these diseases more aggressively with drugs. Another reason for the shortage of pharmacists is the expanded job market. Jobs for pharmacists are no longer restricted to community and hospital practice.

The pharmacist shortage has been noticed overseas, and there has been an influx of foreign pharmacy graduates. *Foreign pharmacy graduates* are

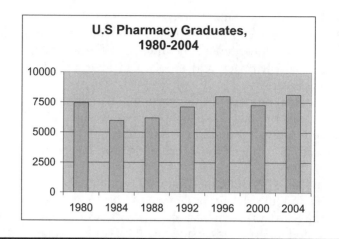

Figure 15.2   U.S. Pharmacy Graduates, 1980–2004. *(Source:* **National Center for Health Workforce Analysis.** *U.S. Health Workforce Personnel Factbook.* **2006.)**

pharmacists whose undergraduate degrees were conferred by recognized schools of pharmacy outside of the 50 United States, the District of Columbia, and Puerto Rico.[4] United States citizens who have completed their pharmacy education outside the United States are considered to be "foreign pharmacy graduates," while foreign nationals who graduated from schools in the United States are not.

For foreign pharmacy graduates to practice in the United States, the person must: (a) complete an application and pass the Foreign Pharmacy Graduate Equivalency Examination (FPGEE), (b) apply for and pass the Test of English as a Foreign Language (TOEFL), and (c) apply for and pass the Test of Spoken English (TSE), before they may apply and sit for the state board exam (NAPLEX).[5]

PHARMACY FACULTY

The work of the schools and colleges of pharmacy gets done by the faculty. In 2005–2006, there were 4206 full-time and 579 part-time pharmacy faculty members and 353 *emerti* at 89 colleges and schools of pharmacy.[2]

Rank

Each faculty member holds a certain academic rank and is a member of a specific academic department. Rank is determined objectively and is based on academic productivity — the quality and quantity of scholarly activity as documented in scientific or clinical publications, research grants and contracts, peer and public recognition, and publications and recognition for teaching.

The ranks (starting with the lowest) are instructor, assistant professor, associate professor, and (full) professor. To achieve the rank of professor, the candidate usually must have achieved national or international recognition. Moving from one rank to the next rank typically takes 7 years or more.

Tenure

Tenure is the right of being in one's position permanently and is the highest achievement in academia. Higher education grants tenure to individuals proven to be academically productive and suitable for permanent status at the university where they teach and perform their research. Unlike rank, tenure is more of a "family" decision of the existing tenured faculty at a school.

Once tenure is granted, the faculty member has a job for life as long as the tenured person does not violate any major rules of the university. Three things should be noted about tenure. First, under the original idea of tenure, most academics are required to develop new knowledge. In doing this, academics explore the yet to be discovered, and some of their ideas can be considered unusual or strange by some, especially if the ideas contradict public or current scientific opinion. However, it is important for civilization that these critical minds explore new knowledge; thus, tenure is available to protect these individual's academic freedom.

The second feature of tenure is that it is not available to all faculty. In most schools of pharmacy, you must hold a certain rank (associate or professor) to apply, and you must be in a *tenure track position*. The Department of Pharmacy Practice, sometimes called the Department of Clinical Pharmacy, may have two tracks, tenure and nontenure. The tenure-track positions in the Department of Pharmacy Practice are for the researcher–teachers, whereas the non-tenure-track positions are for the teacher–practitioners.

The *teacher–researchers* are full-time, pharmacy practice faculty at a school of pharmacy, have the Pharm.D. degree, and probably have completed a specialty residency or a research fellowship in a specific area (e.g., cardiology, infectious disease, or psychiatry). These tenure track pharmacy practice faculty members conduct significant pharmacy research, provide a significant amount of didactic instruction, provide service to the university, and may or may not see patients or provide experiential training for students.

The *teacher–practitioners* are full-time or cofunded (salary partially paid by a practice site) pharmacy practice faculty who have the Pharm.D. degree, and probably have completed a general or specialty residency program, and see patients routinely. These non-tenure-track faculty members do a modest amount of research, do some teaching in the classroom, and provide some service to the university, but mostly provide experiential training to students at clinical sites where they routinely see patients. Teacher–practitioner faculty do not qualify for tenure.

The third feature of tenure is that if you are eligible, you must apply within a certain time frame (which varies from school to school), and if you apply and do not get it, you are provided with a 1-year terminal contract and must leave that school at the end of that year.

The faculty members in the departments, other than those in pharmacy practice, are researcher–teachers. Most have the Ph.D. degree, and some have completed postdoctoral, research fellowships. Researcher–teachers do a significant amount of research and didactic teaching and provide service to the university. All are on the tenure track.

Several other people who help teach pharmacy students are:

Graduate students: Students working toward an M.S. or Ph.D. degree in pharmacy sometimes teach pharmacy students in the classroom and laboratory.

Guest lecturers: An important source of teaching is the use of outside guest lecturers. These guests are able to bring the real world into the classroom. An example is using a practicing pharmacist–attorney into the pharmacy law and ethics course to discuss professional risk.

Residents and fellows: Pharmacists doing postgraduate residency training in pharmacy and pharmacy research fellows can provide "cutting edge" knowledge for students as well.

Adjunct pharmacy practice faculty: Practicing community, hospital, clinical, and consultant pharmacists are the backbone of any school or college of pharmacy's experiential program. Adjunct faculty, many of whom volunteer, feel it is their duty and honor to help train pharmacy students.

Faculty Responsibilities

Academics have three primary responsibilities: teaching, research, and service. How much time a faculty member devotes to each area depends on two things: the appointment (tenure track or nontenure track) and negotiation between the faculty member and the chairperson of the department.

The time of a seasoned, tenure-track faculty member who is conducting a lot of research might be divided as follows: 50% research, 35% teaching, and 15% service. A new, tenure-track faculty member who is just starting his or her research, might have their time divided as follows: 30% research, 50% teaching, and 20% service. Most of the service will be active involvement in various committees of the school and being active in the life of the school.

Non-tenure-track, pharmacy practice faculty who are paid entirely by the college or school of pharmacy might have their time divided as follows: 20% research, 60% teaching, and 20% service. Most of the teaching for non-tenure-track faculty will be for experiential (clinical rotation) teaching. For cofunded (partially paid by a practice site and partially paid by the school of pharmacy) non-tenure-track pharmacy practice faculty, the faculty member's time allocation from the school might be 5% research, 40% teaching, and 55% service. Most of the service part will be maintaining an active practice site and seeing patients there.

Scholarship of Teaching

Teaching, whether it is in the classroom (didactic teaching) or providing practical training (experiential teaching), is an important function of every pharmacy faculty member. Most pharmacy faculty members take their teaching seriously. Even if they do not teach much, pharmacy faculty members seek to improve the content and delivery of the material they are teaching. There is also a priority on being innovative and trying new things.

Each time pharmacy faculty members teach something, they learn and plan what they will do differently next time to be better. Thus, the scholarship of teaching is a continuous quality improvement process. Some authors have offered advice on how to improve and be excellent in teaching pharmacy. The 10 important features of teaching are:[6]

Creativity: In course design and delivery and motivating students.
Knowledge of the discipline: Teaching is more than presenting material.
Course design skills: Being able to design something worthwhile.
Classroom skills: Promoting active, versus passive learning.
Student evaluation skills: Being able to write good test questions.
Empathy for students: Being sensitive, supportive, and firm when needed.
Interface with the curriculum: Teach what every graduate needs to know.
Knowledge of the profession: Being up-to-date about the profession.
Effective self-management: Being able to balance all responsibilities.
Sense of the future: Having students thinking about the future.

Another approach to improving and being an excellent teacher is to concentrate on six qualitative standards[7]:

Having clear goals: Are the basic purposes of the course stated? Are the learning objectives practical and achievable? Are important questions asked and discussed?

Being adequately prepared: An absolute must to be successful.

Using appropriate methods: Do the methods fulfill the goals? Are the methods applied effectively? If something is not working, will there be a change?

Providing an effective presentation: Is the style suitable? Is the delivery organized?

Achieving significant results: How much of an impact will this course have on students?

Undergraduate Teaching

The focus of this chapter is on the Pharm.D. degree. The pharmacy profession is changing so rapidly that the curriculum for the Pharm.D. degree must be dynamic and innovative. Pharmacy schools are not teaching students for practice today, but for practice 10 years from now. To do this, academia needs to keep its finger on the pulse of the profession. How is this done?

One of the strong points about pharmacy academia is its connection to pharmacy practice, to the profession's leadership, to all professional pharmacy organizations, to the government, to the pharmacy industry, and to other health professions. The organization that helps pharmacy schools keep up with new developments is the American Association of Colleges of Pharmacy (AACP).

The AACP is not only a listener to new topics but also cosponsors programs such as "Pharmacy in the 21st Century," a symposium on what pharmacy may be like in the future. Besides a council of deans (all deans of pharmacy schools) and a council of faculty (faculty representatives from each school), the AACP has various academic sections and special interest groups where faculty can come together to discuss various topics of interest and where the profession is headed.

Over the past several years, the AACP has provided leadership and support to schools in moving toward the entry-level and nontraditional Pharm.D. degree and in moving toward ambulatory and pharmaceutical care. The schools are also putting more emphasis on teaching about managed care and improving clinical practice in community pharmacies.[8,9]

The starting point for any undergraduate curriculum is to develop terminal outcome objectives — what every graduate is expected to know.[10] These curriculum outcomes come in two types, professional outcomes and competencies and practice outcomes and competencies.

Each of the competencies may have three advancement levels, with level one being the easiest, but it must be mastered before going to level two competencies. The level two competencies must be mastered before moving to mastering the level three competencies. Figure 15.3 provides

Outcome: The graduate will be able to collect and evaluate patient data to properly assess patients and to determine appropriate courses of action such as prescription drug therapy, nonprescription drug therapy, non-drug therapy, or referral to another health care professional.

Level 1 Competencies:
a. Collect and organize patient data into a format that facilitates making decisions to meet the patient's health care needs.
b. Use appropriate interviewing and patient assessment skills to assess patient's health status.
c. Recommend appropriate non-pharmacological treatment to meet the self-care needs of the patient.

Level 2 Competencies:
a. Select information from the patient record or profile that the pharmacist may need to make decisions on determining a patient's health care needs.
b. Obtain necessary additional information from a health care professional to address a patient's health care needs.
c. Assess pertinent patient data to determine a patient's health care needs related to the presenting problem.
d. Record information related to identification, resolution or prevention of medication-related problems in individual patients.
e. Develop and conduct health screening, promotion and prevention programs.

Level 3 Competencies:
a. Devise a plan for meeting health care needs related to the patient's presenting problem.
b. Devise a methodology for documenting recommendations based on professional and practical considerations.
c. Determine when other health professionals are most appropriate for managing patient's health care needs.

Figure 15.3   An example of a pharmacy practice outcome and the competencies needed to demonstrate the achievement of the outcome.

an example of a pharmacy practice learning outcome and the competencies needed to demonstrate achievement of the outcome.

Once pharmacy faculty agree on curricular outcomes, the next step in building the curriculum is to develop a topic outline on how to teach the various competencies represented in the curricular outcome's document. Once the faculty agree on the topic outline, the topics can be arranged into various courses. Thus, all learning flows from what every graduate needs to know — the curricular outcomes.

Each school and college of pharmacy's curriculum is unique. It is unlikely that any school's curriculum is exactly like another's. The curriculum will be different if one school of pharmacy has a 0 to 6 program (all 6 years of pharmacy in one place) and another has a 2 to 4 program (2 years of prepharmacy and then 4 years of pharmacy school). An example of one pharmacy school's four professional years is shown in Figure 15.4.

A current curricular strategy in a few schools and colleges of pharmacy is to integrate some of the coursework. This means that rather than learning individual topics such as physiology, pathology, pharmaceutical chemistry, pharmacology, pharmacokinetics, and therapeutics, the coursework is divided into various diseases and the student learns all of these topics by disease. This means the courses will be team taught by faculty members from several disciplines and several departments.

For example, when studying cardiovascular disorders, one topic will be angina. Someone from pharmacy administration will discuss the occurrence (epidemiology) of angina. Next, instructors form the Department of Pharmaceutical Science will discuss the anatomy and physiology of the coronary arteries, the pathology of angina, and the chemistry and pharmacology of the drugs used to treat the various forms of angina. Next, members of the Department of Pharmacy Practice will discuss the pharmacokinetics and the therapeutics in treating angina. Last, a faculty member from the Department of Pharmacy Administration will discuss the health outcomes associated with treating angina.

Another new curricular idea is to teach one course at a time rather than have the student be responsible for four to five courses throughout one semester. The one course at a time idea allows the student to be devoted to one learning subject and avoids the problem of students only studying when there is a test.

External Pharm.D. Degree

Because the schools and colleges of pharmacy have made a decision to provide the Pharm.D. degree as the only entry-level degree in pharmacy, there has been a need to provide ways for a practicing pharmacists with B.S. degrees to earn Pharm.D. degrees.[11] As it is difficult for practicing pharmacists to take 4 years out of their lives to attend an on-campus, Pharm.D. degree program, many schools and colleges of pharmacy have developed nontraditional Pharm.D. degree programs for practicing pharmacists. The term *nontraditional* means the learner is an adult and the delivery of the program is nontraditional.

A nontraditional Pharm.D. degree program is a structured, flexible, educational program for practicing pharmacists to earn a Pharm.D. degree. The curricular outcomes of a nontraditional Pharm.D. degree program and an on-campus Pharm.D. degree program are the same — to graduate, the learner or student needs to demonstrate all the competencies to fulfill the outcomes. As most nontraditional Pharm.D. degree students are practicing pharmacists, many already have some of the needed competencies for

First Professional Year	Semester Hours	
Course	**Fall**	**Spring**
Introduction to Pharmacy	3	
Biostatistics, Research Design, Literature Evaluation	3	
Communication Skills for Pharmacists	3	
Biosciences I	4	
Principles of Pharmaceutical Sciences	3	
Patient care I	0.5	
	16.5	
Health Care Organization		2
Pharmacy Law and Ethics		2
Pharmacy Management		4
Biosciences II		4
Pharmaceutics		4
Patient Care II		0.5
		16.5

Second Professional Year	Semester Hours	
	Fall	**Spring**
General Principles of Pharmacotherapy	4	
Nervous System Disorders I	5	
Nervous System Disorders II	4	
Elective	2	
Patient Care III	2	
	17	
Renal and Urologic Disorders		3
Cardiovascular Disorders I		5
Cardiovascular Disorders II		5
Elective		2
Patient Care IV		2
		17

Third Professional Year	Semester Hours	
	Fall	**Spring**
Musculoskeletal Disorders	3	
Endocrine Disorders	4	
Gastrointestinal Disorders	3	
Pulmonary Disorders	3	
Elective	2	
Patient Care V	2	
	17	
Infectious Diseases I		3
Infectious Diseases II		3
Integument and Special Senses		3
Hematology and Oncology Disorders		3
Elective		2
Patient Care VI		2
		16

Fourth Professional Year	Semester Hours	
	Fall	**Spring**
Advanced Practice Experiences	15	15

Figure 15.4   A typical curriculum for the four professional years in pharmacy.

the Pharm.D. degree but need to demonstrate these before they are allowed credit toward the degree. Thus, in some of the nontraditional Pharm.D. degree programs, the course of study is individualized and specific to those competencies needed.[12]

Graduate Education

Besides providing the entry-level Pharm.D. degree, colleges and schools of pharmacy also provide graduate education in various pharmacy disciplines. A majority of the colleges and schools of pharmacy in the United States offer the M.S. and the Ph.D. degrees, usually in pharmacy administration or pharmaceutical science.

In pharmaceutical science, the main areas of concentration are pharmacology, toxicology, pharmaceutics, medicinal chemistry, and pharmacokinetics, but there are other areas as well (Figure 15.5). In pharmacy administration, there can be a concentration on pharmacoeconomics and health outcomes research.

Besides coursework, there is usually a thesis requirement (a formal, lengthy research paper) for the M.S. degree, whereas a dissertation (a formal, lengthy report on exploring original research) is required to earn a Ph.D. degree.

People earning an M.S or Ph.D. degree in pharmaceutical science work in academia (pharmacy schools), as research scientists in the pharmaceutical industry or in the government (U.S. Food and Drug Administration [FDA], Centers for Disease Control and Prevention [CDC], National Institutes of Health [NIH]). A position in academia provides more variety (teaching, research, and service), whereas the other positions are mainly research.

A person holding an M.S. or Ph.D. degree in pharmacy administration usually works in academia (pharmacy schools), or for a pharmaceutical company or private company doing pharmacoepidemiology, pharmacoeconomics, or health outcomes research.

People suited for graduate degrees in pharmaceutical science like science classes and want to pursue a science-based career. These individuals like the laboratory, and they would like to contribute to the health and well-being of society through developing medicines and therapies.[13] An example of a curriculum for a Ph.D. degree in pharmaceutical science is provided in Figure 15.5. To qualify, a person must have earned a previous degree — a B.S. in pharmacy, a Pharm.D. or an M.S. The previous degree requirement varies from school to school.

Core Curriculum	Semester Hours
Introduction to Pharmaceutical Sciences	3
Isotope Techniques	3
Research Techniques I	3
Research Techniques II	3
Quantitative Aspects of Drug Action I	3
Quantitative Aspects of Drug Action II	3
Pharmaceutical Biotechnology	3
Seminar	3
Sub-Total	21
Elective Coursework	14
Dissertation	35
Total	70

Figure 15.5   An example of curriculum for a Ph.D. degree in pharmaceutical science.

Delivery Strategies

Studies have shown that lecturing may be the worst way to teach. The teacher provides words of wisdom, and the student records what the student thinks is important (most students think every word is important). Then most students try to memorize their notes before an examination. Once the exam is over, there is a "brain dump," and the student moves on to studying in the same manner for the next examination. This is no way to learn and to remember what is important.

In higher education today, there is a strong feeling, based on good studies, that active learning and self-learning are the best ways to learn.[14] To do this, the professor should be more of a "guide from the side" than a "sage from the stage."

Active learning means the learning is student rather than faculty focused, which means getting students involved in their learning rather than letting them be passive learners.[13] The goal is to have students doing something and getting them to think critically and problem solve. To do this, students will need to learn most of the course content by reading and by reviewing selected cases before coming to class. In this manner, the professor can take the course and the class to the next level — discussion and application of the course content.

Self-learning can be carried out by reading required texts and journal articles or by learning material placed by a professor on a CD-ROM or on the Internet. The review of case studies and being prepared to discuss the cases in class are also effective learning strategies.

Besides reviewing cases, various techniques can be used to promote active learning in the classroom. Application exercises can be designed for students to work in small groups. The application exercise is used to see if the students have the ability to apply what they have learned from their reading and self-learning.

Another active learning strategy is the use of *problem-based learning* (PBL), which employs a problem as the vehicle for learning. The problem is relevant to future tasks that will be performed as a clinician and serves to guide the student in self-directed learning. Learning results from the process of working toward understanding a clinical problem. This stimulates the student to use reasoning skills and to search for information and possible ways to solve the problem.

The goals of these strategies are to make the learning student focused; to encourage the students to think critically, to solve problems, to learn on their own; and to promote lifelong learning.

For the experiential part of the pharmacy curriculum, it is now recommended (by the ACPE) that there be experiential training in all four professional years of the Pharm.D. degree curriculum. In some schools of pharmacy, students in their first professional year (P1s) gain *introductory pharmacy practice experience* while shadowing students in their fourth professional year (P4s), who spend their entire year on various *advanced pharmacy practice experiences*. However, shadowing is only a descriptive term, as all pharmacy students need to learn by doing during experiential clerkships rather than just observing.

Students in their second professional year (P2s) may gain introductory experience in community pharmacy practice, whereas students in their third professional year (P3s) might gain introductory experience in hospital pharmacy practice. This varies from school to school.

Assessment and Evaluation

Teaching and learning is not complete without good assessment and evaluation of the teaching and learning. The assessment of student learning is accomplished by testing. This is the most objective method of assessment, and if the testing instrument is constructed properly, the assessment is valid. Experiential training, especially those during the fourth professional year, can be assessed by assessing professional and clinical competencies, as stated in the curricular outcomes outlined in the school's curricular outcomes document.

Evaluation of teaching takes two forms — evaluation by the students of the course and evaluation of the faculty teaching the course. Most students underestimate the power of their input and the value schools of pharmacy place on these evaluations. The outcomes of the course evaluation can result in major changes in course design.

Student and peer (other faculty members) evaluations of individual faculty are used by the faculty member's department chairperson to evaluate the faculty member for teaching effectiveness and to address changes the faculty member may need to make to be a more effective teacher. Evaluating a faculty member's teaching is part of the overall, annual evaluation of the faculty member by the chairperson, and the evaluation directly affects the faculty member's merit increase for the coming year.

The Scholarship of Research

Most pharmacy students only think of pharmacy professors as teachers. Many students assume that when they are off from school (spring break and summer vacation), so are their professors. The truth is that most pharmacy faculty members have full-time, year-around appointments. That is because most professors spend less than half of their time teaching. They must also perform research and provide service. Most tenure track faculty spend as much time in research as they do in teaching.

The research performed by a pharmacy faculty member is dependent on the credentials of the faculty member, the position he or she holds (tenure track or nontenure track), and the extent of external funding he or she has for their research. It also depends on how much support (school, graduate students, or fellows) the faculty member has to do the research and his or her agreement with the department chairperson. The time spent on research, teaching, and service is renegotiated each year based on the needs of the school and the wishes of the faculty member.

Pharmacy students need to understand a few things about the research their professors are conducting. First, tuition money is not used to support pharmacy research. The money for research comes form pharmaceutical companies, government agencies, and private foundations. It is the pharmacy faculty's job to find funding for their research, and this is not an easy task. Faculty must write outstanding grant proposals to be funded, and the competition is stiff.

Second, the quality of the research being done by faculty members, and their graduate students and fellows, in the schools and colleges of pharmacy in the United States is high quality, being every bit as good as those working in the pharmaceutical industry and the government.

Third, students benefit a great deal from the research ideas being pursued by their professors. Many times, continuing aspects of research being performed by professors are shared with students. In these situations, the students receive the latest information about a topic. This is because professors must be well read and versed on what everyone else is doing in their area of interest.

The outcomes of research are publishing the results in a reputable journal and presenting the results at professional meetings. To do this, the research is carefully reviewed by a group of peers to ensure that the work was done according to well-accepted research techniques.

Service

Pharmacy faculty members are also obligated to provide service. Service has several components:

Service to the university: To run effectively, a university needs continual input from its faculty. It gets this by having various university committees, many of which are composed of faculty members. Examples of a few university committees are the faculty [House of Delegates], the university benefits committee, and the institutional review board (IRB).

Service to the school of pharmacy: Like the university, a school of pharmacy also has various committees composed of faculty. Some important committees are the curriculum committee, the promotion and tenure committee, and the faculty advisory committee.

Service to the faculty member's department. A faculty member's department may also have several standing committees and *ad hoc* task forces to which faculty members are appointed or volunteer their services.

Service to the profession: Pharmacy faculty members are often active in various international, national, state, and local professional pharmacy organizations as active members, serving as officers, chairpersons, or members of a committee. Faculty members also make presentations at meetings of these organizations. Some faculty members also serve as reviewers of manuscripts submitted to professional publications, including scientific and clinical journals and books.

Service to practice: Some pharmacy-practice faculty will have some of their time assigned to precepting students on introductory or advanced practice experiences. Faculty members who are pharmacists may occasionally practice pharmacy to keep their skills up-to-date and to be able to introduce practical examples when teaching.

Service to the community: Unlike service to the profession, faculty members are not required to provide service to the community. However, universities are a part of a larger community. Therefore, if faculty members perform community service, they receive credit, as it brings honor to the university as well as the faculty members.

FACULTY EVALUATION

Department chairpersons evaluate their faculty members in most schools and colleges of pharmacy on a routine basis. However, the process varies widely from school to school. The criteria for the review are how well the faculty member performed his or her teaching, research, and service. The evaluation document may be a faculty member's plan for the year, as agreed to by the faculty member's chairperson. For example, there may have been agreement on the extent and quality of teaching performed, the amount of research, the number of publications and grants submitted and approved, and the extent of service. This assessment has bearing on annual increases in salary and provides feedback to the faculty member on the possibility of promotion and tenure.

JOB SATISFACTION

One study showed that pharmacy faculty members were basically satisfied with their positions and use of, but not pay for, their skills. For salary, faculty at state and public schools with graduate programs were more satisfied than faculty at private institutions without graduate programs. Those who said service consumed the least amount of their time had a greater general job satisfaction.[15]

Another study measured job stress among school of pharmacy faculty. It was found the highest stress was associated with securing funding for research, having too heavy a workload, and having excessively high self-expectations.[16]

A 2005 report titled "Academia: A Rewarding and Critically Important Career Path" discussed the many rewards of being a pharmacy academic, one of which is collaboration with other pharmacy faculty and other health professionals.[17]

PREPARATION FOR AN ACADEMIC CAREER

Being successful in academia means more than just having the educational and training requirements to be a member of the academy. Successful academics are outstanding teachers, scholars, and service providers. Successful academics like to pursue new knowledge, possess superb library skills, writing skills, and presentation skills. They like dealing with data. They are also lifelong learners, not only in pharmacy and science, but in the arts.

SUMMARY

A career in academia can be challenging and rewarding. Although academia does not offer the financial rewards that come with jobs in practice and in industry, it has other satisfying rewards. Academia offers diversity and flexibility. It also offers satisfaction by seeing students learn and grow and discovering answers to research questions.[18]

Professors are widely respected individuals, who are usually interesting people, in that they are often well read and well traveled, and the academy is a wonderful place for intellectual pursuit, exchange and stimulation.

DISCUSSION QUESTIONS AND EXERCISES

1. Designate your level of interest (1 = low, 10 = high) for the following academic functions:
   a. Didactic, classroom teaching
   b. Research (basic science, clinical, or pharmacy practice)
   c. Experiential teaching (teaching students on pharmacy practice rotations)
   d. Academic administration or service, and/or practice (working with patients)
   e. Practice (working with patients)
2. In regard to teaching, do you like to:
   a. Help people learn new things?
   b. Help people problem solve?
   c. Help people think critically?
   d. Help people apply new knowledge?
3. In regard to research, do you like:
   a. Solving puzzles?
   b. Designing experiments?
   c. Collecting data?
   d. Analyzing data?
   e. Writing?
   f. Making presentations?
4. What proportion (%) of time, if any, would you like to spend working with patients?
5. If you were a pharmacy faculty member, how would you prefer to spend your time? For the following five areas, assign percentages of time to each. The total must add to 100%. Didactic teaching (___%), experiential teaching (___%), research (___%), service (___%), and practice (___%).

6. Faculty members of a school of pharmacy are supposed to be academics, and academics are supposed to be scholars. What do these terms mean?

7–8. Make an appointment to interview at least two of the following:
a. A tenure-track basic science faculty member
b. A tenure-track faculty member in pharmacy administration
c. A tenure-track faculty member in pharmacy practice
d. A non-tenure-track faculty member in pharmacy practice

9. What do you see as the pros and cons of academic pharmacy?

10. Based upon what you know and have read thus far, does academic pharmacy interest you? Why? Why not?

CHALLENGES

1. Pharmacy needs more students in graduate programs (pharmaceutical science and pharmacy administration). For extra credit, and with the permission of your professor, look into the graduate courses at your college of pharmacy and write a concise paper on how schools of pharmacy can attract more undergraduate students into their graduate programs.

2. You will never really know what it is like to be a professor of pharmacy unless you take a didactic elective or senior rotation in academic pharmacy. If your school of pharmacy does not have either of these experiences available, for extra credit, and with the permission of your professor, find an interested pharmacy professor you can shadow for at least eight hours and write a concise report on your experience.

WEB SITES OF INTEREST

American Assocociation of Colleges of Pharmacy: www.aacp.org
Accreditation Council for Pharmacy Education: http://www.acpe-accredit.org/
American Foundation for Pharmaceutical Education: http://www.afpenet.org

REFERENCES

1. Bender, GA, and Thom, RA. *Great Moments in Pharmacy: The Stories and Paintings in the Series, a History of Pharmacy in Pictures, by Parke Davis & Company*. Northwood Institute Press. Detroit, MI, 1965.

2. American Association of Colleges of Pharmacy. *Academic Pharmacy's Vital Statistics*. Institutions and Programs. Updated September, 2005.

3. National Center for Health Workforce Analysis: *U.S. Health Workforce Personnel Factbook*. Available at http://bhpr.hrsa.gov/healthworkforce/reports/factbook.htm. Accessed May 7, 2006.

4. Rajayya, M. Pharmacy graduates from foreign countries flooding US job market. *Am J Pharm. Ed.* 2003. Available at http://www.findarticles.com/p/articles/mi_qa3833/is_200301/ai_n9175915. Accessed May 7, 2006.

5. Foreign pharmacy graduates. Available at http://www.immigration.com/student/pharmacy.html#definition. Accessed May 7, 2006.

6. Kinnard, WJ. Teaching and its encouragement (some post-decanal ramblings). *J Pharm Teach.* 1994;4(2):3–18.

7. Draugalis, JR. The scholarship of teaching as career development. *Am J Pharm Ed.* 1999;63:359–363.

8. Kennedy, DT, Ruffin, DM, Goode, JV, and Small, RE. The role of academia in community-based pharmaceutical care. *Pharmacotherapy.* 1997:17:1352–1356.

9. Vogenberg, FR. Academia and the challenge of managed care. *Hosp Pharm.* 1997;32:170–178.

10. Francisco, GE, and White, CA. Model for curricular assessment. AACP Annual Meeting. 2000;01(Jul):110.

11. Kelly, WN, Chrymko, MM, and Bender, FH. Interest and resources for non-traditional PharmD programs in Pennsylvania. *Am J Pharm Ed.* 1994; 58:171–176.

12. Kelly, WN, Francisco, GE, Brooks, PJ, and Marquess, JG. Development of a non-traditional PharmD program offered jointly between a private and public university. *Am J Pharm Ed.* 2000;64:59–61.

13. American Association of Pharmaceutical Scientists. Is a career in the pharmaceutical sciences right for me? Available at www.aapspharmaceutica.com/products/career/careerinps.htm. Accessed May 20, 2001.

14. Brandt, BF. Effective teaching and learning strategies. *Pharmacotherapy.* 2000;20:307S–316S.

15. Stajich, GV, Murphy, JE, and Barnett, CW. Job satisfaction of pharmacy faculty: a preliminary examination. *Am J Pharm Ed.* 1988;52:64–67.

16. Wolfgang, AP. Job stress and dissatisfaction among school of pharmacy faculty members. *Am J Pharm Ed.* 1993;57:215–221.

17. Cobaugh, DJ. Academia: a rewarding and critically important career path. *Am J Health Syst Pharm.* 2005;62:1204.

18. Murphy, N. Exploring your choices for the future: perspectives in pharmacy-academia. *Wash Pharm.* 1992;34:21.

16

PHARMACY ORGANIZATIONS

From its beginning, pharmacy formed groups that share common interests and concerns. At first these groups (mostly in Europe) were called guilds. Guilds eventually became associations. Now these groups are called professional organizations. Pharmacy organizations are important to current and future practitioners, as they help define, defend, and promote the profession.

This chapter will provide some brief history about pharmacy organizations, explain what they do, the kinds of organizations, and why they are important. The importance of pharmacists joining pharmacy organizations will be discussed, and several pharmacy organizations will be highlighted.

LEARNING OBJECTIVES

After reading this chapter, you should be able to:

- Define a professional pharmacy organization
- Discuss some brief history of pharmacy organizations
- Provide two roles for pharmacy organizations
- State the importance of joining pharmacy organizations
- Name the types of pharmacy organizations

A BRIEF HISTORY

Before the colonization of America, various trade professions in Europe banded together into groups called *guilds*. Pharmacy guilds were a way for apothecaries and chemists to gather to discuss items of common interest, share medicinal recipes, settle on how young apprentices should be trained, and keep the profession together. Pharmacy guilds often received royal or city sanction.[1] Associations formed from guilds and were organized for economic, social, professional, and scientific purposes. Thus, it was natural for the first chemists and apothecaries in this country to form associations when they came here from Europe.

Few chemists and apothecaries existed during colonial times in the United States. Physicians dispensed most of the medicine. In early 1821, J. Redmond Coxe, a prominent professor at the University of Pennsylvania, was concerned with the varying skills among chemists, apothecaries, and druggists in Philadelphia.[2] He made a suggestion "to which 16 prominent Philadelphia druggists affixed their signatures, proposing that an honorary degree be granted to such apothecaries 'as they have taken every measure to become perfect masters of their profession'...."[2] This action by the University of Pennsylvania roused the indignation of those druggists not granted the honorary degree.

A committee was appointed by the university to look further into this matter. One of the committee's recommendations was to set up a college of apothecaries. This college was founded on March 13, 1821, as the first recognized professional pharmacy organization in the United States. About 1 year later (March 20, 1822), the name was changed to the Philadelphia College of Pharmacy.

Soon cities such as Boston (1823) and New York (1829) formed their own local pharmacy associations.[3] In 1852, the American Pharmaceutical Association (APhA) became the first national pharmaceutical organization in the United States (Figure 16.1).[4] Under the APhA, statewide pharmacy organizations started to grow; the first one in Maine in 1867.

National pharmacy organizations that followed the APhA included the National Wholesale Druggists (NWDA) in 1882, the National Retail Druggists Association (NRDA) in 1883, and the National Association of Retail Druggists (NARD) in 1898. The National Association of Boards of Pharmacy was formed in 1904, the Chain Store Association (NCSA) in 1933, the American College of Apothecaries in 1940, and the American Society of Hospital Pharmacists in 1942. Relatively new national pharmacy organizations include the American Society of Consultant Pharmacists formed in 1969, the American College of Clinical Pharmacy in 1979, and the Academy of Managed Care Pharmacy in 1988.[3,5]

THE ROLE OF PHARMACY ORGANIZATIONS

Most pharmacists do not have the time or the financial resources to attend to the current conflicts or opportunities facing the profession. This is where pharmacy organizations can help. "Organized associations are to pharmacists what government is to its citizens. They represent, protect, and propagate the profession of pharmacy."[6]

Each pharmacy organization has a constitution, bylaws, a statement of beliefs, a mission statement, and sometimes a vision statement to govern

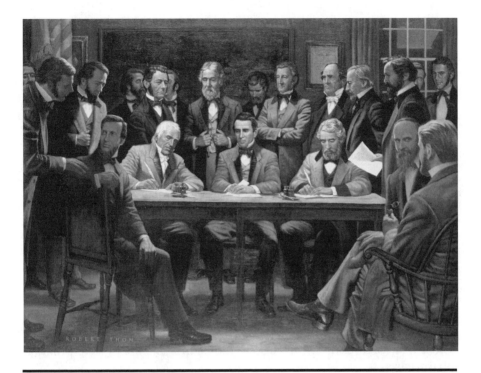

Figure 16.1 The American Pharmaceutical Association, 1852. (From Bender, GA and Thom, RA. *Great Moments in Pharmacy. The Stories and Paintings in the Series, a History of Pharmacy in Pictures,* by Parke Davis & Company. Pfizer, Inc. and Northwood Institute Press, 1965.)

the organization. Most pharmacy organizations are member driven and have elected officers and full-time staff members.

Zellmer has set forth the argument that national pharmacy organizations play a role in transforming the profession, and he uses pharmaceutical care to state his case.[6] Zellmer's view is that national pharmacy organizations have played a critical role in diffusing the idea of pharmaceutical care deeply into the profession, and that time will show that pharmacy organizations are effective change agents for pharmaceutical care.

THE IMPORTANCE OF MEMBERSHIP

It is important for pharmacists to belong to pharmacy organizations. "After investing time and money in pharmacy school, pharmacists should ensure their place on the health care team by joining a professional association," says Patricia Poole, who was a pharmacy student at the time she wrote that statement.[6]

As reported in *American Pharmacy* in 1986, and based on information from Schering Laboratories' "Inside Pharmacy: The Anatomy of a Profession," pharmacists belonging to a national pharmacy association said they were very satisfied with work in general (52%) compared to with non-members (31%).[7] Members of pharmacy organizations were also satisfied in dealing with patients and had status and pride as pharmacists. When asked about their reasons for joining a national pharmacy organization, pharmacists cited education and training, financial benefits, social benefits, and influence on legislation.[8]

PHARMACY ORGANIZATIONS

Pharmacy organizations can be divided into: (a) practitioner organizations, (b) educational organizations, (c) special interest organizations, (d) trade organizations, (e) pharmacy technician organizations, and (f) other organizations. The following is a comprehensive, but not exclusive, descriptive summary of various national pharmacy organizations.

Pharmacy Practitioner Organizations

These are organizations in which the active members are primarily pharmacists.

American College of Apothecaries (ACA)

> 2830 Summer Oakes Drive
> Bartlett, TN 38134-3811
> http://acainfo.org
> (901) 383-8119
> (901) 383-8882 (fax)

The ACA's mission is to translate and disseminate knowledge, research data, and recent developments in professional pharmacy practice for the benefit of pharmacists, pharmacy students, and the public. The ACA has about 700 members. There are qualifications for membership.

American College of Clinical Pharmacy (ACCP)

> P.O. Box 458
> Glastonburg, CT 06033
> http://www.accp.com
> (203) 281-4322
> (860) 633-6023 (fax)

The ACCP is a professional and scientific society that provides leadership, education, advocacy, and resources enabling clinical pharmacists to achieve excellence in practice and research. Currently, more than 7000 pharmacists belong to ACCP.

Academy of Managed Care Pharmacy (AMCP)

100 North Pitt Street, Suite 400
Alexandria, VA 22314
http://www.amcp.org
(703) 683-8416
(800) 827-2627
(703) 683-8417 (fax)

The AMCP is the national professional society dedicated to the idea and practice of pharmaceutical care in managed care environments. Currently, 4800 pharmacists belong to AMCP.

American Pharmacists Association (APhA)

2215 Constitution Avenue, NW
Washington, DC 20037-2985
http://www.aphanet.org
(202) 628-4410
(800) 237-2742
(202) 783-2351 (fax)

The APhA is the national professional society for pharmacists. The APhA is dedicated to improving public health by helping its members and strengthening the profession of pharmacy. Currently, the APhA has more than 50,000 members.

American Society of Consultant Pharmacists (ASCP)

1321 Duke Street
Alexandria, VA 22314-3563
http://www.ascp.com
(703) 739-1300
(703) 739-1321 (fax)

The ASCP is the international professional association that provides leadership, education, advocacy, and resources to advance the practice of senior care pharmacy. Currently, the ASCP has more than 7000 pharmacist members.

American Society of Health-System Pharmacists (ASHP)

> 7272 Wisconsin Avenue
> Bethesda, Maryland 20814
> http://www.ashp.org
> (301) 657-3000
> (301) 652-8278 (fax)

The ASHP represents pharmacists who practice in hospitals and other parts of health care systems. The history of the organization has been documented.[10] Currently, the ASHP has about 30,000 members.

International Academy of Compounding Pharmacists (IACP)

> P.O. Box 1365 Sugar Land, TX 77487
> http://www.iacprx.org
> Phone: 281-933-8400
> Toll-Free Referral Line 800-927-4227
> Fax: 281-495-0602

Since 1991, the IACP has fought to protect, promote, and advance the art and skill of the compounding pharmacy profession. IACP represents more than 1800 pharmacists, physicians, technicians, and patients who are committed to practicing quality pharmacy compounding.

National Community Pharmacists Association (NCPA)

> 100 Daingerfield Road
> Alexandria, VA 22314
> http://www.ncpanet.org
> (703) 683-8200
> (800) 544-7447
> (703) 683-3619 (fax)

The NCPA represents the pharmacist owners, managers, and employees of nearly 25,000 independent community pharmacies across the United States.

National Pharmaceutical Association (NPhA)

107 Kilmayne Drive, Suite C
Cary, NC 27511
http://npha.net
(800) 944-6742
(919) 469-5870 (fax)

The NphA is dedicated to representing the views and ideas of minority pharmacists on critical issues affecting health care and pharmacy. The NPhA seeks to serve as a role model, through its members, for minority youth and vigorously supports their recruitment into the profession. Currently, NPhA has about 200 pharmacist members.

Joint Commission of Pharmacy Practitioners (JCPP)

D.C. Huffman, Corresponding Secretary
Executive Director of ACA
5788 Stage Road
Suite 206
Bartlett, TN 38134
Web page not available
(901) 383-8819
(901) 383-8882 (fax)

The JCPP, created in 1977, is a federation of national pharmacy practitioner organizations: AMCP, ACA, ACCP, APhA, ASCP, ASHP, and NCPA. Non-practitioner organizations, including AACP, NABP, and NCSPAE, are liaison members. The JCPP meets quarterly to examine current issues facing the profession and explore if they wish to collaborate on any issues.

Educational Organizations

These organizations are exclusively involved with education or the accreditation of education for students in pharmacy schools or pharmacists.

Accreditation Council for Pharmaceutical Education (ACPE)

20 North Clark Street, Suite 2500
Chicago, IL 60602-5109
http://www.acpe-accredit.org
(312) 664-3575
(312) 664-4652 or (312) 664-7008 (fax)

The ACPE is the national agency for the accreditation of professional degree programs in pharmacy and providers of continuing education. The ACPE is an autonomous and independent agency whose board of directors is drawn from AACP, APhA, NABP, and the American Council on Education (ACE).

American Association of Colleges of Pharmacy (AACP)

1426 Prince Street
Alexandria, VA 22314
http://www.aacp.org
(703) 739-2330
(703) 836-8982 (fax)

The AACP is the national organization representing the interests of pharmaceutical education and educators. It is composed of all 89 U.S. pharmacy colleges and schools including more than 4,000 faculty, 36,000 students enrolled in professional programs, and 3,600 individuals continuing graduate study.

American Foundation for Pharmaceutical Education (AFPE)

One Church Street, Suite 202
Bethesda, MD 20850
http://www.afpenet.org
(301) 738-2160
(301) 738-2161 (fax)

The AFPE is the only U.S. organization whose sole purpose is funding undergraduate research projects, graduate education, and faculty research at schools and colleges of pharmacy.

Special Interest Organizations

These organizations are for pharmacists interested in a certain aspect or specialty practice in pharmacy.

American Association of Homeopathic Pharmacists (AAHP)

5112 Wilshire Drive
Santa Rosa, CA 95404
http://www.homeopathicpharmacy.org
(800) 478-0421
(800) 478-0421 (fax)

The AAHP is a not-for-profit corporation representing the interests of homeopathic manufacturers, distributors, and individual pharmacists in cooperative efforts with regulatory agencies and other organizations nationally.

American Association of Pharmaceutical Scientists (AAPS)

2107 Wilson Blvd., Suite 700
Arlington, VA 22201-3042
http://www.aaps.org
(703) 243-2800
(703) 243-9650 (fax)

The AAPS represents more than 12,000 members employed in academia, industry, government, and other research institutes worldwide.

American College of Veterinary Pharmacists (ACVP)

2830 Summer Oaks Drive
Bartlett, TN 38134-3811
http://www.vetmeds.org
(877) 838-6337
(901) 383-8882 (fax)

The ACVP, a subsidiary organization of ACA, supports the efforts of independent pharmacists who provide services for animals and veterinarians.

American Institute of the History of Pharmacy (AIHP)

777 Highland Avenue
Madison, WI 53705-2222
http://www.aihp.org
(608) 262-5378

The AIHP is a nonprofit national organization devoted to advancing knowledge and understanding of the place of pharmacy in history. It is composed of pharmacists and pharmacy historians.

American Society for Automation in Pharmacy (ASAP)

492 Norristown Road, Suite 160
Blue Bell, PA 19422-2359
http://www.asapnet.org
(610) 825-7783
(610) 825-7641 (fax)

The ASAP helps its members in advancing the application of computer technology in the pharmacist's role as caregiver and in the efficient operation and management of a pharmacy.

American Society of Pharmacognosy (ASP)

> 3149 Dundee Rd. #260
> Northbrook, IL 60062
> David J. Slatkin, PhD, treasurer
> http://www.phcog.org
> (623) 202-3500
> (847) 656-2800 (fax)

The ASP is an international group that brings together men and women dedicated to the promotion, growth, and development not only of pharmacognosy but also to all aspects of those sciences related to and dealing in natural products.

American Society for Parenteral and Enteral Nutrition (ASPEN)

> 8630 Fenton Street, Suite 412
> Silver Spring, MD 20910-3805
> http://www.clinnutr.org
> (301) 587-6315
> (301) 587-2365 (fax)

The ASPEN represents members who are involved in the provision of clinical nutrition therapies, including parenteral and enteral nutrition. Physicians, pharmacists, nurses, dieticians, and other health professionals belong to ASPEN.

American Society for Pharmacy Law (ASPL)

> 1224 Centre West, #400B
> Springfield, IL 62704
> http://www.aspl.org
> (217) 391-0219
> (217) 793-0041 (fax)

The ASPL is an organization of pharmacist–lawyers, whose members are pharmacists who are interested in the law as it applies to pharmacy, lawyers who are interested in the subject of pharmacy law, and students of these disciplines.

Food and Drug Law Institute (FDLI)

1000 Vermont Avenue, N.W., Suite 200
Washington, DC 20005
http://www.fdli.org
(202) 371-1420
(800) 956-6293
(202) 371-0649 (fax)

The FDLI is a nonprofit institute dedicated to advancing public health by providing a neutral forum for critical examination of the laws, regulations, and policies related to drugs, medical devices, other health care technologies, and foods.

International Society for Pharmacoepidemiology (ISPE)

5272 River Road, Suite 630
Bethesda, Maryland 20816
http://www.pharmacoepi.org
(301) 718-6500
(301) 656-0989 (fax)

The ISPE is a nonprofit international professional membership organization dedicated to promoting pharmacoepidemiology, the science that applies epidemiological approaches to studying the use, effectiveness, value, and safety of pharmaceuticals.

International Society for Pharmacoeconomic and Outcomes Research (ISPOR)

3100 Princeton Pike
Building 3, Suite E
Lawrenceville, NJ 08648
http://www.ispor.org
(609) 219-0773
(609) 219-0774 (fax)

The ISPOR is an international organization promoting the science of pharmacoeconomics and health outcomes research.

Parenteral Drug Association (PDA)

Bethesda Metro Center, Suite 1500
Bethesda, MD 20814
http://www.pda.org

(301) 656-5900
(301) 986-0296 (fax)

The PDA is a nonprofit, international association of scientists involved in the development, manufacture, quality control, and regulation of pharmaceuticals and related products.

Society of Veterinary Hospital Pharmacy (SVHP)

Starr Miller, President
School of Veterinary Medicine
Tuskegee University
Tuskegee, AL 36088
http://www.svhp.org

The purpose of the SVHP is to further the interests and continuing education for veterinary hospital pharmacists.

Pharmacy Technician Organizations

These organizations are for pharmacy technicians, educators of pharmacy technicians, or accreditation of pharmacy technician programs.

American Association of Pharmacy Technicians (AAPT)

P.O. Box 1447
Greensboro, NC 27402
http://www.pharmacytechnician.com
(336) 333-9356
(877) 368-4771
(336) 333-9068 (fax)

The AAPT provides leadership and represents the interests of its members to the public as well as health care organizations.

National Pharmacy Technician Association (NPTA)

3707 FM 1960 RD W
Suite #460
Houston , TX 77068
http://www.pharmacytechnician.org/
(888) 247-8700
(281) 866-7900
(281) 895-7320 (fax)

NPTA is the leading provider of technician-specific CEs in the United States. You can access CE online with immediate grading and certificate issuance.

Pharmacy Technician Certification Board (PTCB)

2215 Constitution Avenue, NW
Washington, DC 20037-2985
http://www.PTCB.org
(800) 363-8012
(202) 429-7596 (fax)

The PTCB is the organization that oversees the process of pharmacy technician certification.

Pharmacy Technician Educators Council (PTEC)

1426 Prince Street
Alexandria, VA 22314-2841
http://www.pharmacy.org/pharmtech.html
(703) 683-9493

The PTEC is an organization for educators of pharmacy technicians.

Pharmacy Trade Organizations

These organizations represent the interests of owners of corporately owned drug companies, wholesalers, and pharmacies, rather than pharmacists.

Chain Drug Marketing Association (CDA)

43157 W. Nine Mile Road
P.O. Box 995
Novi, MI 48376-0995
http://www.chaindrug.com
(248) 449-9300
(248) 449-4634 (fax)

The CDA's sole purpose is to support chain drug owners' marketing and merchandising efforts.

Food Marketing Institute (FMI)

655 15th Street, NW
Washington, DC 20005
http://www.fmi.org
(202) 452-8944
(202) 429-4519 (fax)

Generic Pharmaceutical Association (GPhA)

2300 Clarendon Blvd., Suite 400
Arlington, VA 22201
http://www.gphaonline.org
(703) 647-2480
(703) 647-2481 (fax)

The GPhA represents the generic drug manufacturers and shares a commitment to improving consumer access to high-quality, affordable medicine.

Healthcare Distribution Management Association (HDMA)

901 North Glebe Road
Suite 1000
Arlington, VA 22203
http://www.healthcaredistribution.org
(703) 787-0000
(703) 935-3200 (fax)

The HDMA is the only trade association representing pharmaceutical and related health care product distributors (e.g., drug wholesalers) in the Americas.

National Pharmaceutical Council (NPC)

1894 Preston White Drive
Reston, VA 20191-5433
http://www.npcnow.org
(703) 620-6390
(703) 476-0904 (fax)

The NPC is supported by more than 20 of the nation's major research pharmaceutical companies. It sponsors various research and education projects aimed at showing the correct use of pharmaceuticals that improve both patient treatment outcomes and the cost-effective delivery of overall health care services.

National Association of Chain Drug Stores (NACDS)

413 N. Lee Street
P.O. Box 1417-D49
Alexandria, VA 22313-1480
http://www.nacds.org
(703) 549-3001
(703) 836-4869 (fax)

The NACDS represents chain drugstore owners including supermarket chains, traditional chain drugstores, and mass merchandisers.

Pharmaceutical Care Management Association (PCMA)

601 Pennsylvania Ave, NW
Seventh Floor
Washington, DC 20004
http://www.pcmanet.org
(202) 207-3610
(202) 207-3623 (fax)

The PCMA represents managed care pharmacy and its health care partners in pharmaceutical care: managed care organizations, PBMs, HMOs, PPOs, third-party administrators, health care insurance companies, drug wholesalers, pharmaceutical manufacturers, and community pharmacy networks.

Pharmaceutical Research and Manufacturers of America (PhRMA)

1100 15th Street NW, Suite 900
Washington, DC 20005
http://www.phrma.org
(202) 835-3400
(202) 835-3414 (fax)

The PhRMA represents the country's leading research-based pharmaceutical and biotechnology companies, which are devoted to developing medicines that allow patients to live longer, healthier, happier, and more productive lives.

Other Organizations

Board of Pharmaceutical Specialties (BPS)

2215 Constitution Avenue, NW
Washington, DC 20037-2985
http://www.bpsweb.org
(202) 429-7591
(202) 429-6304 (fax)

The BPS improves the public health through recognition and promotion of specialized training, knowledge, and skills in pharmacy and certification of pharmacist specialists.

Commission for Certification in Geriatrics Pharmacy (CCGP)

1321 Duke Street
Alexandria, VA 22314-3513
http://www.ccgp.org
(703) 535-3038
(703) 739-1500 (fax)

The CCGP tests and certifies pharmacists in geriatric pharmacy.

International Pharmaceutical Federation (FIP)

2517 JP The Hague
The Netherlands
http://www.pharmweb.net/fip.html
(31)(70) 302-1970
(31)(70) 302-1999 (fax)

The FIP is a worldwide federation of national (professional and scientific) associations, which has a mission to represent and serve pharmacy and pharmaceutical sciences around the globe.

National Association of Boards of Pharmacy (NABP)

1600 Freehanville Drive
Mount Prospect, IL 60056
http://www.nabp.net
(847) 391-4406
(847) 391-4502 (fax)

The NABP is the only professional association that represents the state boards of pharmacy in all 50 states, the Virgin Islands, New Zealand, nine Canadian Provinces, and the four Australian states.

United States Pharmacopeia (USP)

12601 Twinbrook Parkway
Rockville, MD 20852-1790
http://www.usp.org
(301) 881-0666
(800) 227-8772
(301) 816-8148 (fax)

The USP sets up standards to ensure the quality of medicine for human and veterinary use. The USP also develops authoritative information about the correct use of medicines. National health care practitioner reporting programs support U.S. public health standards and information programs.

SHOULD PHARMACY ORGANIZATIONS CHANGE?

An article entitled "Restructuring America's Pharmacy Associations" asks whether pharmacy organizations adequately represent and address the concerns of the profession.[9] The main thrust of this editorial is that many pharmacy organizations are in decline because of the restructuring of health care that has caused reduced memberships, especially at the state level. Another thought is that enormous energy is being used to fight undesirable changes in health care that take place anyway. The author calls for a strategic assessment of the organizational structure of American pharmacy.

Another question is whether there are too many pharmacy organizations. Currently, no one organization can speak for the practice of pharmacy. Donald E. Francke, during his 1953 A.K. Whitney Award lecture, wrote:

> It is my firm conviction that American pharmacy will not come into its own until we have a majority of our pharmacists actively supporting their national professional organization. Someone has defined an organization as a medium for the efficient movement of groups of men towards goals to which they aspire. How can we move American pharmacists towards professional goals until we enroll them in our association? Only when this is done will the Association, its ideals, its ethics, its concepts of professional service be ingrained in all who practice our profession.[10]

The JCPP represents the seven pharmacy organizations that represent practicing pharmacists. This is a good start; however, this group only works by consensus, is not known by many pharmacists, and does not have trumping power over the minority opinions of its member organizations. At this point, one voice for pharmacy seems far off, but it remains a dream of many pharmacists.

SUMMARY

There are over 30 professional organizations in pharmacy. They are divided into practitioner, educational, special interest, technician, trade, and other types of organizations. Pharmacy organizations play a critical role in representing their members, and they are important change agents in moving pharmacy forward. Therefore, it is important for every pharmacist to be a member of at least one pharmacy organization.

DISCUSSION QUESTIONS AND EXERCISES

1. Why are professional pharmacy organizations important? Of all of these reasons, which reason is most important to you? Why?
2. It is recommended (by this author) that all pharmacists belong to at least one national, one state, and one local professional pharmacy organization. Why?
3. Using the listing of professional organizations in this chapter, select one organization that interests you from each type of organization.
   a. Practitioner organizations
   b. Educational organizations
   c. Special interest organizations
   d. Pharmacy technicians organizations
   e. Trade organizations
   f. Other organizations
4. Using your answers to question 3, visit those organizations' Web sites (they are listed in this chapter). Which organizations impress you the most? Why?
5. Investigate when and where local pharmacy organizations meet in your area. Attend two different meetings.
6. Before you graduate from pharmacy school, attend one state and one national pharmacy meeting.
7. In your opinion, what is the most important thing a professional pharmacy organization can do for its members?
8. Make an appointment to interview a pharmacist working for a professional pharmacy organization.

9. Based upon what you know and have read, what are the pros and cons of working for a professional pharmacy organization?

10. Is working for a professional pharmacy organization something you think you may want to do? Why or why not?

CHALLENGES

1. Some believe the pharmacy profession has too many pharmacy organizations speaking for it and that the messages sent to the public and congress are diluted and sometimes conflicting. For extra credit, and with the permission of your professor, prepare a concise report on this issue. Are there too many pharmacy organizations speaking for pharmacy? What can be done about it? Are there other models available to follow?

2. For extra credit, and with the permission of your professor, write a concise report debating the pros and cons of belonging to a national, state, and local pharmacy organization. Discuss how your dues money should be apportioned and why.

WEB SITES OF INTEREST

The web site for each pharmacy organization is in the text for each organization listed.

REFERENCES

1. Cowen, DL, and Helfand, WH. The Renaissance. In *Pharmacy: An Illustrated History*. Abrams, New York, 1990, chap. 4.

2. Kremers, E, and Urdang, G. The growth of associations. In *History of Pharmacy: A Guide and a Survey*. Lippincott, Philadelphia, 1951, chap. 13.

3. Wroblewski, JJ. Your associations and their roots. *Drug Top*. 1983;127:49–52.

4. Bender, GA, and Thom, RA. *Great Moments in Pharmacy: THE Stories and Paintings in the Series, a History of Pharmacy in Pictures*, by Parke Davis & Company. Northwood Institute Press, Detroit, MI, 1965.

5. Posey, LM. *Pharmacy Cadence*. PAS Pharmacy/Association Services, Athens, GA, 1992.

6. Zellmer, WA. Role of pharmacy organizations in transforming the profession: the case of pharmaceutical care. *Am J Health-Syst Pharm*. 2001;58:2041–2049.

7. Anonymous. Pharmacists in national associations more satisfied with work, Schering report shows. *Am Pharm*. 1986;26:12, 14.

8. Harris, RR, and McConnell, WE. The American Society of Hospital Pharmacists: a history. *Am J Hosp Pharm*. 1993;50:S3–S45.

9. Johnson, RC. Restructuring America's pharmacy associations. *J Am Pharm Assoc*. 1998;38:402, 404.

10. Francke, DE. Hospital pharmacy looks to the future. In *Harvey A.K. Whitney Award Lectures, 1950–1992*. ASHP Research and Education Foundation. Bethesda, MD, 1992.

17

HOW DRUGS ARE DISCOVERED, TESTED, AND APPROVED

It is exciting to read in the newspaper about a scientific "breakthrough" in developing a new drug, especially if you or a loved one has a debilitating or terminal disease. However, on further reading, you discover the product is still several years away from being available for use. Your exhilaration suddenly turns to frustration. Frank E. Young, former commissioner of the U.S. Food and Drug Administration (FDA), believes this happens because of the way the media reports the news and the public's unclear understanding of drug development, testing, and approval.[1]

Pharmacy is about patients, drugs, caring about the patient, and about the patient receiving the best drug for them. Therefore, it is important to understand how drugs are discovered, developed, tested, and approved for use.

This chapter will focus on new drug development in the United States. It will begin with a brief history of drug discovery and then move on to how drugs are discovered. Next will be information on drug design, drug testing, drug standards, and the critical step of drug approval. All of this takes time. This process will be discussed along with the associated developmental costs. The chapter ends with information on the postmarketing surveillance of drugs, generic drugs, over-the-counter drugs, and the future of drug discovery and development.

LEARNING OBJECTIVES

After this learning session, you should be able to:

- Discuss how drugs are discovered

- Discuss how drugs are tested
- Outline the drug approval process in the United States
- Explain the terms *IND*, *NDA*, and *IRB*
- Discuss drug standards and the USP
- Define the term *CGMP*
- Discuss generic and OTC drugs
- Discuss the importance of postmarketing surveillance

A BRIEF HISTORY OF DRUG DISCOVERY AND DEVELOPMENT

Although many small steps took place in discovering and developing modern drugs, the first breakthrough was by Swedish pharmacist Carl Wilhelm Scheele, who in the early 1800s, isolated organic plant acids. In 1816, a young German apothecary, Friedrich Sertuner, gave the world its first class of organic substances — the *alkaloids* — by isolating morphine from opium. Soon to follow (1817 to 1820) was the discovery of emetine from *ipecacuanha*, strychnine from *nux vomica*, and quinine from cinchona bark by two French pharmacists, Pierre-Joseph Pellitier and Joseph-Bienaime Caventou.[2]

These drug discoveries provoked concern about standardizing drug formulas. In 1820, the *United States Pharmacopeia* (USP) was started to develop drug standards. Following this was a surge in discovering new medicinal plants from various parts of the world including jungles, forests, and mountainous areas. These excursions to find new drugs continued at a brisk pace until 1940 and then slowed down.

In the late 1800s and early 1900s, scientists were discovering *biological products* such as diphtheria antitoxin. Horses were inoculated with diphtheria toxin. After the horse developed diphtheria antibodies, the horse's serum was collected and purified to make diphtheria antitoxin. Soon to follow were other biological products of animal origin.

Ernest Fourneau (1872 to 1949), a French pharmacist at the Pasteur Institute, discovered that bismuth and arsenic compounds could be used to treat syphilis, developed sulfa drugs, and discovered the properties of antihistamines. These discoveries signaled the arrival of modern chemotherapy. In 1883, German scientists *synthesized* (made in a test tube) antipyrine. This dramatically changed drug discovery, design, and development from this point forward.

Research in pharmacy rapidly evolved between 1925 and 1945. The biggest step forward took place in 1929 when Alexander Fleming discovered penicillin. However, it was the pharmaceutical manufacturers — under the pressure of World War II — who developed mass production and purification methods for penicillin and made it affordable and widely available to physicians.

The last breakthrough to be discussed in this chapter is considered to be one of the greatest in medical science. In 1952, James Watson and Francis Crick, working at the Cavendish Laboratory in Cambridge, U.K., solved the puzzling structure of deoxyribonucleic acid (DNA).[3] This achievement was preceded by the work of Erwin Chargaff and Rosalind Franklin.[4] This event and the discovery of what makes up the human genome in 2000 will have a major impact on treating disease over the next 30 years.

HOW NEW DRUGS ARE DISCOVERED

Developing a new drug is complex and time consuming. Some feel it is like finding a needle in a haystack or a diamond in the rough. Drug discovery and development all starts with a human need and is based on *good science*. Good science uses proven scientific methods and avoids shortcuts in designing and developing new drugs.

The object of *drug discovery* is to find new active ingredients or to modify the chemical structures of existing active ingredients of drugs to form the basis of a new drug. The object of *drug development* is to provide superior dosage forms and ways of delivering effective drugs into the body.

The discovery of a new drug (the active ingredient of a drug product) and development of one or more dosage forms are so complex and technical that no one individual is qualified to carry out the operation from beginning to end. Thus, drug discovery, development, and approval take the services of many scientifically and administratively trained workers skilled in applying their knowledge to the problems of pharmacy.[5]

Pharmaceutical development is mostly done by scientists — usually those with a Ph.D. — working for pharmaceutical companies where extensive research laboratories, sophisticated equipment, and resources are available to do the research. However, pharmaceutical research is also conducted in the 89 colleges of pharmacy. Most bench (laboratory) research on drugs is performed by basic science faculty members. Pharmaceutical companies often contract with a college of pharmacy or an independent research institute to conduct some of their drug research.

DRUG DISCOVERY

The active ingredients of drugs are extracted from plants, mammalian hormones, microorganisms, and various semisynthetic and synthetic compounds. Today, some of the synthetic compounds are genetically engineered.

Plant Poisons

Before it was discovered that drugs could be synthesized, plants were the main source of physiologically active substances that could be tested for therapeutic properties. Some examples of drugs still used today that were first found from plants are morphine (from the opium poppy), quinine (from cinchona bark), digitalis (from foxglove), and belladonna (from deadly nightshade). These alkaloids are not present in these plants to supply humans with medicines but probably are present to discourage predators. The problem of using alkaloids from plants as drugs is a matter of purity and being able to produce enough quantity. Not all plants of the same species are grown under the same conditions. Thus, the alkaloid within each plant will vary in potency.

Inorganic Chemicals

The body's fluids and tissues contain various inorganic substances — chemicals such as potassium, sodium, chloride, and calcium — to help maintain homeostasis. Disease can cause the body to have either too much or too little of these substances. Fortunately, these chemicals are plentiful in nature and can be purified and made into sterile medicinal preparations for use by physicians.

Drugs from Animal Sources (Biologics)

Administering substances from animals dates from ancient Egypt. Apothecaries of old used substances from crayfish, earthworms, frogs, lizards, scorpions, snails, swallows, toads, vipers, and wood lice to compound powders, oils, and syrups.[6] Products drawn from animal sources such as thyroid, insulin, estrogen hormones, epineprhine, and diphtheria antitoxin are still used today.

Drugs from the Seas

Natural product researchers have recently been discovering interesting raw plant material as a source of new drugs in the tropical rain forests. However, the latest frontier for finding new sources of drugs is in the tropical seas.[7] Researchers at the National Cancer Institute's (NCI) natural products branch and at about 15 other laboratories throughout the country are screening such organisms as algae, invertebrates, and sponges. They are hoping to discover compounds that will lead to new drugs with antitumor, anti-inflammatory, antibacterial, and antiviral potential.

As of this writing, four substances from marine life are in clinical trials as anticancer drugs and four others are in preclinical trials — two as anticancer agents and two as anti-inflammatory agents.

Screening for New Natural Drug Products

Screening is the discovery of new drugs that might be of use later in clinical medicine.[8] Various approaches are used for screening compounds for pharmacological activity. All pharmacological screening is dependent on test methods that have a significant bearing on the disease they are to match in the laboratory.[9] Finding compounds and then testing them in various diseases is not considered to be a practical or fruitful approach to drug discovery.

The initial testing of drugs is always carried out in laboratory glassware (an *in vitro* experiment) rather than in an animal model (an *in vivo* experiment). A screening test must be selected that a skilled technician can perform easily and that will alert the technician to any potential the compound may have for the targeted disease selected. An example would be a potential drug substance inhibiting an enzyme associated with the disease. Once the experiments are set up, hundreds of potential compounds can be screened using these methods. Today, some screening of potential drug compounds is automated.

Synthetic Substitutes

Because of the variance in the potency of medicinal substances found in plants, it was necessary to see if these substances could be made in a test tube. The first drug for which synthetic substitutes were sought was quinine. Next came morphine and cocaine.[6] Once the structural formula is discovered for a new drug, an attempt is made to synthesize it, as this is the fastest and most inexpensive way to make a drug. This is how most drugs are produced today. However, sometimes the basis of a drug comes from a natural product and then is altered in the laboratory to become a *semisynthetic drug.*

Biotechnology

The latest approach to developing new drugs is *biotechnology.* The science of biotechnology is defined as the process of *in vitro* (in a test tube) change of genetic material for the purpose of creating new gene combinations or changes.[8] It relies on living systems to produce biological materials. Sometimes this process is called *molecular biology* or *genetic engineering.* The biotechnological approach to new drugs has been limited to proteins. Recombinant hepatitis B vaccine and recombinant insulin were two of the first biotechnological drugs.

NEW METHODS OF DRUG DESIGN

Until recently, most new drugs were discovered through random screening or through molecular change. However, new and exciting methods of drug discovery are starting to be employed. Rational drug design, using powerful computers, computational chemistry, x-ray crystallography, nuclear magnetic resonance spectroscopy, and three-dimensional structure activity relationship analysis is creating specific, biologically active molecules by virtual reality modeling.[9]

Sophisticated screening methods, using the latest technology, are used to remove all but the most promising lead compounds. These new methods should provide more efficacious, safer, and more cost-effective drugs while lessening development time and cost.

THE DRUG RESEARCHER

It takes a team of scientists to develop a new drug. These scientists come from several disciplines, mainly pharmaceutical chemistry, clinical pharmacology, clinical pharmacokinetics, clinical toxicology, and pharmaceutics. Once out of animal testing, development will involve clinical pharmacy and clinical medicine.

Pharmaceutical Chemistry

If the active ingredient is a natural product, pharmaceutical chemists will try to synthesize the parent compound. Once this is completed, these scientists may alter the parent compound by molecular change to decide if any of the compound's analogues are more active. After animal testing, they will discover if any are less toxic.

Clinical Pharmacology

The next step in the development of a drug is to see how the potential drug works in animals —preferable in animals with the disease for which the drug is intended; however, this is rare.

Biopharmaceutics and Clinical Pharmacokinetics

Before a drug dosage form can be tested in animals, it first must be determined how long it takes to dissolve and be available to the body.

This involves testing the drug's *bioavailability*. The results vary based on the drug's chemical makeup and pH (acidity and alkalinity) and on other nondrug components of the drug's *dosage form* (e.g., capsule, tablet, liquid). During testing in animals, the drug's absorption, distribution, metabolism, and excretion (ADME) is carefully measured using serum drug levels — or levels of other body fluid levels — and mathematical models to see how the drug is being handled (pharmacokinetically) in the body.

Clinical Toxicology

When testing in animals, an initial dose, then a usual dose, then a maximum dose is established for the substance. These form the basis for a starting dose for human testing.

Pharmaceutics

The active ingredient must be delivered in the proper dosage form to arrive at the intended site of action. This process will involve selecting the best routes of administration and drawing up the product so it dissolves and is absorbed into the patient's circulation at the correct time. The drug may be in any one of the many dosage forms available: capsules, compressed tablets, liquid oral dosage formulations, a *parenteral* (injectable) product, a controlled-release product, an ointment or cream, or a *transdermal* medication. Unlike ointments (oil-soluble semisolids) and creams (water-soluble semisolids), where the drug in the cream or ointment base is passively absorbed into or through the skin, transdermal medication is actively transported through the skin with the help of a *catalyst*.

DRUG TESTING

A potential new drug must pass many tests before it will be considered for licensure by the FDA and marketed in the United States. These tests begin in the laboratory. If the potential drug continues to show promise, it will move into animal testing. If it continues to show promise, it will move into limited and then expanded human testing.

Animal Testing

During the animal testing phase of a potential new drug, researchers try to use as few animals as possible, and they always handle the animals with care. Two or more species are typically tested, and the testing is mainly to assess the drug for toxicity.

Some other goals of animal testing are to see how and how much of the drug is absorbed (biopharmaceutics), how it is handled (pharmacokinetics), how it is broken down in the body (metabolized), and how it is eliminated (excreted). Scientists may add other chemicals to the active ingredients in the dosage form (the drug) to heighten its dissolution, absorption, or distribution in the body.

In the process of animal testing, many drugs stop showing any promise and are eliminated from further consideration. A representative of the former Upjohn Pharmaceutical Company has estimated that of every 2000 chemical substances studied, only 200 (10%) show any potential in early tests.[10] Of these, only 20 may be tested in humans, and only 1 may be found to be safe and effective enough to be approved by the FDA. Other estimates are gloomier. The Pharmaceutical Manufacturers Association (now the Pharmaceutical Research and Manufacturers Association) puts success at 1 in 10,000.

Testing in Humans

Once the preclinical testing (laboratory and animal studies) is complete and a drug continues to show promise, it is tested in humans. Although drug testing is performed by the drug company sponsoring the drug rather than the FDA, the FDA has developed different phases of testing in humans (Table 17.1). These are called phases I, II, III, and IV. Each phase uses progressively more humans for testing. Drug companies arrange with physicians, hospitals, and clinical pharmacy faculty to conduct these clinical trials.

However, before a pharmaceutical company can start testing an *investigational drug* — a drug only approved for investigation by the FDA — in humans, it must provide the FDA with the results of laboratory and animal research. It also must file a detailed plan on how the clinical trials will be performed — how many people, how they will be selected, where the studies will be done, how the drug's safety and effectiveness will be evaluated, and what findings would cause the study to be changed or halted.[10] All of this goes to the FDA in the form of an *investigational new drug application* (an IND).

Phase I Clinical Trials

Testing of a potential new drug in humans starts with a low dose in a small number (20 to 100) of healthy volunteers. The volunteers are tested in a secure environment and carefully checked. Doses are slowly raised until there is a *dose response* — when the intended effect can be measured. The main objective of phase I testing is to find the initial dose in humans and

Table 17.1   How Experimental Drugs Are Tested in Humans[13]

Phase	No. of Patients	Length	Purpose	% of Drugs Successfully Completed[a]
1	20–100	Several months	Mainly safety	70
2	Up to several hundred	Several months to 2 years	Some short-term safety, but mainly effectiveness	33
3	Several hundred to several thousand	1–4 years	Safety, effectiveness, and dosage	25–30

[a] For example, of 100 drugs for which investigational new drug applications are submitted to the FDA, about 70% will successfully complete phase I trials and go on to phase II; about 33% will complete phase II and go to phase III; 25 to 30 will clear phase III (and, on average, about 20 of the original 100 will ultimately be approved for marketing).

Source: U.S. Food and Drug Administration, Center for Drug Evaluation and Research. *From Test Tube to Patient: Improving Health Through Human Drugs.* Department of Health and Human Services, Rockville, MD, 1999.

to see if a human can tolerate the drug. The patients take the drug for approximately a month. Other important things to learn during phase I are how the drug is absorbed, distributed, metabolized, and excreted (pharmacokinetics), which organs are affected by the drug (pharmacology), how the drug is tolerated (toxicology), and if there are any side effects.

Phase II Clinical Trials

If the drug continues to show promise — there is a definite dose response in humans and the drug appears to be safe — the drug enters phase II testing. In this phase, the drug is tested in patients — a few hundred — who have the disease or condition for which the drug is intended. During this phase, extensive pharmacologic, toxicological, pharmacokinetic, and clinical monitoring takes place. The initial dosing and usual dosing is usually determined during this phase. Phase II is the critical phase in the clinical testing process. Many potential drugs do not make it past this point.

Phase III Clinical Testing

If the drug makes it out of phase II testing, it will be tested in phase III to discover the drug's efficacy — how good it is in treating the disease or condition for which the drug is intended. This phase will also reveal short-term side effects and risks in people whose health is impaired.

The investigational drug will be used in several randomized, controlled studies in various clinical research facilities — usually Veterans Administration and university teaching hospitals — throughout the United States. In recent years, the use of outside contractors for clinical drug development has been expanding. Sponsors are outsourcing more clinical studies to contract research organizations(CROs).[11] These fee-for-service, independent *clinical research organizations* have emerged because of the need to speed the development process and get drugs approved sooner. Academic health centers, which traditionally have performed most of the phase III work for the drug companies, produce high-quality work but are not known for their speed.[12]

CROs work as partners with the pharmaceutical companies from submitting the IND application to submitting the *new drug application* (NDA), but even they are subject to competition. The newest players in this business are site management organizations (SMOs).[12] SMOs work to bring investigators to a sponsor during site selection and work as a conduit for central contracting and quick patient uptake. Some SMOs are led by pharmacists.

During phase III testing, several thousand patients receive the investigational drug during a randomized, controlled study. A *randomized, controlled study* is a scientifically designed study with two patient groups that are randomly assigned — one group receives the drug and the other receives a placebo. A *placebo* is a drug that looks exactly like the real drug but does not contain the active ingredient of the drug. The nurse, patient, and physician are *blinded* — they do not know whether the patient received the real drug or the placebo. However, the pharmacist in the research facility does know and therefore is usually in charge of randomizing patients.

WHO OVERSEES RESEARCH ON INVESTIGATIONAL DRUGS?

Research on investigational drugs is controlled by the FDA and by local, independent, *investigational review boards* (IRBs). Federal rules and regulations govern IRBs. For example, the IRB can be part of an organization, such as a hospital or university, but must act independently of that organization. The composition of the IRB is also dictated by federal regulation. For example, IRBs must be composed of at least five people with varying backgrounds who are knowledgeable in the research areas to be covered. Racial, ethnic, and other interests must be represented. There also must be a nonscientific person on the board. Most IRBs are composed of a combination of medical investigators, medical practitioners, a layperson, a clergyman, an attorney, a pharmacist, and a nurse, and some have an ethicist. The chairperson of the IRB is usually a medical practitioner, but can be a pharmacist. The secretaries of many IRBs are pharmacists.

The FDA works closely with the drug companies and makes sure the sponsor is fulfilling the agency's requirements. The sponsor is responsible for:

- Fulfilling all FDA requirements
- Selecting investigators and study monitors
- Informing investigators
- Reviewing ongoing investigations
- Keeping and retaining records
- Inspecting the sponsors' records and reports
- Disposing of any unused supply of investigational drugs

The responsibilities of the clinical investigators (the primary investigator is held accountable) are:

- Fulfilling all IRB requirements
- Controlling the investigational drug
- Receiving IRB approval to perform the investigation
- Receiving IRB approval for a patient consent form
- Obtaining patient consent
- Following the study protocol — the research plan
- Keeping and retaining records
- Inspecting the investigator's records and reports
- Filing necessary reports with the IRB and sponsor

The overall responsibility of the IRB is to ensure that risks to study subjects are minimized. The specific responsibilities of the IRB are to:

- Review and approve the qualifications of the investigators
- Review and approve the study protocol
- Make sure the selection of study patients is fair and equitable
- Review and approve the patient consent form
- Review and approve the procedure to obtain patient consent
- Routinely review the progress of the study
- Review and make substantial changes to the study protocol
- Routinely review patient outcomes

DRUG STANDARDS

It is important that drugs be made according to high standards. As it turns out, most standards are not established by the FDA, but by the United States Pharmacopeia (USP). The USP was started in 1820 over concern about drug purity and consistency. The USP helps ensure that consumers receive medicines of the highest possible quality by setting the standards that manufacturers must meet to sell their products in the United States. The standards set by the USP concern purity and the amount of active ingredients, when and how quickly oral dosage forms of a drug are bioavailable (dissolves and is absorbed) to the body, and the drug's labeling and safe use.

The USP is an independent, not-for-profit organization but works closely with the FDA and drug companies. It makes *reference standards* — pure, accurately measured samples of the drug — available for drug companies to calibrate their analytical equipment and, in turn, to measure samples of the drugs they produce to ensure accuracy. Being able to put "USP" on a drug's label shows the drug meets all USP requirements.

HOW DRUGS ARE APPROVED FOR USE

The FDA only approves drugs it feels are safe and effective. However, the drug may not be absolutely safe. There is always some risk with every drug. In addition, every individual's physical makeup is different. Thus, the drug may not be handled by the body the same way in all people. The FDA's Center for Drug Evaluation and Research (CDER) carefully evaluates the drug for efficacy and risk.[13] However, when the FDA's advisory committees, composed of various outside experts, and the FDA feel that the benefits of the drug outweigh its risks, the drug is approved.

The FDA has 180 days to approve a new drug once it receives an NDA. However, this time is extended if the FDA needs more information from the sponsor, which is normally the case. Thus, it may take as long as 10 to 18 months to approve the drug. This will vary by how the FDA classifies the new drug.

FDA's Classification of New Drugs

The FDA classifies NDAs to assign review priority on the basis of the drug's chemical type and potential benefit.[14]

Chemical Type

The chemical types are:

New molecular entity: An active ingredient that has never been marketed before

New derivative: A chemical derived from an active ingredient already marketed

New formulation: A new dosage form or new formulation of an active ingredient already on the market

New combination: A drug that contains two or more compounds, the combination of which has not been marketed together

Already marketed drug product: A product that duplicates another firm's already marketed drug product

Potential Benefit

Types of potential benefit are:

Important gain: May effectively treat or diagnose a disease not adequately treated or diagnosed by any marketed drug.

Modest gain: Offers a modest, but real, advantage over other marketed drugs.

Little or no gain: Essentially the same medical importance and use as a marketed drug.

Orphan drug candidate: A product that treats a rare disease affecting fewer than 200,000 Americans. There are an estimated 2000 rare diseases.

Thus, a new drug that is a new molecular entity and represents an important therapeutic gain (classified 1A) receives the highest priority review. An overview of the regulatory approval process is available.[15]

TIME AND COST OF DRUG DEVELOPMENT

It takes times to do good research, and it takes time to develop a new drug. Developing a new pharmaceutical agent may take more than a decade, but usually takes 8 to 15 years. Some high-priority drugs, like those for the human immunodeficiency virus (HIV), have been approved much faster. Most of the time spent is in clinical trials (2 to 10 years).[10] Figure 17.1 shows the typical timeline for the new drug development process.[16] The average time for FDA approval in 1992 was 29.9 months. In 1996, the time dropped to 17.8 months and now is even shorter.[12]

In 2005, members of the Pharmaceutical Research and Manufacturers of American (PhRMA) claimed to have invested an estimated $39.4 billion in discovering and developing new medicines. Industry-wide research and investment reached a record $51.3 billion in 2005.[17] Yet the total expenditures for drug research and development is a matter of some controversy, since the pharmaceutical industry claims have not been subject to independent validation.

The biggest single item driving up research and development costs is contract studies, mainly in the clinical area and also the preclinical area

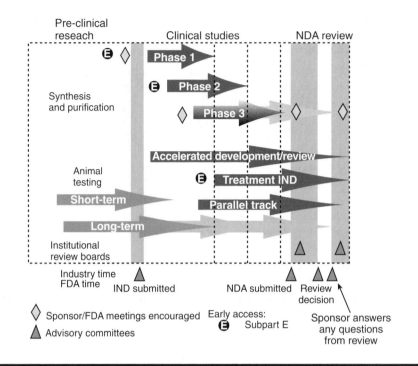

Figure 17.1   Timeline for the development of a new drug in the U.S. (From U.S. Food and Drug Administration, Center for Drug Evaluation and Research, *Report to the Nation 2004*.)

such as toxicology studies or analytical sample costs. One vice-president and chairman of research at a major drug company was quoted as saying, "We'd take a lot of cost out if we could develop drugs with two or three clinical trials and few thousand people, instead of 20 trials and 20,000 patients."[18] The total per patient cost to a pharmaceutical company for a good recruiting site (for patients), including monitoring and data processing fees, approaches $6000 ($3000 for the investigator or site and $3000 for the patients).[12]

These costs are putting a premium on innovation and spurring a profound shift in research strategies. Drug companies that do not have the means to develop successful new drugs may find themselves forced into mergers or takeovers to carry growth, or even to survive.[19]

DRUG MANUFACTURING

Once a drug company has its NDA approved by the FDA, they can start marketing and producing the drug. The production process for a drug is beyond the scope of this text. However, it is important to know that the drug manufacturer must follow *current good manufacturing practices* (CGMP).[20] If they do not, the FDA can claim the drug is *adulterated* and can stop the manufacturer from making further quantities of the drug until CGMP is restored.

GENERIC DRUGS

A generic drug is a drug product that is an identical copy in active ingredients, formulation, and strength that is marketed by a company other than the company that did the original research on the drug product (the innovator).[21] These drugs are sometimes called "me too" drugs. The innovator firm would have completed many years of research and spent much money before getting approval from the FDA to market the drug. Innovator firms are allowed to patent and provide a trade name for their newly approved drug. The patent gives the innovator about 20 years to market the drug without competition.[13]

At the end of the patent period, other drug companies may develop a generic version of the innovator's product and may do so without extensive clinical testing by applying for an *abbreviated new drug application* (ANDA) with the FDA. If approved, the company marketing the generic version of the innovator's product must use the drug's generic — common — name rather than a trade name.

Because competition enters the picture when a patent expires, generic drugs usually sell for 20 to 75% less than the brand name product. But are generic drugs safe? Are they as effective as the brand name products? The answers to these two questions are yes and yes. Drug companies — both brand name and generic firms — making generic drugs must test the drug's bioavailability. This *bioavailability* is dependent on the drug's dissolution, disintegration, and absorption into the body. With only a few exceptions, generic drugs are as bioavailable and as safe as their trade name counterparts.

DESI DRUGS

Drug Efficacy Study Implementation (DESI) drugs are drugs that were approved solely on the basis of their safety prior to 1962. Thereafter, Congress required drugs to be shown to be effective as well. The FDA initiated a DESI to evaluate the effectiveness of those drugs that had been previously approved on safety grounds alone. These drugs, and those identical, related, and similar to them, may continue to be marketed until the administrative proceedings evaluating their effectiveness have been concluded, at which point continued marketing is only permitted if an NDA is approved for such drugs.[22]

HOMEOPATHIC DRUGS

> Homeopathy is a system of medicine based on the observation
> that high doses of pharmacologically active substances cause
> symptoms when administered to adults. These same substances,
> when prepared in very dilute form, may relieve similar symp-
> toms in conditions resulting from different etiologies.[23]

Homeopathic drugs, unlike dietary supplements, are subject to the Food,
Drug, and Cosmetic Act and regulations issued by the FDA. However,
instead of the new drug approval process, premarket approval for homeopathic drugs is by way of monograph approval of the Homeopathic
Pharmacopeia Convention of the United States.

NONPRESCRIPTION DRUGS

The FDA has always applied the same standards to nonprescription drugs
as it does to prescription ones when the proposed *over-the-counter* (OTC)
drug meets the criteria for a new drug. The problem with OTC drugs has
not been safety, but effectiveness. Do all of them work? Over the past 20
years, the FDA has systematically evaluated all OTC products for the safety
and effectiveness of their active ingredients.[14] Some OTC drugs are similar
to prescription only (Rx) drugs but have smaller amounts of the active
ingredients than the Rx version.

Sometimes an approved prescription drug is considered safe enough
for self-use and is switched to OTC status. For a switch to occur, the drug
must be safe at the dose recommended on the label. In addition, the
answer to the following four questions must be yes: (a) Can the consumers
read the label? (b) Can they understand the label? (c) Do they follow the
label? (d) Do they achieve the desired outcome?

A manufacturer wanting to switch a prescription-only product must
provide substantial evidence to the FDA the switch is reasonably safe and
is in the public's best interest.

POSTMARKETING SURVEILLANCE OF NEW DRUGS

All drugs have some degree of risk, and this risk is not evenly distributed
throughout the population. These risks are described as side effects or
adverse drug reactions (ADRs).

Side effects are minor, predictable, unwanted effects of the drug. These
effects stem from the drug's pharmacology. Therefore, they are experienced by most people taking the drug — some more than others. These
effects go away when the drug is discontinued. An example would be
drowsiness associated with some antihistamines used for hay fever.

ADRs are moderate to severe, sometimes life-threatening, unwanted, usually unpredictable, effects of the drug. Predictable ADRs are based on the drug's pharmacology and are dose related. An example would be respiratory depression associated with narcotic analgesics. Unpredictable ADRs are the most troubling and can be the most severe. These reactions are considered to be bizarre, as they are not based on the drug's pharmacology and are not dose related. An example would be thrombocytopenia (decreased platelets) associated with the use of heparin — an anticoagulant.

Even the most extensive premarket testing of a new drug can never uncover all of the potential side effects, ADRs, or *drug interactions* (one drug affecting the action of another drug). Testing 3000 people over a period of months or even a few years will not always detect a rare reaction. The effect may occur in just one person in 10,000.[13] However, once the drug is approved, literally thousands of all types of patients receive the drug in a short period of time. This is when new effects of the drug may be discovered.

To help monitor the serious adverse effects of drugs, the FDA has a reporting system called *MedWatch*. Serious ADRs are fatal, life-threatening, cause hospitalization, prolong hospitalization, or result in disability. ADRs are reported to the FDA by health care personnel or patients through MedWatch. The FDA quickly puts all reports into a computer system and then searches for any significant patterns. There is a similar program for the reporting of serious ADRs for vaccines. This program is cosponsored by the FDA and the Centers for Disease Control and Prevention (CDC) and is called the *Vaccine Adverse Event Reporting System* (VAERS).

Should an important, new adverse event emerge and be confirmed, the FDA and the drug manufacturer have several options. One is to change the directions for the product to reduce the dose or warn certain vulnerable groups of people. In urgent and unusual circumstances products can and have been withdrawn from the market either voluntarily by the manufacturer or by FDA order.

CURRENT ISSUES IN DRUG DEVELOPMENT

Drug companies have complained that the drug approval process takes too long and have lobbied the U.S. Congress to do something about it. This has resulted in legislation requiring the FDA to speed up the approval process. The FDA, although concerned about this, has done a remarkable job in speeding up the process. In fact, there is recent evidence that the FDA is now approving new drugs too quickly, as many drugs have had to be removed fro the market because of safety issues.

More and more new drugs are being removed from the market.[24] Under pressure, the FDA adopted a faster approach that sometimes disregarded the warnings of its own experts. Further concern is that the agency is moving too quickly on switching prescription-only drugs to OTC status. Drug companies like to switch their drugs to OTC status, as it is more profitable.

Another new development is that drug companies are starting to test their drugs overseas where there is less delay and less scrutiny.[25] Companies looking for lucrative drugs are turning to poorly paid foreign physicians and looking for a faster turnaround on drug testing. The FDA is only capable of inspecting a small number of foreign test sites, and thus there is concern.

The FDA under Fire

The FDA is always under public scrutiny, but no more so than because of what has happened after refecoxib (Vioxx) was pulled from the market because of a heightened risk of myocardial infarction. The FDA has been accused of making drug safety a much lower priority than approving drugs. The FDA's drug safety section resides under the office of new drug approval and has a much smaller staff and budget.

The FDA is also under fire for having advisory panels with experts who have conflicts of interest because they receive grants or receive financial honorariums for speaking on behalf of drug companies. Many drugs were approved by the FDA with the understanding that the drug's manufacturer would study the drugs (primarily for safety) after they were approved, but rarely did this happen, and the FDA rarely checked to see that the studies were done.

FUTURE OF DRUG DISCOVERY

In 2000, a major scientific event took place. The human genome was mapped. The human genome is the basis for understanding the blueprint that directs our external appearance and behavior, as well as the quality of our internal organs. The human genome project is changing, dramatically, how drugs are discovered and developed. We are now on the verge of possessing genetic information on various diseases and the custom designing of drugs for patients with a certain genetic makeup. Although this is exciting, it is also complex. How all of this will affect the approval process for new drugs and the practice of pharmacy is unknown.

At the time of this writing (2006), everyone in drug development was excited about using *surrogate markers* — a kind of clinical trials "crystal ball." Surrogate markers are tests or patient milestones that researchers can use as stand-ins to predict longer-term results, such as survival.[26] Also at this time, drug researchers are optimistic about *metabolomics* — studying the changes in concentrations of metabolites within the body's cells to find unique patterns or profiles, and a screening tool for disease.[27]

SUMMARY

Consumers and patients in the United States can be confident and proud of the drug discovery, development, and approval process for new drugs. They are less confident that once drugs and vaccines are approved, that the medications are continually monitored for safety. Unfortunately, not all patients respond the same to medication, and some patients are harmed. Many pharmacists work in the drug discovery, development, and approval process for drugs and vaccines in the United States. Some work in pharmaceutical companies, some perform drug research in colleges of pharmacy and in hospitals, whereas others work for the FDA and CDC and help with the drug approval process or help perform postmarketing surveillance.

DISCUSSION QUESTIONS AND EXERCISES

1. What intrigues you about:
   a. The drug discovery process?
   b. The drug investigation and testing process?
   c. The drug approval process?
2. Put the following in order of your interest: drug discovery, drug investigation and testing, and drug approval.
3. Which do you think is better — a drug designed to take once a day or one to be taken three times a day? Why?
4. A patient comes up to you (the pharmacist) and is concerned that animals are being used to test drugs. How would you handle this?
5. How do you feel about giving people with an active disease a placebo (no active drug) because they were selected for the control group in a study?
6. How do pharmacists find the results of new studies on drugs?
7. The FDA approves drugs as generally safe and effective. However, five drugs approved during the past 3 years have been removed from the market. Why do you think this has happened?
8. What would you do if a patient told you (the pharmacist) he or she was receiving and taking drugs ordered over the Internet that are not approved for use by the FDA?

9. What do you think the advantages and disadvantages are in doing drug research for a drug company versus doing drug research in a school of pharmacy?
10. Interview someone who does drug research. Ask them what they like and do not like about their job.

CHALLENGES

1. There are still some highly prevalent diseases throughout the world that have no drugs or vaccines to prevent them. For extra credit, and with the permission of your professor, investigate and prepare a concise report about two or three major diseases in this category. Make predictions about what would happen if vaccines or drugs were available to prevent these diseases throughout the world. Also, explore why these vaccines and drugs are not available and what can be done about this problem.
2. The number of students pursuing graduate degrees (MS or PhD) in pharmacy that would allow them to do drug research has declined. For extra credit, and with the permission of your professor, explore and write a concise report about this problem. Why does the problem exist? How bad is it? Advance at least five plausible arguments on how this problem can be solved for society.

WEB SITES OF INTEREST

Food and Drug Administration: http://www.fda.govs
United States Pharmacopeia: http://www.usp.org
Pharmaceutical Research and Manufacturers of the United States: http://www.phrma.org/
Generic Pharmaceutical Association: http://www.gphaonline.org//AM/Template.cfm?Section=Home
Homeopathic Pharmacopeia: http://www.hpus.com/

REFERENCES

1. Young, FE. From test tube to patient: new drug development in the United States. Part 1: The reality behind the headlines. *FDA Consum.* 1987;21:4–5.
2. Bender, GA, and Thom, RA. *Great Moments in Pharmacy.* Parke Davis. Northwood Institute Press, Detroit, 1965.
3. Brooks, M. *Get a Grip on Genetics.* Time-Life Books, Alexandria, VA, 1998.
4. Gonick, L, and Wheelis, L. *The Cartoon Guide to Genetics.* Harper Perennial, New York, 1991.

5. Deno, RA, Rowe, TD, and Brodie, DC. Pharmaceutical research. In *The Profession of Pharmacy*. Lippincott, Philadelphia, 1966, chap. 8.
6. Sneader, W. *Drug Development: From Laboratory to Clinic*. Wiley, New York, 1986.
7. Dybas, CL. Study of marine creatures yields human benefits. *Wash Post*. December 18, 2000.
8. Hamner, CE. *Drug Development*. CRC Press, Boca Raton, FL, 1990.
9. Wanke, LA, and DuBose, RF. Designer drugs: the evolving science of drug discovery. *Pharm Pract Manag Q*. 1998;18(2):13–22.
10. New drug development in the United States. An FDA Consumer Special Report. HHS Publication No. (FDA) 88-3168. January, 1988.
11. Vogel, JR, and Getz, KA. Factors driving the increased use of outside contractors in drug development. *Clin Res Regul Affairs*. 1997;14(3–4):177–190.
12. Vlasses, PH. Clinical research: trends affecting the pharmaceutical industry and the pharmacy profession. *Am J Health-Syst Pharm*. 1999;56:171–174.
13. U.S. Food and Drug Administration, Center for Drug Evaluation and Research. *From Test Tube to Patient: Improving Health Through Human Drugs*. Department of Health and Human Services, Rockville, MD, 2006.
14. Farley, D. Benefit vs risk: how FDA approves new drugs. *FDA Consumer Special Report*, January, 1995.
15. Chow, SC, and Pong, A. An overview of the regulatory approval process in drug development. *Drug Inf J*. 1998;32(4 suppl):1175s–1185s.
16. FDA Center for Drug Evaluation and Research. *CDER Handbook*. Available at http://www.fda.gov/cder/handbook/index.htm. Accessed May 10, 2006.
17. Pharmaceutical Research and Manufactures of America. R&D Investments by America's Pharmaceutical Research Companies Near Record $40 Billion in 2005. Available at http://www.phrma.org/news_room/press_releases/r%26d_investments_by_america%92s_pharmaceutical_research_companies_nears_record_%2440_billion_in_2005/. Accessed May 11, 2006.
18. Anonymous. Pharmaceutical companies confront high-cost of drug development. *R&D Magazine*. 1996;38:17A.
19. Weber, J. Drugmakers are discovering the high cost of cutting costs. *Bus Week*. 1994;3394:204–207.
20. Willig, SH, and Stoker, JR. *Good Manufacturing Practices for Pharmaceuticals: A Plan for Total Quality Control*, 4th ed. Mercel Dekker, New York, 1997.
21. Juhl, RP. Prescription to over-the-counter switch: a regulatory perspective. *Clin Ther*. 1998;20(suppl C):C111–117.
22. U.S. Food and Drug Administration. US Food and Drug Administration. Questions and answers on the unapproved drug compliance policy guide (CPG). Available at http://www.fda.gov/cder/compliance/CPG_QandA.htm. Accessed May 11, 2006.
23. Borneman, JP. Regulation of homeopathic drug products. *Am J Health-Syst Pharm*. 2006;63:86–91.
24. Change in FDA approved policy led to 7 deadly drugs. *St. Petersburg (FL) Times*, December 28, 2000.
25. Testing tidal wave hits overseas — on distant shores, drug firms avoid delays — and scrutiny. *Wash Post*. December 18, 2000.

26. Mundell, EJ. Coming soon: faster, yet still safe, clinical trials. *Health Day.* March 29, 2006. Available at http://www.healthday.com/view.cfm?id=531771. Accessed May 11, 2006.

27. Bren, L. Metabolomics: working toward personalized medicine. *FDA Consumer Magazine.* Nov-Dec, 2005. Available at http://www.fda.gov/fdac/feactures/2005/605_metabolmics.html. Accessed May 11, 2006.

18

PHARMACEUTICAL INDUSTRY

Not that long ago, the usual choices for new pharmacy graduates were to practice in community or hospital pharmacy. Over the past 15 years, the opportunities for pharmacists have expanded. One of these opportunities is working in the pharmaceutical industry.

There have always been pharmacists in the pharmaceutical industry. Indeed, several pharmaceutical companies were founded by pharmacists. However, in the past, most pharmacists working in the pharmaceutical industry were used as salespeople to convince physicians to use their company's products. Today, pharmacists work in a wide variety of positions within pharmaceutical companies.

This chapter discusses how pharmaceutical companies are organized and highlights those areas within a pharmaceutical company where pharmacists work. Information will be presented on the various titles pharmacists hold with the industry, the transition from practice, career development, and the pros and cons of working for a pharmaceutical company.

LEARNING OBJECTIVES

After reading this chapter, you should be able to:

- Discuss how pharmaceutical companies are organized
- Identify the departments in the pharmaceutical industry where pharmacists work
- Name three job titles held by pharmacists in the pharmaceutical industry
- Discuss some of the issues associated with going from practice to the pharmaceutical industry

- Explain how pharmacists can grow within the pharmaceutical industry
- Contrast the pros and cons of working as a pharmacist in the pharmaceutical industry

PHARMACEUTICAL COMPANIES

The pharmaceutical industry is large, diverse, and important. It produces chemicals, over-the-counter and prescription drugs, and other health products. Over 100 pharmaceutical companies are involved in the research of new drugs in the United States. Research-based pharmaceutical and biotechnology companies are devoted to discovering medicines to allow patients to live longer, be healthier, be happier, and lead more productive lives.

These companies invested more than $28 billion in 2005 developing new medicines.[1] Much of the high cost is because only one of every 10,000 potential medicines makes it through the research and development pipeline and is approved for use by the Food and Drug Administration and because of the amount of money used for sales and marketing.

Table 18.1 shows the top 10 pharmaceutical and biopharmaceutical companies ranked by revenue in 2004.[2] Because of merger mania occurring, it is important to keep in mind the top 10 listing is constantly under revision.

All pharmaceutical companies employ pharmacists — some more than others. Pharmacists enjoy working in various positions within pharmaceutical companies. Some have become presidents or chief executive officers (CEOs) of these large corporations.

Table 18.1   Top 10 Pharmaceutical and Biopharmaceutical Companies Based on 2004 Revenues in Millions

Rank	Pharma Company	Revenue	Biopharma Company	Revenue
1	Pfizer	$46,133	Amgen	$9,977
2	GlaxoSmithKline	$31,417	Genetech	$3,749
3	Sanofi-Aventis	$29,596	Serono	$2,178
4	Johnson and Johnson	$22,128	Biogen Idec	$2,112
5	Merck	$21,494	Genzyme	$1,479
6	AstraZeneca	$21,426	Gilead	$1,242
7	Novartis	$18,497	Medimmune	$1,124
8	Bristol-Myers Squibb	$15,482	Chiron	$990
9	Roche	$13,840	Millenium	$349
10	Eli Lilly	$13,059	Intermune	$147

Source: From Contract Pharma. 2005 Top Companies. Adapted with permission.

Organizational

Although individual pharmaceutical companies are organized differently, most have some of the same features. The most common areas in pharmaceutical companies where pharmacists work are research and development, government or regulatory affairs, manufacturing and production, medical affairs, sales and marketing, trade and professional relations, and management and administration.

Research and Development

The research and development (R&D) division is responsible for the discovery and development of new drug products, dosages, and dosage forms.

Basic research is where breakthrough products are first imagined. Basic research involves studies of diseases and the synthesis of new drugs to treat these diseases. If a promising new drug is identified, it must go through rigorous acute and chronic toxicity studies in animals before it can be tested in humans (see Chapter 17, How Drugs Are Discovered, Tested, and Approved).

Basic research is also the area where improvements are made to existing drugs. Pharmaceutical companies are always looking for ways to improve the effectiveness of and reduce any side effects of their approved drugs.

Pharmaceutical development is closely related to research. It involves testing the chemistry, stability, and compatibility of a new compound. Development also is the place where formulation of the dosage form, pharmaceutics, takes place. "In a nutshell, pharmaceutical development bridges the gap between research and production. The product is taken from a research level to an intermediate level before being taken into full-scale manufacturing."[3]

Clinical research follows new products from the beginning through the four phases of clinical studies (see Chapter 17, How Drugs Are Discovered, Tested, and Approved). Clinical research involves planning, implementing, monitoring, and reporting clinical trials in humans.

Regulatory Affairs

This department is responsible for representing data for drug products to the U.S. Food and Drug Administration (FDA). People working in government affairs monitor legislation and regulations. They also testify before state and federal legislatures, and present the company's views on a piece of legislation or a regulation to professional groups.[4]

Government affairs must keep executive management up-to-date on key developments in legislation and health care and represent the company in public and professional meetings. Personnel working in regulatory affairs must also recommend actions the company should take on particular issues.

Manufacturing, Production, and Quality Control

Manufacturing, production, and quality control are closely related, but in most companies, these are separate departments.

Manufacturing includes the buying of raw materials and the transformation of these materials into the finished product. At all levels, the goal is to ensure the production of a quality product.[3]

To do this, pharmaceutical companies must comply with regulations called *good manufacturing practices* (GMPs).[4] Manufacturing is influenced by new technologies that are often changing.

Production involves producing the right amount of product at the right time. Production includes heading production units, supervising production employees, planning schedules, preparing budgets, and working to modernize equipment and procedures.[5]

Quality control involves conducting tests to ensure that the product meets precise quality standards. People working in quality control are committed to meeting high manufacturing standards and quality assurance.

Medical Affairs

Sometimes a part of medical services or operations, medical affairs supports many parts of the company through drug information, medical writing, and communication with various health care professionals, including pharmacists. In most cases, this department focuses on adding value to existing products or funding new publications. Medical operations may include all or some of the following disciplines: clinical applications, clinical development, disease state research, epidemiology, postmarketing surveillance, trade and professional relations, and medical affairs.[6]

Sales and Marketing

Major pharmaceutical companies employ large numbers of people in their sales and marketing divisions. *Sales* is one of the largest areas of most pharmaceutical companies. Sales representatives are employed to discuss the features and benefits of the company's drug products with physicians, pharmacists, and other health care professionals. Anyone who may increase the use of the company's drugs is a potential client.

Marketing involves positioning the company's drugs to maximize sales. The marketing department matches the benefits of the drug with the needs of patients and physicians and develops marketing information for the company's sales representatives. This information is also used in advertising the drug in medical journals;,subject to approval by the FDA.

Trade and Professional Relations

This area within a pharmaceutical company provides services to the various health professions, chiefly medicine, pharmacy, and nursing. This department works to develop close relationships with the leadership and key opinion leaders of the health professions. Examples are the provision of continuing education, help in sponsoring speakers or support for national and state meetings of various health professional groups, and attending these meetings when possible.

Management and Administration

"Managers and administrators make sure that their department works smoothly and is in line with the rest of the company. Hard work, dedication, and consistent success in each position of higher responsibility marks the company executive."[3]

PHARMACISTS IN THE PHARMACEUTICAL INDUSTRY

Pharmacists have been associated with the pharmaceutical industry since its beginning. Most companies recognize that the pharmacist's education and training provide an excellent background for work within the industry. Most pharmacists working in the pharmaceutical industry work for sales and marketing, and some work in management and administration, research and development, and in production and quality control.[3]

Working in Sales

Pharmaceutical companies need knowledgeable sales representatives to promote the use of their products. Some companies, most notably, Eli Lilly and Merck and Company, use many pharmacists as sales representatives, although individuals with business, science, or other backgrounds are also employed. Other companies use college graduates with business or other backgrounds as sales representatives. The advantage of using pharmacists is their education and their ability to communicate with other health care practitioners. Pharmacists also understand the health care delivery system and what is important to patients.

All sales representatives receive intensive training in the life sciences (if they are not pharmacists), communication, sales techniques, and the company's strategic goals before they start work. Once oriented, sales representatives usually start their jobs working with "seasoned" sales representatives, and the learning continues as long as the person holds the job.

Starting as a local sales or field representative is considered to be an entry-level position, but one that is important if the pharmacist would like to advance to marketing or managerial positions with increased responsibility in the company. Each sales representative has a territory to cover. The territory can be a large metropolitan area, part of a state, or several states. Thus, travel varies from company to company.

The major responsibility of a sales representative is to call on physicians to discuss the features and benefits of the company's products. Thus, sales representatives must have a clear understanding of the indications, contraindications, dosing guidelines, side effects, and drug interactions of the products they detail.

There are also hospital sales representatives who call on the physicians, nurses, pharmacy managers, and clinical pharmacists working in hospitals. Hospital sales representatives usually work as local sales representatives before they become hospital representatives.

Each sales representative reports to a district sales manager, who supervises a group of sales representatives. District sales representatives work for regional sales managers, who in turn usually report to a vice-president of sales.

Managed care has dramatically changed how pharmaceutical companies conduct business. Today, account mangers interact with managed care accounts to maximize access to a company's products. One goal is to get the company's product on the managed care formulary with as few limitations as possible. Account managers report to regional account managers, who are responsible for all managed care plans within a larger area. Regional account managers report to a national account director, who is responsible for a single national account such as Aetna, United Health Care, or Kaiser Permanente.

For those interested, some testimonials have been written by pharmacists who are pharmaceutical sales representatives.[7,8]

Working in Marketing

A successful track record in sales can lead to opportunities for increased responsibility in marketing. Marketing is composed of product, price, promotion, and place.[8] The perspective a previous sales representative can bring to the marketing area is important. The marketing department conducts research, planning, the development of distribution channels, pricing, advertising, and support for sales representatives. Pharmacists fill these roles well, especially if they also have an M.B.A. or MS degree in pharmacy.

Within the marketing division are product managers, who are responsible for the overall marketing strategy of a single product. They make decisions such as whether money should be spent in direct-to-consumer advertising or on sales ads in professional journals. Product managers report to the director of marketing, who has overall responsibility for multiple products.

An excellent reference, written by a pharmacist who has worked in the marketing area for a pharmaceutical company, is available for those seeking more information on this field.[8]

Working in Advertising

The pharmaceutical industry has been criticized for its aggressive promotion of its products to physicians, pharmacists, and the public.[9,10] The industry's direct to consumer advertising is accused of spending an inordinate amount of time pointing out the benefits of its drugs and little time talking about its drug's risks. Some pharmaceutical companies have overstepped their bounds in promoting their company's products to physicians. This has resulted in tighter federal guidelines for the pharmaceutical industry's relationship with doctors.[11]

Working in Management and Administration

Management positions exist in sales in the field (district sales managers) or in the administration of the company. Managers make sure their department works smoothly and is in line with the company's strategic plan.

Moving into management takes excellent people and organizational skills. "The R.Ph. on your business card is very important when you start out in sales, but not that important later on. You are looked at for what you are and the knowledge you have, not for the title of pharmacist."[5]

Some pharmacists have advanced through the ranks of pharmaceutical companies to become high executives. A reference providing more insight on this is provided.[5]

Working in Research and Development

Pharmacists working in the basic research areas of a pharmaceutical company usually need a graduate degree (M.S. or Ph.D.) in the physical–chemical areas. These areas include working at the research bench in pharmaceutics, pharmacokinetics, pharmaceutical chemistry, and toxicology. These pharmacists conduct and lead the early research on new drugs.

Pharmacists working in clinical research have a chance to develop and oversee clinical trials testing the safety and efficacy of new drugs. Pharmacists working in this area usually need a Ph.D. or Pharm.D. and sometimes a research-based clinical fellowship in a specific area of drug therapy.

Two references on pharmacists working in the basic and clinical research areas of pharmaceutical companies are provided for those interested in learning more about this interesting work.[5,12]

Working in Medical Affairs

Medical affairs, sometimes called the medical department, medical services, or medical operations, usually provide various functions.

Working as a Medical Science Liaison

Pharmaceutical companies have found a need to have knowledgeable medical science liaisons (MSLs) who are trained technical experts on the company's products and related disease states. MSLs provide the latest information to opinion leaders in medicine and pharmacy, often well before a drug is approved by the FDA. Their goals are to support product utilization and formulary adoption.

These positions require a Pharm.D., M.D., or Ph.D. degree along with extensive clinical experience (usually five years), typically in a specialty area of drug therapy (e.g., infectious disease, cardiology, respiratory diseases).

Working in Drug Information

There is a need within a pharmaceutical company to provide accurate and up-to-date drug information in response to inquiries from health care professionals, consumers, and other departments within the company. This job requires skills in drug information retrieval, drug literature evaluation skills, communication, and knowledge of the company's products. Most companies hire pharmacists with Pharm.D. degrees, and most prefer someone who has also completed a residency in drug information.

Working in Medical Writing

Medical departments of pharmaceutical companies write product monographs (written summaries on the technical details of a drug) and sales training manuals to support the sales and marketing division. They also prepare scientific manuscripts for publication in medical and pharmacy journals and write technical documents for submission to the FDA. Pharmacists have the scientific and clinical background to do this job well; however, candidates for these positions also need good writing skills.

Working in Outcomes Research

Medical practice has advanced to measuring the success of drugs by the health outcomes they produce rather than their theoretical value based on the drug's pharmacology. Health outcomes include clinical outcomes, humanistic outcomes, and economic outcomes (see Chapter 10, Managed Care Pharmacy). Pharmaceutical companies understand they now have to perform outcome studies to prove to practitioners (physicians and pharmacists) that their drug affects positive outcomes.

Outcome researchers develop and conduct outcome studies to support their products. Some will work with customers (mostly managed care organizations and some large hospitals) to develop the means of assessing some research question the customer wants answered. Most pharmaceutical companies hire those with Pharm.D. degrees who have completed a pharmacoeconomics fellowship or pharmacists with graduate degrees (M.S. or Ph.D.) in health outcomes or pharmacoeconomics to do their health outcomes work.

Working in Drug Safety

Drug safety is responsible for maintaining a database of postmarketing adverse drug events and reporting serious events to the FDA. These reports may come to the company's attention via consumers, health care professionals, or the company's MSLs or sales representatives.

Another role of the medical operations department is to conduct additional clinical studies following a drug's approval by the FDA (phase IV studies). These postmarketing studies may be performed to answer additional questions about a drug or its place in therapy or may be required by the FDA as a condition of a drug's approval. Formal, postmarketing surveillance can be performed by pharmacists if they have added training in pharmacoepidemiology. Such training can be gained by earning a masters of science (M.S.) degree in biostatistics and epidemiology or by completing a fellowship in pharmacoepidemiology.

One reference is provided on careers for pharmacists in the medical affairs departments of pharmaceutical companies.[13]

Working in Manufacturing, Production, and Quality Control

The manufacturing and production of pharmaceuticals is an ideal job for pharmacists interested in using their technical knowledge and getting involved in the rapidly changing world of technology. The pharmacist in the manufacturing and production area must be task oriented, have a sound understanding of people, and have strong managerial skills.

"Because pharmaceutical operations are specialized, high-level careers in this area almost always need an advanced degree."[3]

Working in Trade and Professional Affairs

Pharmacists are ideally suited to work in the trade and professional affairs sections of pharmaceutical companies. After all, they understand the profession, and they know the needs and concerns of hospital, clinical, community, managed care, and consultant pharmacists. Pharmacists working in the trade and professional affairs departments are well-known and well-liked individuals, because it is their job to help pharmacists, and pharmaceutical companies are generous with resources to the profession.

Working in Regulatory Affairs

Pharmacists working in the regulatory affairs divisions of pharmaceutical companies help prepare investigational new drugs (INDs) and new drug applications (NDAs) for submission to the FDA. Before writing these, they must analyze data from animal, laboratory, and clinical studies. This division must also monitor all health care legislation and regulations. Thus, an interest in legal affairs is a plus.

Regulatory affairs is a sophisticated and complex process; thus, there are M.S. programs at two colleges of pharmacy, and certification by examination is available.[12] An excellent reference is provided for readers interested in this field.[12]

Moving from Practice to the Industry

There is usually some concern when a pharmacist is faced with a decision to give up practice to go to work for a pharmaceutical company. Some of this concern is about losing touch with patients and some is about losing some autonomy. One pharmacist has documented his concerns, thought process, and the pros and cons of making the transition to the pharmaceutical industry.[14]

Female Pharmacists in the Pharmaceutical Industry

Women, particularly female pharmacists, have made great strides in the pharmaceutical industry. A survey showed that women like the personal growth and interesting responsibilities.[15] Despite these findings, the industry recently sponsored a brainstorming meeting designed to help raise awareness of the need to have more women in top positions and to increase the understanding of the challenges women face.[16]

SATISFACTION AND CAREER ADVANCEMENT

Pharmacists working in the pharmaceutical industry are satisfied with the work and enjoy knowing that what they do helps people improve their quality of life by using their company's drugs. Working for a pharmaceutical company can be exciting as new drugs work themselves through the discovery, development, and clinical trial process and then are approved for use and launched.

Pharmacists working for pharmaceutical companies find the salaries, benefits, and incentives attractive. The downside for some pharmacists is missing direct patient care, and the long hours add to the stress and pressures that can come with working for a major corporation.

At the same time, career advancement can be rapid. The following would be a typical career path to becoming vice-president of marketing[17]:

1. Professional sales representative
2. District sales manager
3. Product manager
4. Director of marketing and sales
5. Vice-president of marketing

The following is an example of how someone in a pharmaceutical company could advance to be the president of the company[17]:

1. Professional sales representative
2. Coordinator of sales training
3. District sales manager
4. Product manager
5. Regional sales manager
6. Vice-president of sales
7. Vice-president of marketing
8. President

"Hard work, dedication, and consistent success in each position of higher authority marks the company executive."[17] Pharmacists, with their backgrounds and training, are contributing much to the success of the pharmaceutical industry, and they have the ability to rise to high levels within the corporate structure of these companies.

CASE STUDIES

There are three interesting case studies of pharmacists: one pharmacist who has spent his entire career in the pharmaceutical industry, another pharmacist who started out in practice and then switched to a career in the pharmaceutical industry, and one pharmacist who went from practice to the pharmaceutical industry and back to practice.[18–20] These case studies provide more insight into what it is like the work for a large pharmaceutical company.

CRITICISMS OF THE INDUSTRY

The pharmaceutical industry provides many new and wonderful drugs. However, to provide a balanced view of the pharmaceutical industry, one must provide some current criticisms. Here are just a few from a previous editor of the *New England Journal of Medicine* and a well-known academic physician at the Harvard Medical School:[21,22]

- The pharmaceutical industry claims to be a high risk industry but every year has higher profits than any other industry.
- The pharmaceutical companies are not that innovative — most drugs are "me too" drugs.
- Many of the most innovative drugs are researched by academic medical centers, financed by the federal government (NIH), and then acquired by pharmaceutical companies.
- Drug companies promote diseases to match their drugs.
- The drug companies have a too much influence over medical education and practice.
- Big drug companies spend far more on sales and marketing than on research.

Other criticisms include having influence over many members of the FDA's drug advisory panels by funding many of these members' research or paying honorariums for speaking on behalf of the pharmaceutical companies or being on their advisory boards, and having unbalanced direct-to-consumer advertising.

Whether these criticisms are valid should be investigated and determined by the reader.

SUMMARY

Today, a variety of positions within the pharmaceutical industry are available for pharmacists. Some positions require a Pharm.D. degree, others require advanced training (a residency or fellowship), and other positions require an M.S. or Ph.D. degree in a basic science. A career in the pharmaceutical industry can be rewarding, and advancement is possible. However, like any job, it has it cons as well.

DISCUSSION QUESTIONS AND EXERCISES

1. Put the following areas where pharmacists work in the pharmaceutical industry in order of your preference, for example, sales>marketing>medical services>research>manufacturing/production.
   a. Sales
   b. Marketing
   c. Medical services
   d. Research
   e. Manufacturing and production
2. In some areas of the pharmaceutical industry where pharmacists work, it is recommended that the pharmacist have education and training beyond the Pharm.D. degree. What are these areas?
3. Pharmaceutical companies vary considerably. Some are large and some are small. Some are more research based, whereas others are based more in sales and marketing. Comment on your preferences and why.
4. How do salaries and benefits for pharmacists working in the pharmaceutical industry compare with positions for pharmacists outside the pharmaceutical industry?
5. If you do a good job, new opportunities and promotions are commonly available in the pharmaceutical industry. However, a promotion sometimes means relocating to a different city. How comfortable are you with this possibility?
6. Do you think there might be ethical dilemmas when working as a pharmacist in the pharmaceutical industry?
7. Do you feel there is any stigma associated with working as a pharmacist for the pharmaceutical industry?
8. Make an appointment to interview a pharmacist working for a pharmaceutical company.
9. What do you feel are the pros and cons of working for the pharmaceutical industry?
10. Based on what you know and have read about working within the pharmaceutical industry, is this something you may want to do? Why or why not?

CHALLENGES

1. The goal of pharmaceutical companies is to stay within the law and make as much money as possible for their investors. They do this by trying to produce the safest, most effective drugs and heavily marketing these drugs to those who have control over their use.

For extra credit, and with the permission of your professor, write a concise report on the methods you will use as a pharmacist to determine if the merits of the drugs promoted by drug companies are valid and if there is evidence of a drug's efficacy and safety.

2. For extra credit, and with the permission of your professor, prepare a concise report comparing and contrasting the pros and cons of working in the pharmaceutical industry as a pharmacist with another career choice.

WEB SITES OF INTEREST

Pharmaceutical research and manufacturers: http://www.phrma.org/
Generic Pharmaceutical Association: http://www.gphaonline.org
Parenteral Drug Association: http://www.pda.org/
Biotech Industry Organization: http://www.bio.org/

REFERENCES

1. Pharmaceutical Research and Manufacturers of America. Search for Cures. Available at http://www.phrma.org/searchcures/ and http://www.phrma.org/who/. Accessed May 15, 2006.
2. Contract Pharma. 2005 Top Companies. Available at http://www.contractpharma.com/top_comp.php. Accessed May 15, 2006.
3. Bendis, I. What it takes to have a career in industry. *Pharm Times.* 1997;63:86–90.
4. Kanarek, AD. *A Guide to Good Manufacturing Practices*, 2nd ed. D&MD Publications. Westborough, MA, 2004. Available at http://www.bio.com/industryanalysis/product.jhtml?id=prod2390028. Accessed May 14, 2006.
5. Anonymous. Pharmacists in industry. *Am Pharm.* 1981;NS21:11–26.
6. Sogol, EM. Career paths: Pharmacists in industry. *US Pharm.* 1991;16:35–35–37, 59.
7. Lecca, V. Manufacturer representative. *Tex Pharm.* 1998;117:16.
8. Singletary, JC. Alternative practice: sales and marketing. *J Pharm Pract.* 1989;2:117–122.
9. Rubin, R. Spotlight falls on drug ads. *USA Today.* December 11, 2001, Section 9D.
10. Schmit, J. Drugmakers likely to lob softer pitches. *USA Today.* March 16, 2005, Section 3B.
11. Chimonas, S, and Rothman, DJ. New federal guidelines for physician-pharmaceutical industry relations: the politics of policy formation. *Health Affairs*, 2005;24(4)949–960.
12. Edwards, SA. Pharmacist roles in industrial clinical research and regulatory affairs. *J Pharm Pract.* 1996;9:444–466.
13. Korberly, BH, Mann, KV, and Denisco, MJC. Careers for pharmacists in the pharmaceutical industry: perspective on medical affairs. *J Pharm Pract.* 1989;2(Apr):105–109.

14. Vanderveen, TW. Perspectives of a pharmacist in industry. *Am J Hosp Pharm.* 1986;43:2757–2759.

15. Lear, JS, and Kirk, KW. Women pharmacists in the pharmaceutical industry: their preparation, satisfaction, and outlook. *Am Pharm.* 1987;NS27:34–39.

16. Madell, R. Structure and strategy for women's career advancement in the pharmaceutical industry. *Pharm Exec.* 1998;18(suppl):4–5.

17. Monen, F. Exploring your choices for the future: perspectives in pharmacy-pharmaceutical industry. *Wash Pharm.* 1992;34:18.

18. Pfizer Pharmaceuticals. Industry-based pharmacist. Pharmacy Guide. Available at http://www.pfizercareerguides.com/default.asp?t=article&b=pharmacy&c=practiceAreas&a=IndusPharm. Accessed May 14, 2006.

19. Riggins, JL. Pharmaceutical industry as a career choice. *Am J Health-Syst Pharm.* 2002;59:2097–2098.

20. Lawrence, KR. Journey to the pharmaceutical industry and back: my experience as a medical science liaison. *Am J Health-Syst Pharm.* 2002;59:2098–2090.

21. Avorn, J. *Powerful Medicines.* Random House, New York, 2005.

22. Angell, M. *The Truth About the Drug Companies: How They Deceive Us and What to Do About It.* Random House, New York, 2004.

19

OTHER OPPORTUNITIES FOR PHARMACISTS

Most pharmacists work in community pharmacy, and this is the first choice of new graduates. Other common choices for pharmacists are hospital pharmacy, managed care pharmacy, and consultant pharmacy. There are, however, many more opportunities for pharmacists.

This chapter is about some of those other opportunities. Some of these jobs are well known, whereas others may come as a surprise to the reader. There is no way of knowing exactly how many pharmacists work in each of these areas. What is known is that pharmacists working in these other areas enjoy what they do.

LEARNING OBJECTIVES

After reading this chapter, you should be able to:

- Identify and explain at least eight nontraditional career pathways for pharmacists
- Provide one positive feature and one negative feature of each of the following nontraditional pathways listed under the major headings

ALTERNATIVE MEDICINE

Alternative medical therapies are defined functionally as interventions that are neither widely taught in medical schools nor widely available in U.S. hospitals.[1] *Alternative medicines* include herbal medicines, folk remedies, megavitamins, and homeopathy.

439

Herbal Medicines

Herbal medicines are the various parts (seeds, barks, leaves, berries, or roots) of naturally growing plants. These plant parts are thought to contain one or several active ingredients that help relieve various ailments. Herbal products can be sold in the United States as "dietary supplements," which is a restriction of the FDA. The maker cannot make claims that a dietary supplement can be used to treat, cure, diagnose, or mitigate a specific disease. Only structure–function claims can be made, for example, "improves breathing" or "reduces blood pressure."

Folk Remedies

The use of folk remedies, which are remedies handed down from generation to generation in various ethnic groups, has existed in the United States for hundreds of years. Various Native American tribes still use these remedies, and folk medicine cures are still commonly used by some people in New England and in mountainous areas of the southeastern United States.

Megavitamins

Megavitamin use involves taking large doses (many times the normal daily requirement set by the government) of vitamins and minerals. The theory is that if a little is good, more should be better. However, there is little or no scientific evidence that this theory is true. Although regulated by the FDA, most vitamins and minerals are over-the-counter products that can be sold in any retail outlet. Thus, health food stores and mass merchandisers can sell these products, and no pharmacist is available to advise patients.

Homeopathy

Homeopathy was founded by a German physician, Samuel Hahnemann, over 200 years ago.[2] It is based on stimulating the body to recover itself. Homeopathy is also based on likes curing likes. This is done by using minute dilutions (as small as 1 part per million) of a mineral, botanical substance, animal part, microorganism, or other source that, in larger doses, will produce the very symptoms the patient is experiencing.

Homeopathic medicines are drug products made by homeopathic pharmacists under the processes described in the *Homeopathic Pharmacopeia of the United States* (HPUS), the official manufacturing manual recognized by the FDA. There are about 1200 homeopathic substances in the HPUS.

Although many doubt the effectiveness of homeopathy, there is some scientific evidence that it works better than a placebo in at least one condition — perennial allergic rhinitis.[3] However, the study was conducted in only a few patients.

Use of Alternative Medicines

The use of alternative medicines has increased greatly in the United States chiefly because of an increase in the population seeking alternative therapies.[4] The alternative medicines increasing the most are herbal medicines, megavitamins, folk remedies, and homeopathy.

Pharmacists and Alternative Medicines

The increased use of alternative medicines affects the pharmacist in several ways. First, every practicing pharmacist must be knowledgeable about these products — their uses, effectiveness, and adverse effects. Second, the sale of effective alternative products, and counseling patients on their use, can supplement a practice or become full-time work.

Of the 400 pharmacists responding to a survey, 94% said they believed many alternative medicines can be helpful to the health of patients.[5] Their concern was about the unregulated nature of the products, including concerns about toxicity, and the need for more evidence that alternative medicine works.

Despite misgivings some pharmacists have about the use of alternative medicines, pharmacies are stocking more and more of the products. Independent community pharmacies are taking more interest in this niche market, and some community pharmacies are starting to include homeopathic products.[6] One pharmacist is Bob Hoye, owner of Hoyes' Natural Pharmacy and Wellness Store in Tampa, Florida. Another is Donna Lee, owner of Natural Alternatives in Greensboro, North Carolina, whose only business is in natural medicines.[7]

It is recommended that pharmacists wanting to specialize in alternative medicines learn more about these products by studying professional journals, taking some coursework (e.g., at Columbia University and the University of Arizona), and completing continuing education programs.[7]

ASSOCIATION MANAGEMENT

Pharmacy associations are to pharmacists what government is to its citizens.[8] These professional organizations represent, protect, and promote the profession.

Why Consider This Opportunity?

Pharmacists working in association management speak of the opportunity for professional growth and personal satisfaction.[9] Other reasons include the diversity and the opportunity to have a direct impact upon the future of the profession.

What Do Association Pharmacists Do?

More than 140 pharmacists work for state and national pharmacy associations in the United States.[9] Pharmacists working in professional pharmacy organizations work in the management structure or as staff members of the organization.

Pharmacists working in the administrative part of a professional association use a broad range of administrative skills to help achieve the organization's mission. Working with the association's elected leadership, association executives help set up goals and objectives for the association, and continue their achievement by carrying out effective strategies.

A few specific functions pharmacists are providing in associations today include editing; writing; public relations; government affairs; developing practice standards; educational programming; practice information resources; residency and technician training inspections; providing advice on patient safety, drug shortages, and counterterrorism; and developing student leaders.

Pharmacist staff members of professional pharmacy organizations use skills in law, clinical pharmacy, journalism, education, and public relations to help serve the profession and its members.[9]

Getting Started

Pharmacy students interested in association management can start exploring this opportunity by visiting a state or national pharmacy organization and asking the pharmacists who work there about jobs. Some schools of pharmacy also offer elective classes in management and pharmacy administration that can help.

Some pharmacy organizations, such as the American Pharmaceutical Association (APhA) and the American Society of Health-System Pharmacists (ASHP), and some national pharmacy fraternities and sororities offer association management internships in the summer. The ASHP, the APhA, and the American Society of Consultant Pharmacists (ASCP) also offer 12-month postgraduate residencies in association management.[10]

CONSULTING

Since pharmacy is knowledge based, pharmacists possess knowledge and know-how about pharmacy, drugs, and drug therapy that can be valuable to others. Pharmacists with specific knowledge and experience can consult on a part or full-time basis.

Pharmacists have always consulted. However, modern pharmacy consulting started in the early 1970s when federal requirements for pharmacy consulting in long-term care was mandated.[11] Today, the American Society of Consultant Pharmacists (ASCP) represents pharmacists interested in pharmacy consulting.

Few pharmacists start out as consultants. Most work for years in traditional or clinical practice and gain valuable experience.[12] Some pharmacists become bored with what they are doing, or they become tired of working for somebody else. They start looking around for something different to do. The same happens when some pharmacists retire from what they have been doing most of their lives. They still would like to work, but not necessarily full-time. Consulting fills this need if the pharmacist feels he or she has knowledge needed by others and if the pharmacist is bold enough to take the step of not having a guaranteed source of income at first.

Services and Clients

To be successful at consulting, the entrepreneurial pharmacist must have some knowledge or know-how needed by others. The following is a list of services some pharmacists who perform consulting offer, the skills needed to offer these services, and some potential clients for these services.

Education

Many organizations need education that can be provided by a pharmacist or those who can organize educational sessions. The client for these services is usually the pharmaceutical industry. The education is needed within the company, or the company sponsors educational programs for various professional groups such a physicians, nurses, or pharmacists.

Pharmacists organizing educational programs for the pharmaceutical industry need strong organizational skills, and they need to know who can speak, and speak well, on certain topics needed. Thus, the educational consultant pharmacist needs to be well networked with others to be successful.

Public Speaking

Pharmacists who have knowledge in an area of interest to others always have opportunities to be hired as public speakers. The clients are professional health care organizations, who are always looking for interesting speakers for the various educational meetings they sponsor. Speaker bureaus of pharmaceutical companies always need good speakers, and they keep a pool of available speakers who can talk on interesting topics. Public speaking is a good way for consultant pharmacists to keep visible, and it is a chance for pharmacists to display and market their expertise. However, pharmacists who want to be good speakers must be good teachers, proficient in audiovisual preparation, and entertaining.

Professional Writing and Editing

Good writers are always needed in the health care field. The clients are book publishers, journal editors, and companies that publish manuals and educational materials for health care professionals.

The essential skills needed include good writing and communication skills, intellectual curiosity, the willingness to take risks, being open to new ideas and perspectives, and having a fresh approach to subjects.[13] To be a good writer you need to read — a lot. As Stephen King and Ernest Hemingway said, "if you do not have time to read, you do not have time to write."[14,15]

Many journals and magazines have a set range of fees for writing certain types of articles. The person submitting the article can name his or price but should be willing to accept less in the beginning. This field is low in pay to begin, but fees can become higher once writers get established and become known for their good writing.

Consultant to the Pharmaceutical Industry

Some pharmacists are hired as consultants, on a project basis, by the pharmaceutical industry.[16,17] Most of these pharmacists have technical knowledge in a basic science or in an area such as regulatory affairs. Some clinical pharmacists are hired as consultants to help with phase III and IV clinical trials.

Some pharmaceutical companies also have community or hospital pharmacy advisory boards that hire well-known pharmacists to help the company market its new products or to advise the company on how it should be approaching physicians and pharmacists about its products.

Patient Self-Care

Some pharmacists have set up consulting practices that help patients with self-care.[18,19] Some of this consulting is done outside the retail pharmacy setting, and pharmacists are paid to aid patients with their self-care needs. The key to this business is having access to a supply of patients who have a high priority for keeping healthy or who have poor access to care. It is also important that the self-care pharmacist knows what products and services patients need. Marketing services to physicians for referrals and to patients for new and repeat business is critical.

Setting Up Services and Providing Staffing

Some pharmacists have developed consulting services based on their pharmacy practice expertise. Some provide expertise in setting up systems such as unit-dose or IV additive services, performing drug use evaluations (DUEs), setting up pharmaceutical care, or developing specialized clinical services. Some pharmacists have also gone into the staffing business and supplying pharmacists and pharmacy technicians on a short-term or long-term basis.

The clients for these services are hospitals and managed care organizations. Sometimes these organizations also need education and training. To be a consultant in pharmacy practice, the pharmacist must have expertise in a needed area, strong organizational and time management skills, and the ability to keep on top of everything.

Home Health Services

Many pharmacists have started out by offering their expertise in nutritional support and providing home infusions.[20] The clients are home care agencies, hospices, and home infusion facilities. The knowledge needed is that of nutritional support. The skill needed is to convince others that your expertise will strengthen the services they provide to patients.

Proposals

Often, the client will want the pharmacy consultant to provide a proposal for services. These proposals need to be carefully developed. The ASCP provides examples and advice on business proposals. It is important for the proposal to be concise, clear, and letter perfect.

Fees

It is important that the consultant pharmacist be paid a fair fee for the services delivered. Fees need to be competitive; thus, the consultant pharmacist must find out what others are charging for similar services even if it is outside pharmacy. Usually, pharmacists charge too little, although some start low and then charge more as experience is gained.

Contracts

If possible, it is always important to have a contract or letter of agreement for consulting jobs. These can be basic, but they must specifically list the work to be performed, the time frame, and the consideration for the work.

Incorporation

For pharmacists deciding to be consultants on a full-time basis, it is strongly advised that they seek counsel of a certified public accountant (CPA) and incorporate their business.[21] There are several options for doing this, each with pros and cons. This decision adds the greatest layer of protection and the most flexibility.

Hire a Good Accountant

Hiring a good accountant is a must because you will have to pay your own payroll and income taxes and keep detailed records of your expenses.

Getting Started

For those serious about being a full-time pharmacy consultant, some good advice is offered in Table 19.1. The full article should be consulted for a view of what it takes to be a successful, self-employed consultant pharmacist.[12]

Risks

The risks of trying to do full-time pharmacy consulting involve not knowing when the next paycheck is coming, and more importantly, how much it will be for. This can be stressful. Many people are not willing to take these risks.

Rewards

Successful, entrepreneurial pharmacists repeatedly use words like *challenging, stimulating,* and *rewarding.* What they enjoy is solving problems and

Table 19.1   Ideas on Getting Started in a Career in Pharmacy Consulting

Contact ASCP or a seasoned pharmacy consultant information, support and resources.

Try to learn the ropes from someone already in the business.

Make a long list of potential customers, especially those you know.

When you do get work, continue to market yourself.

Start small and keep your expenses low.

Keep your rates low to start.

Show your willingness to have your brain picked for free.

Hire a good accountant.

Don't get in over your head by overpromising on a job.

Develop and focus on your area of expertise.

Get an associate to share the load as the work starts to increase.

Source: Adapted and reprinted with permission from Garel, E. Selling your pharmacy know-how. *Pharm Pract.* 1998;14(5):60–64.

seeing their ideas carried out. They also enjoy working for themselves, making their own decisions, setting their own schedules, and being their own bosses.

COMPOUNDING PHARMACY

Compounding pharmacy is defined as practicing as a dispensing community pharmacist with an emphasis on preparing customized dosage forms and prescription medication to meet individual patients' or physicians' needs. Compounding prescription medications started at the birth of the profession, grew until the 1960s, died, and then was reborn in the 1990s. In 2003, 1% of all prescriptions dispensed were compounded.[22]

Compounding pharmacies prepare medications that are not commercially available or are not stable for long periods of time and commercially available medications that need to be altered to serve the needs of the patient.

For those interested, there is an article that offers insight into a day in the life of a compounding pharmacist.[23]

FORENSIC PHARMACY

Some pharmacists have knowledge of pharmacology, pharmacokinetics, therapeutics, or drug safety and can be hired as consultants and expert witnesses to provide reviews of legal cases, provide depositions, or testify in trials involving medication. The clients are usually attorneys. This practice is known as *forensic pharmacy* — the application of medication sciences to legal work.[24]

Forensic pharmacists engage in litigation and the regulatory process and sometimes in the criminal justice system. To do this work, one must study, be prepared for anything, be unbiased, be knowledgeable about the legal system, and be able to stand the pressure of long depositions and cross examinations by attorneys.[25]

INFORMATION TECHNOLOGY

Pharmacists with a good working knowledge of computers, information technology, or pharmacy automation and who understand how this technology can improve pharmacy or patient care are often employed by sellers of these products. Hardware and pharmacy software companies often need pharmacists to make improvements to their products and to help sell and set up their products in pharmacies.

MEDICAL EDUCATION AND COMMUNICATIONS

Some pharmacists work for companies that produce various written medical communications. Some of these communications can be package inserts for pharmaceutical companies, documentation and manuals for computer software, drug therapy newsletters (e.g., *The Medical Letter*), brochures, handbooks, and advertisements for drugs.

Medical communicators review the literature, explore developments, and interact with medical experts. They must know how to write in an interesting way to keep the reader's attention. Pharmacists going into medical writing also need above-average writing skills and should be able to find information, balance several projects at once, and meet deadlines.[26]

There are some interesting articles about being a pharmacist in the medical education and communication fields.[27–29]

MAIL-ORDER PHARMACY

Patients can mail their prescriptions or have their physician call in a prescription for them to a remote pharmacy. After dispensing, the mail-order pharmacy mails the medication to the patient. This is usually legally permissible, even between most states, as long as the pharmacist can reasonably determine that the prescription is legal, is for an FDA-approved drug, and the prescriber is licensed to prescribe in the state where the prescription was written.

Value of Mail-Order Pharmacies

The value of mail-order pharmacies is continuously debated by pharmacists. Those in the business feel they are meeting patients' needs and providing a fine service both legally and ethically. Patients use and like mail-order pharmacy services for the savings they gain by buying their medication in this manner. However, patients sometimes get anxious about receiving their medication on time. Some community pharmacists are quick to point out the lack of face-to-face, personal attention and ask if there is a relationship between the pharmacist working at the mail-order pharmacy and the patient.

What Is it Like inside a Mail-Order Pharmacy?

Mail-order pharmacies are large operations with cutting-edge technology. Here is a description of what you might see inside a mail-order pharmacy.

> Inside this pharmacy, vacuum tubes pop the exact quantity of pills required for an individual's prescription into a procession of plastic trays filled with bottles. Machines screw the caps onto the bottles with a force just right for handling by an arthritic senior. Robotic arms zero in on the correct bottle for a patient from thousands of trays and drop it into a waiting, addressed envelope. Conveyor belts carry the envelopes to mail-sorting stations, where they slide off sloped trays into large bags, ready to be taken to the nearby postal depot.[30]

Largest Mail-Order Pharmacy Provider

Many people are surprised to learn that the first (early 1950s) and largest provider of mail-order prescriptions in the United States is the Department of Veteran's Affairs — the VA hospitals and medical centers. The VA mails approximately 100 million prescriptions a year, of which 65% is dispensed through automation. How the VA does this is fascinating (see Chapter 6, Information Technology and Automation).

The VA has regionalized and automated its large outpatient medication refill program. Instead of each VA medical center refilling and mailing prescriptions, the refills are electronically sent to a regional commercial mail-order pharmacy (CMOP).

Commercial Mail-Order Pharmacies

The American Association of Retired Persons (AARP) started commercial mail-order pharmacy in the 1950s.[31] Today, there are over 200 commercial mail-order pharmacy programs.[32] Some of the major commercial mail-order pharmacies are Express Scripts, Caremark, Medco, and Walgreens.

Although mail-order pharmacies have been gaining on the retail pharmacy market share, the use of mail-order is starting to drop (see Chapter 8, Ambulatory Pharmacy). This may be because most health plans only allow 90-day fills of prescriptions through mail-order pharmacies. The Medicare Part D prescription benefit has leveled the playing field by allowing 90-day fills at any pharmacy.

Mail-Order Practice

Pharmacists working in mail-order pharmacies share the same dedication to patients as their retail counterparts.[33] They dispense and consult with professionalism while meeting productivity goals. Their functions include screening prescriptions, calling physicians, answering calls from physicians and patients, dispensing, checking prescriptions for accuracy, calling patients, and improving patient compliance.

Mail-order pharmacies provide toll-free telephone numbers and patient advisory leaflets with every new and refilled prescription. Other safety features include pharmacists' checking each other on certain types of prescriptions, such as those for warfarin. There are also standards for when patients receive their medication. For example, the AARP mail-order pharmacy service expects that patients will receive their medication within 6 days of mailing in a prescription.[31]

There are pros and cons of every pharmacist position, and this is true of working for a mail-order pharmacy. The pros of working for a mail-order pharmacy include flexible schedules — sometimes no weekends, evenings, or holidays; the chance to discuss matters with patients; informal dress codes; and advancement. The major disadvantages are lack of face-to-face contact with patients and the stigma sometimes felt because of competition with retail pharmacists. Other concerns include standing all day and repetition.[33]

NUCLEAR PHARMACY

Many students are not aware of the field of nuclear pharmacy, as only a few schools of pharmacy offer elective courses in this subject. The practice of nuclear pharmacy involves tagging, which is attaching low-level radioactivity to a drug.[34] The new product becomes a *radiopharmaceutical*. Radiopharmaceuticals are chiefly employed to aid diagnosis of a disease and to monitor the outcome of drug therapy.[35] The radiopharmaceutical is injected into a patient, and the drug localizes in a target organ depending on which drug is used. A camera is placed over the patient's organ, and the radiation from the radiopharmaceutical exposes the film in the camera. Nuclear medicine physicians read the film to see if the patient's organ is functioning normally.

Most radiopharmaceuticals are prepared fresh each morning; therefore, a nuclear pharmacist's day starts early in the morning. Early tasks involve reviewing the schedule of patients for the day, preparing the radiopharmaceuticals, record keeping, consulting with referring physicians and the nuclear medicine physicians, perhaps some teaching, and some committee work.

The Nuclear Regulatory Commission (NRC) requires a minimum of 700 contact hours of training (typically 200 hours of didactic instruction and 500 hours of experiential training) to become an "authorized user" of radioactive material. This training can be obtained from some colleges of pharmacy, through residency training or from one of the three major companies (Mallinckrodt, Nicomed-Amersham, and SynCor) that employ nuclear pharmacists.[35]

Nuclear pharmacy was the first specialty area recognized by the Board of Pharmaceutical Specialties (BPS) in 1978.[36] In 2005, there were 495 board certified nuclear pharmacists.

Nuclear pharmacists are satisfied with what they do. One nuclear pharmacist has stated, "I am very happy with my career in nuclear pharmacy. New drugs, better technology, and the demand for improved diagnostic techniques make this industry dynamic. I find the changes mentally stimulating because they put my knowledge of the pure sciences to use."[34]

Several excellent references are provided for those seeking more information about nuclear pharmacy.[37,38]

PHARMACY BENEFIT MANAGEMENT

Pharmacy benefit management companies (PBMs) manage the pharmacy benefit provided by health plans. PBMs provide clients with accessible retail pharmacy networks, process drug claims, and review utilization, and some provide mail-order pharmacy services.

Most PBMs hire several pharmacists to undertake numerous functions such as interpreting which drugs represent a covered benefit, supervising drug formulary content and revision, negotiating rebates with manufacturers, and directing drug utilization review programs. Pharmacists also help market contracts that enlist pharmacies that will accept payment from the plan for each prescription dispensed to covered individuals and maintain relations with participating pharmacists and enrolled patients.

PHARMACY LAW

Another interesting area of practice is pharmacy law. Pharmacists who earn a law degree can specialize in pharmacy and drug laws. Colleges of pharmacy, drug companies, and professional pharmacy organizations often employ pharmacists with a law degrees.

Many articles have been written about being a pharmacist attorney.[39–47] Pharmacist attorneys make major contributions to the profession by being up-to-date, writing, and presenting to practicing pharmacists on new drug and pharmacy laws and regulations and on the movement of the law through legal case reviews.

PHARMACOECONOMICS AND OUTCOMES RESEARCH

Pharmacoeconomics is a tool designed to provide users and decision makers with information about the cost-effectiveness of different pharmacotherapies.[48] This is an emerging field of study for pharmacists. Some colleges of pharmacy offer graduate studies, and there are also residencies and fellowships.

Outcomes research is the process by which different therapies or drug regimens are evaluated in order to measure the extent to which a goal of therapy or desirable outcome can be reached.[48] As with pharmacoeconomics, graduate studies, residencies, and fellowships are available.

PHARMACOEPIDEMIOLOGY

Pharmacoepidemiology focuses on pharmaceutical care outcomes and the identification of potential or realized drug problems.[49] Pharmacoepidemiology measures the source, diffusion, use, and effects of drugs in a population and determines the frequency and distribution of drug use outcomes in that population. Pharmacists who are interested in pharmacoepidemiology need strong backgrounds in biostatistics and epidemiology.

PHARMACY MANAGEMENT

Pharmacy management is another opportunity for pharmacists. Pharmacy managers are found in community pharmacy, hospital pharmacy, managed care pharmacy, and other companies where pharmacists work. The roles of a pharmacy manager are to plan and manage operations, people, facilities, equipment, information systems, and fiscal resources.

To become a pharmacy manager, it is recommended that the person receive supervisory and management training. These can be obtained by earning more academic credit, completing a residency, or receiving more training supplied by the employer.

VETERINARY PHARMACY

Imagine having patients who cannot verbalize what is wrong with them and are therefore unable to be counseled about their medication. That is what it is like being a veterinary pharmacist — challenging, to say the least.

The difference between a regular pharmacy practice and a veterinarian pharmacy practice is that the patients are unique and the treatment diverse. Patients can be birds weighing 5 g or elephants weighing over 2000 pounds. Other challenges include varying dosages and responses to the same drug in different species of animals, the names of the drugs being different from those for humans, and a lot of compounding. However, pharmacists can come up to speed through self-learning and on-the-job training.[50]

Veterinary pharmacists provide value by having a broader knowledge of drug therapy than most veterinarians, being able to compound medications, develop formularies, control inventory, and set up safe systems of medication distribution. Veterinary pharmacists have also set up a computer network to share information between veterinary pharmacists in the United States and even outside the country.[52]

The job of a veterinary pharmacist is rewarding. "In working together, the pharmacist and veterinarian can establish a good professional relationship."[50] "It is rewarding to have a relationship with veterinary practitioners that allows me to be intimately involved with the drug product selection. It is very satisfying, both professionally and personally, to know that a pharmacist can make a difference in the success of drug therapy."[51]

For those who would like to learn more about the diseases and regulatory issues of veterinary pharmacy, Creighton University School of Pharmacy offers an on-line veterinary continuing education course.[52]

SUMMARY

Although most pharmacists work in community and hospital pharmacies, plenty of opportunities exist beyond these traditional practice sites to use the knowledge they gain in their education, training, and practice experience. Some nontraditional areas pharmacists are working can be fulfilling.

DISCUSSION QUESTIONS AND EXERCISES

1. Rate your interest (1 to 10) for the following opportunities in pharmacy (1 = low interest, 10 = high).
   a. Alternative medicines _____
   b. Consulting _____
   c. Homeopathic pharmacy _____
   d. Jobs with no patient contact _____
   e. Jobs outside pharmacy _____
   f. Mail-order pharmacy _____
   g. Pharmacy management _____
   h. Pharmacy benefit management _____
   i. Self-care pharmacy practice _____
   j. Veterinary pharmacy _____

     k. Medical communications _____
     l. Nuclear pharmacy _____
     m.Pharmacy law _____

2. Circle your top three choices in question 1.
3. 3–5. Make appointments to interview pharmacists working in each of your top three areas of interest.
4. From what you know and have read about the three top areas you selected in question 2, what are the pros and cons of each?
5. Which of the three areas you discussed in question 6 interests you most. Why?
6. How does your choice in question 7 compare with other interests you have in pharmacy?
7. Name three pharmacist positions that require no patient contact.
8. Name three areas outside the pharmacy profession where pharmacists can work and still use their education and training in pharmacy.

CHALLENGES

1. For extra credit, and with the permission of your professor, select one of the careers described in this chapter and investigate and prepare a concise report about this career. Include the pros and cons of this opportunity and describe what it would take for you to pursue this career. End your report by making a convincing argument as to why you may pursue this option.
2. Some pharmacists work in jobs where being a pharmacist is not a requirement. For extra credit, and with the permission of your professor, investigate and prepare a concise report with three cases studies where pharmacists are working in such situations and include why they did this and why they like their jobs.

WEB SITES OF INTEREST

Alternative medicine: http://www.pitt.edu/~cbw/altm.html
Association management: See Web addresses in Chapter 16
Compounding pharmacy: http://www.iacprx.org
Consulting: http://www.ascp.com
Forensic pharmacy: http://hometown.aol.com/PAnder7291/forensic-pharmacist.index.html
Medical education and communications: http://www.shsinc.com/meded_jobs.htm
Mail-order pharmacy: http://rxinsider.com/mail_order_pharmacy_jobs.htm
Nuclear pharmacy: http://nuclear.pharmacy.purdue.edu/what.php

Pharmacy benefits management: http://www.nhpf.org/pdfs_ib/IB749_
ABCsofPBMs_10-27-99.pdf

Pharmacoeconomics: http://www.ispor.org/

Pharmacoepidemiology: http://www.pharmacoepi.org/

Pharmacy law: http://www.aspl.org

Pharmacy management: http://www.pharman.co.uk/

Veterinary pharmacy: http://pharmacyonline.creighton.edu/pha380/

REFERENCES

1. Eisenberg, DM, Kessler, RC, Foster, C, et al. Unconventional medicine in the United States. *N Engl J Med*. 1993;328(4):246–252.
2. Stehlin, I. Homeopathy: real medicine or empty promises? *FDA Consumer*. 1996;30:15–19.
3. Taylor, MA, Reilly, D, Llewellyn-Jones, RH, et al. Randomised controlled trial of homoeopathy versus placebo in perennial allergic rhinitis with overview of four trial series. *Br Med J*. 2000;321:471–476.
4. Eisenberg, DM, Davis, RB, Ettner, SL, et al. Trends in alternative medicine use in the United States, 1990–1997. *JAMA*. 1998;280:1569–1575.
5. Portyansky, E. Alternative medicine. *Drug Top*. 1998;142:44–50.
6. Levy, S. Welcome, homeopathy. *Drug Top*. 2000;144:74–78.
7. McCormick, E. Natural medicines: new career for pharmacists? *Pharm Times*. 1998;64:52–55.
8. Poole, P. How pharmacy associations protect members' livelihood, future. *Calif Pharm*. 1988;35:20.
9. Temple, TR. Pharmacy association management. *J Pharm Pract*. 1989;2:70–76.
10. Zetzl, SE. Preparing for a career in association work. *Am J Hosp Pharm*. 1988;45:2495.
11. Guidry, T. Practice alternatives: consulting. *VA Pharm*. 1998;82:14.
12. Garel, E. Selling your pharmacy know-how. *Pharm Pract*. 1998;14(5):60–64.
13. D'Achille, KM. Living on the edge: nontraditional consulting practices. *Consult Pharm*. 1991;6:888–902.
14. King, S. *On Writing*. Pocket Books, New York, 2000.
15. Hemingway, E. *On Writing*. Touchstone, New York, 1984.
16. Ptak, LR. Consulting in pharmaceutical research. *J Pharm Pract*. 1996;9:471–476.
17. Gebhart, F. Superpharmacists finding cash rewards in nontraditional practice. *Drug Top*. 1999;143:111.
18. Srnka, QM. Ten ways to build a self-care consulting practice. *NARD J*. 1993;115:75–79.
19. Srnka, QM. Implementing a self-care-consulting practice. *Am Pharm*. 1993;NS33:61–71.
20. McPherson, ML, and Ferris, R. Establishing a home health care consulting practice. *Am Pharm*. 1994;NS34:42–49.
21. Baker, KR. Necessary lessons for the entrepreneur pharmacist. *Drug Store News Pharm*. 1996;6:25.
22. Torrie, YC. Pharmacy compounding is flourishing once again. *Pharm Times*. November, 2005. Available at http://www.pharmacytimes.com/article.cfm?ID=2780. Accessed April 21, 2006.

23. LeClaire, J. Compounding pharmacists on cutting edge. Monster.com. Available at http://www.healthcare.monster.com/pharm/articles/compounding/. Accessed April 21, 2006.

24. Anderson, PD, and O'Donnell, JT. The forensic pharmacist. In *Drug Injury: Liability, Analysis, and Prevention,* 2nd ed. Lawyers and Judges Publishing Company, Tucson, AZ, 2005, chap. 42.

25. Van Dusen, V, and Pray, WS. The hospital pharmacist as an expert witness. *Hosp Pharm.* 2000;35:1296–1303.

26. Price, KO. Career alternative: medical communications. *Pharm Stud.* 1992;22(4):13–15.

27. Connelly, SB. Continuing medical education: a view from the inside. *Am J Health-Syst Pharm.* 2003;60:1901–1902.

28. McConnell, KA. Am I still a pharmacist? *Am J Health-Syst Pharm.* 2003;60:1898–1899.

29. Moghadam, RG. Scientific writing: a career for pharmacists. *Am J Health Syst Pharm.* 2003;60:1899–1900.

30. Duvall, M. Strong medicine: big companies think automatic mail-order pharmacies like Medco help cure rising drug costs. That remedy won't make retail giants like Walgreens and CVS feel better. *Baseline.* 2005;1(43):50.

31. Hitchens, K. A day in the life of a mail-order pharmacist. *Drug Store News Pharm.* 1994;4:18.

32. Personal correspondence with Will, B. *Info USA.* August 13, 2001.

33. Heller, A. The real face of mail-order pharmacy. *Drug Store News Pharm.* 1996;6:17–19.

34. Trisko, CD. Exploring your choices for the future: perspectives in pharmacy–nuclear pharmacy. *Wash Pharm.* 1992;34:22.

35. Shaw, SM. Introduction to nuclear pharmacy. *Int J Pharm Compound.* 1998;2(6):424–25,469–470.

36. Ponto, JA. Nuclear pharmacy and the Board of Pharmaceutical Specialties (BPS). *J Pharm Pract.* 1989;2:299–301.

37. Laven, DL, and Hladik, WB. Radiologic pharmacy: forward. *J Pharm Pract.* 1989;2:267–321.

38. College of Pharmacy, the University of Arkansas for Medical Sciences. The Nuclear Pharmacy. Available at http://nuclearpharmacy.uams.edu. Assessed January 1, 2001.

39. Fink, JL. Law school for pharmacists? *Am Pharm.* 1981:NS21(8):52–53.

40. Anonymous. Information about law school. *Pharmacy Law Digest. Facts & Comparisons.* 1991;July:I20–I21.

41. Chesser, J. Prescription for legal education. *Bus Record.* 1989;Dec 18–24:4.

42. Brushwood, DB. Career opportunities for lawyer-pharmacists. *Tomorrow's Pharm.* 1986;8(2):4–5.

43. Steeves, RF. Pharmacist-lawyers. *J Am Pharm Assoc.* 1967;7(3):145, 151.

44. Woods, WE. Career opportunities as a pharmacist-attorney. *Squibb Rev Pharm Students.* 1965;4:1–4.

45. Fink, JL. Pharmacist-lawyers. *J Am Pharm Assoc.* 1974;14(10):565–569.

46. Brushwood, DB, and Cole, MG. The case for pharmacy law as a career. *Legal Aspects Pharm Pract.* 1985;8(6):1–2.

47. Anonymous. Pharmacist who are lawyers. *Am Drug.* 1974:Oct 1:34–40.

48. Basskin, LE. What is the difference between pharmacoeconomics and outcomes research. In *Practical Pharmacoeconomics*. Advanstar Communications, Inc., Cleveland, OH, 1998, chap 1.

49. Waning, B, and Montagne, M. In *Pharmacoepidemiology: Principles and Practice*. McGraw-Hill, New York, 2001, chap 1.

50. Rivkin, L. Expanding opportunities in veterinary pharmacy. *Tomorrow's Pharm*. 1983;5:4–6.

51. Jones, JW. Career alternatives: veterinary pharmacist. *Pharm Stud*. 1992;22(2):30–31.

52. Anonymous. Creighton offers online veterinary CE course. *AACP News*. May, 2002.

20

CAREER DEVELOPMENT

Few pharmacists stay in the same position their whole career. In 1986, the average American changed jobs every 3.8 years, and the average hospital pharmacist every 4 years.[1] This means that throughout your pharmacy career, you will probably change jobs, and you may even change the type of work you do as a pharmacist.

This is a great time to be a pharmacist. There is an unprecedented number and variety of career opportunities for pharmacists. Despite the many opportunities for pharmacists, finding a good job or changing to another job is something that should be done with care.

This chapter is about career planning for pharmacists beginning a career in pharmacy or for veteran pharmacists looking for a job change. The chapter will present information about careers, career development, how to assess strengths and preferences, and about being prepared for the next job. It also will cover how to find opportunities, how to assess job offers, and how to make a career change.

LEARNING OBJECTIVES

After this reading this chapter, you should be able to:

- Define a career
- Describe the pitfalls of planning for your career
- Identify the steps in finding a job as a pharmacist
- Describe how to differentiate yourself from others to find the job you want
- Write a convincing letter of application and develop a CV
- Explain some dos and don'ts in interviewing

A CAREER

Having a job and having a career are not the same. Anyone can have a job, but not everyone can have a career. *Webster's Dictionary* defines a career as "a pursuit of progressive achievement, especially in public, business, or professional life."[2] *Webster's Dictionary* goes on to say, under the word *career*, "a profession for which one trains and is undertaken as a permanent calling."

Pharmacy is more than a job and more than work for hire. Pharmacy is a profession that should be pursued as if you will never learn enough. Members of the pharmacy profession chose pharmacy, learned a body of specialized knowledge, and prepared for a life pursuit of their profession. Pharmacists are lifelong learners who continually are improving their practice skills and are proud to be a part of a noble profession.

CAREER PLANNING

To be the most successful, careers need to be planned versus drifting from opportunity to opportunity. Planning involves selecting goals and deciding how to achieve them.

Common Mistakes Students Make

Pharmacy students often make mistakes when it comes to career planning.[3] The first mistake is procrastination. Many students become so involved in coursework that they do not think about or plan what they would like to do with their degree until it gets close to graduation. Ideally, pharmacy students should be thinking about what they would like to do as pharmacists as soon as they decide to be pharmacists. They should also be exploring various opportunities throughout their time as a students.

Every pharmacy student should be introduced to and should investigate the pros and cons of graduate work in pharmacy during the first year of pharmacy school. The two tracks available are in the social–administrative and pharmaceutical science domains.

The second mistake pharmacy students often make in career planning is to be too passive. Many students wait for the jobs to come to them in the form of interviewers who come to the campus on "career day" rather than actively looking for good opportunities. Because there are so many opportunities available for new graduates, some students are not challenged to think about their careers.

The third mistake is for students to make assumptions about what is available in the workplace. Students may only assume positions are available in independent, chain, or hospital pharmacy or that the only positions available are the ones being recruited during campus career day.

The fourth mistake is letting the pressure of paying off schools loans overcome the value of pursuing a pharmacy residency, which some students think is just another year of senior clerkships — it is not. A 1-year pharmacy residency is the equivalent of 2 to 3 years of practice experience, and provides training in being a pharmacy leader. It provides increased knowledge and confidence and puts the resident in a position to obtain the best new jobs — the ones that are the most satisfying.

Avoiding Common Pitfalls

The author of an article entitled "Choosing Your Career Direction — Before It Chooses You" offers some don'ts for students thinking about their careers as a pharmacists:[3]

- Don't be driven by what others think you should do with your life.
- Don't assume there is only one right choice.
- Don't assume that career planning is something you do once, and then it is over.
- Don't assume the decision you make just out of pharmacy school will be your only decision about your career.
- Don't wait for an opportunity to find you. Continually seek opportunities and learn all you can about them.

FINDING YOUR JOB AS A PHARMACIST

The first decision to be made, as early as possible, is to decide what will happen after graduating from pharmacy school. Will you pursue more education or added training or gain employment?

More Education

Many good opportunities exist for pharmacists with education beyond a Pharm.D. degree. Many opportunities in the pharmaceutical industry require an M.S. or Ph.D. degree (see Chapter 17, How Drugs are Discovered, Tested, and Approved and Chapter 18, The Pharmaceutical Industry). An M.S. or Ph.D. degree in a specific science discipline (pharmaceutical chemistry, pharmacology, pharmacokinetics, or pharmaceutics) can also be obtained and used to find a job in academics (see Chapter 15, Pharmacy Academia).

Some pharmacists also find that seeking a master's degree in business administration (M.B.A.) provides more flexibility in finding the ideal job. Other educational degrees that work well with the Pharm.D. degree are the master's of public health (M.P.H.) or a law degree (J.D.).

More Training

Some of the best opportunities in pharmacy are for pharmacists who have advanced training provided by a pharmacy residency or fellowship. Pharmacy residencies provide 1 to 2 years of intense training in the practice of pharmacy and pharmaceutical care. Pharmacy fellowships provide 2 years of intense training in performing clinical research (see Chapter 2, The Pharmacist). Residencies and fellowships help distinguish one pharmacist from another.[4] Many of the top leaders in the pharmacy profession have completed a postgraduate residency or fellowship.

Gaining Employment

Another possibility is to go directly into the workforce after graduating from pharmacy school. Endless opportunities abound for new pharmacy graduates. However, selecting the correct job is not an easy task. In finding the first or next job, it is important to take charge and put in the necessary time to locate the best job available. Finding a good job takes planning and assessment.

Planning

Planning starts with identifying career goals. Most important is putting the goals into written statements. If the goals are not written, they will just become wishes, and few, if any, of these, will be achieved.

Goals should be practical, achievable within a certain time frame, and as specific as possible. One way to do this is to make two or three short-term goals (achievable within 2 years), two or three intermediate goals (achievable within 10 years), and two or three long-term goals (achievable over a career). Once drafted, goal statements need to be revised and refined over several days and revised annually. Table 20.1 is an example of some goal statements written by one new pharmacy graduate.

Assessment

To set realistic and achievable goals involves knowing yourself and the opportunities available. Learning about the two should take place as close together as possible, but the process starts with self-assessment.

Self-Assessment

There are different ways of examining yourself for your likes and dislikes and your strengths and weaknesses. Several tools are available that can help makes self-assessment easier. The first approach is to read *What*

Table 20.1 Professional Goals for One New Pharmacy Graduate

Goals Achievable within 2 Years

Work in a thriving, independent community pharmacy

Learn about owning and running a small business

Get involved in professional organizational work locally

Goals Achievable within 10 Years

Identify the type of pharmacy I would like to purchase

Seek advice from a pharmacy administration professor in pharmacy ownership

Evaluate three to five independent community pharmacies for their potential

Purchase one store

Become an officer in the state pharmacy association

Goals Achievable within My Career

Make the first store into a professional pharmacy where patients and pharmaceutical care are the priorities

Make the pharmacy successful from business and patient viewpoints

Be elected president of the state pharmacy association

Color is Your Parachute?[5] This is an inexpensive, short, easy to use manual that has been in print for over 30 years. An excellent workbook is also available. These will help answer important questions such as What do I like to do? What am I good at? Where do I want to do it?

The other tool recommended for self-assessment and job assessment is the APhA Pathway Evaluation Program, first developed by Glaxo Pharmaceutical Company to help pharmacy professionals, especially pharmacy students, in career planning.[6] The program consists of three parts.

Briefing document: Pre-workshop, self-assessment exercises; a combination of written and online exercises

Workshop workbook: Materials and exercises to use during a live workshop

Follow-up materials: Exercises and resources to use after completing the workshop

It is highly recommended that the student use this program during his or her first year of pharmacy school, especially while taking an introduction to pharmacy course. There is even a virtual mentor program. The Web site for this program is listed at he end of this chapter.

As far as getting to know a job better, there is nothing like finding out about it firsthand. Pharmacy students who can handle coursework and a part-time job should work as pharmacy interns or as pharmacy technicians to become familiar with what various pharmacy jobs have to offer. While in school, students should also try to schedule their practice experiences at various places where pharmacists work.

Another good way to find out the pros and cons of various jobs in pharmacy is to attend professional pharmacy meetings — local, state, or national — to network with pharmacists. Never fail to ask pharmacists where they work, what they do, and what they like and do not like about their job. Most pharmacist love helping pharmacy students find their way.

Finding Opportunities on Your Own

Finding opportunities on your own can be daunting if you are seeking to go beyond finding a job by word-of-mouth. Here are some tips:

- Attend local, state, and national pharmacy meetings.
- Sign up for ASHP's personnel placement service.
- Attend ASHP's mid-year clinical meeting in December.
- Go to the Monster.com site.
- Go to Pharmacist.com.

Pharmacist.com has many tools for seeking a good job in pharmacy including: (a) choosing the right employer, (b) 25 tactics for negotiating with your potential employer, (c) networking for career success, (d) successful job interviews, and (e) typical interview questions.

Developing Your CV

Putting It Together

Once you identify a preferred job, the next step is to develop a resume, which in pharmacy is more commonly referred to as a *curriculum vitae* (CV). The CV is a critical document used during job searches. A CV tells employers who you are and what qualifications you have to perform a job. CVs must be carefully composed, and the presentation should journalistically perfect and attractive.

CVs usually consist of seven categories: the heading, the job objective, education and training, work experiences, honors and awards, activities and interest, and references.[7]

Heading: Include your formal and complete name (first, middle initial, and last).

Job objective: Include a brief description of your career objective for the job being sought. This needs to be carefully thought out and crafted. It should not include clichés such as, "I want to be a valuable member of the health care team." Be honest and write this section from your heart.

Education and training: Include all formal college education, special coursework, and any residencies and fellowships.

Work experiences: Include any work experiences, paid or unpaid, that would contribute to gaining the job being sought. This section should list the job title and a brief summary of a few key responsibilities.

Honors and awards: This needs to be carefully considered. Include only the most worthy accomplishments.

Hobbies and interests: This is a chance to show that you have well-rounded interests. List only two or three.

References: For new graduates, it is important to list two job references, a professor who knows your classroom work, and a clerkship preceptor who knows your clinical abilities.

Contact information: Addresses, phone numbers, and e-mail addresses should be listed last.

Students may think their CVs do not show much. At this point in your pharmacy career, the quality and presentation of the information are more important than the quantity of information. The CV should be produced using a word processor with average font size (12 point) using boldface type for major section headings, be printed on high-quality, off-white paper, and be letter perfect. The writer and several others should carefully proofread the CV before it is used to find a job and look for these five mistakes commonly made on CVs.[7]

Aiming too high, too soon: Do not use words like leader, manager, or supervisor unless you have the background to support their use. Employers favor people who like to start in entry-level jobs and prove they can handle more responsibility.

Giving all education, training, and work experience equal billing: The education, training, and work experiences should point to your ability to do the job for which you are being considered. Directly related items should receive top billing. Those not related to the job being sought should not be stressed.

Burying crucial information: Formatting the CV is critical. The readers should not have to hunt for the information they are after, such as who are you and why they should hire you. The information should be laid out in such a way that it plays like a symphony. It should start out with an attention-getting statement (most likely the job objective statement), flow from movement to movement, and end with a finale. The CV merely gets your foot in the door. Therefore, the CV writer's goal is for the reader not to throw the CV into the trashcan, but to place it in the small pile of "candidates to be interviewed."

Highlighting the irrelevant: This goes back to selecting what needs to be stressed — the special skills the employer may want.

Keeping the employer in the dark: When the CV is written in such a way as to leave questions in the employer's mind, the applicant may never get a chance to interview and provide those answers.

Some final recommendations for preparing a CV include reading, rereading, and rewriting drafts. Also share the draft CV with others, especially friends who have experience hiring professional people. Finally, answer this key question: Why should someone hire me?

Assessing the Opportunities

As soon as there are a few good jobs to consider, the job seeker should turn his attention to the 20 critical job factors (from the APhA's Career Pathways Program) the job seeker scored when job seeking began. Each of the job opportunities should be assessed for each critical job factor and matched to the importance placed on each job factor by the candidate. For example, let's say "security" was marked as important (score of 8 or higher) by the job seeker. The question is, for each of the opportunities being considered, how good is job security?

Not all the job factors will be listed in the employment advertisement. When this happens, the job seeker should write out specific questions that can be asked when interviewing for the job. Before accepting a job offer, all of the job factors important to the job seeker should be assessed.

After going through the job factors for all job opportunities, scoring can be used to see which job provides the best fit for you as an individual. Once this process is complete, you can begin applying for the best-fitting jobs.

Salary is not the most important feature of a job. Having an opportunity to show what you can do is just as important. In addition, the benefit package must be carefully considered even if you are a new graduate and this is your first job as a pharmacist. It is recommended that you look for a benefit package that has the following features[8]:

■ Provides benefits that are important now

- Provides enough flexibility to meet future needs
- Is stable and secure
- Is economically rewarding
- Is within your employer's ability

When handed a list of benefits with explanations, make sure you read it and understand it. People who have worked a long time can be consulted to explain what you may not understand. Next, identify which of the benefits are most important to you now and identify the quality of each benefit important to you. Last, compare the benefits for one job versus other jobs being considered. Benefits can represent as much as 30% of the total compensation for a job. Therefore, benefits need to be considered with the salary and other job factors important to you.

The quality of the work you will be doing, growth in the job, expectations the employer has for you, and the work environment and culture are important considerations that are often overlooked until it is too late and you have been hired. How you think you will be treated by the employer or a supervisor is a critical consideration. Do the people working at the place you are considering seem happy? Do they feel comfortable working there? How are they treated? What is the downside of the job, and how important is that to you?

THE LETTER OF APPLICATION

The letter of application is as important as a well-written CV. It must be done carefully. The letter of application should not say, "I read your advertisement for a pharmacist position. I am a pharmacist. Enclosed is my CV." The letter of application must grab the attention of the reader but not be so overwhelming that the reader thinks you are too good to be true. Here are ten tips for writing an outstanding letter of application. The reference provided has more detail on each tip.[9]

- Keep it accurate and concise.
- Express interest in the specific position and the company.
- Sell your value.
- Tie your qualifications to the needs of the company.
- Project your potential.
- Request an interview.
- Ask more than one person to read it.
- Print it on high-quality paper.
- Keep it flat
- Spend extra on delivery

The letter of application should have the correct spelling and title of the person who will read the letter. Time should be taken to find out as much as possible about this person. What does this person value? The letter of application needs to be clear, concise, and organized. Most importantly, the letter should be composed in such a way that the reader cannot wait to read your CV that is enclosed with the letter.

The goal of writing a letter of application and sending your CV is to gain an interview. A carefully crafted letter of application and a good-looking CV with good references can do that.

THE INTERVIEW

Interviewing is hard work and not enjoyed by many people. That may be because they do not understand the interviewing process. The interviewer and the person being interviewed have different goals that need to be satisfied to have a successful interview.

The goal of the interviewer is to find out if the person being interviewed is qualified to do the job. If the candidate is qualified, the next goal of the interviewer is to find the strengths and weaknesses of the candidate. The interviewer will try to discover the quality of work performed and how well the candidate will fit with other employees. If the interviewer is satisfied with the candidate's responses, the interviewer may shift to telling the candidate about the job and why he or she should work there. This is a good sign during the interview.

The primary goal of the person being interviewed is to find out as much as possible about the job. If the job sounds good, the other goal is to impress the interviewer that you are the right person for the job, but not in a boastful way.

The interviewer has all the power in the interview and will conduct the interview the way the interviewer sees fit. A good interview is when there is a two-way conversation rather than questions by the interviewer and answers by the job candidate. If the interview is conducted using the latter method, time may expire before the candidate's goals can be achieved. If this is the case, about two-thirds of the way through the interview, the candidate should be assertive and start asking questions about the job.

It is a good idea to have a list of questions. Ask if it is okay to take notes. It is always good to ask if there is a *job description* available. It is the job of the person being interviewed to understand the job and to get a feel for the employer. The person being interviewed also needs to feel he or she has convinced the interviewer that he or she (the candidate) is able to get the job done and is the best person for the job.

CHANGING JOBS

After working as a pharmacist for some time, your job may no longer be challenging or the environment may have changed and be no longer to your liking. Perhaps you would like to try something new and different. You ideally should be moving from a negative experience to a positive experience or from a positive experience to an even more positive one. No matter how bad your current job may get, it is ill-advised to jump into another job right away without some self-assessment and planning. It is important to go through the same steps as previously listed for finding the first job. However, there needs to be more reflective thinking about the jobs you have had as a pharmacist. What did you like? What did you not like?

The potential job change may be coming at an important point in your career. What is it that you want to do in pharmacy? Are you headed in the right direction? Do you want to make a major change such as moving from community to hospital pharmacy? Some unhappy pharmacists are just in the wrong setting.

One approach is to list all jobs you know pharmacists do. The Pathways Program mentioned earlier can help. Make sure the list is comprehensive. Circle those jobs you think you would like to explore further.[10] You should be open minded and should not discount opportunities that you may not be qualified for now.

After brainstorming about potential career choices, put the jobs in order of preference, and for the first three, ask yourself these questions:[10]

- What skills are necessary for this job?
- Which of these skills do I possess now?
- Which skills do I need?
- Where can I learn these skills?
- How long will it take me to learn these skills?
- How much will it cost to invest in my future?
- When will I start to learn these skills?
- Will it be worth it?

If a major change is what is needed, do you need more education or training? If you have a B.S. pharmacy degree, what about applying for a nontraditional Pharm.D. program? What about doing a mid-career residency?[11]

Differentiation

The best jobs go to the people with the most education and experience or to those with a special set of skills. The key to finding the best jobs is to differentiate. "Differentiation is the development of competencies which collectively create a quality distinction."[4] What will set you apart from others who are seeking the same job? It might be completing a residency or fellowship. It might be some specific experience or certification in a specialized area.[12] Diversification, knowing a little bit about many different areas of pharmacy practice, also works.[13]

What about Just Changing from One Job to a Similar Job?

Some pharmacists just change job sites rather than thinking about changing the kind and quality of the work they do. One wonders whether this fits the definition of a career. For this strategy to work, you must like the quality of the work you are doing, like the environment, and like the salary and benefits.

Finding a New Job

Finding opportunities when you would like to make a change is similar to when you seek a first job. You hunt the newspapers, professional journals, go to local pharmacy meetings, and, most of all, seek out friends who may be aware of good opportunities. There is also one other avenue usually not used by new graduates — the use of an *employment agency*. Using a good employment agency that specializes in health care opportunities can be invaluable.[14] There might be a small application fee to use an employment agency; however, the employer usually pays the agency for connecting you to the employer. A well-designed, up-to-date CV will be needed no matter the approach used to find a new job.

CHANGING CAREERS

What if you wake up one day and find that you no longer like dealing with sick people? Or you no longer like being a pharmacist? The short answer? There is plenty you can do.

Many jobs pharmacists hold have no patient contact. Many management positions, most positions in the pharmaceutical industry, and those in the government have no patient contact. Companies that make and sell pharmacy software, companies that publish information about drugs, and professional pharmacy organizations need pharmacists, and none of these positions involve patient contact.

What can you do if you are a pharmacist and do not want to practice pharmacy at all? Donald Rucker, Professor Emeritus at the University of Illinois College of Pharmacy, wrote an interesting book about jobs in pharmacy.[15] This book contains useful information for pharmacists in the predicament of no longer wanting to practice pharmacy, yet wanting to use their background to do something useful and rewarding. Dr. Rucker was able to identify 260 nonpharmacist job titles held by pharmacists.

Some examples of nonpharmacist jobs being done by pharmacists include developing cosmetics, buying drugs for a drug wholesale company, editing a pharmacy journal, performing legal work as a pharmacist–attorney, and working in a pharmacy library.

FOR MORE INFORMATION

For those interested in more information about career opportunities, Pfizer Pharmaceuticals has published an interesting book that covers 70 job titles held by pharmacists.[16] Each job is described by someone doing the job at the time the book was published. These stories are invaluable to someone wanting to know more about a specific pharmacist job. Another excellent publication, *Strategies for Survival in Your Career*, has been published by the ASHP.[17]

SUMMARY

Being a pharmacist means being a part of a profession. Being a professional means that you have a career rather than just a job. Having a career means continually striving to improve in your chosen profession and taking your oath seriously. This does not mean you need to continue doing the same job forever. Growth sometimes means having to go on to different and perhaps more challenging opportunities. When this happens, good planning and self-assessment make the change easier and success more likely.

DISCUSSION QUESTIONS AND EXERCISES

1. Rate your interest in the following areas (10 = high, 1 = low):
   a. Caring for patients
   b. Interpreting and using data
   c. Presenting information
   d. Problem solving
   e. Teaching
   f. Discovering new knowledge
   g. Helping others
2. Circle your top three choices in question 1. Which areas in pharmacy do you feel best match your top three interests?

3. Review a newspaper and two pharmacy journals listing jobs for pharmacists.
4. Make an appointment to interview a pharmacy resident by telephone or in person.
5. From what you know and have read about pharmacy residencies, what are the benefits of doing a residency?
6. Make an appointment to interview someone who interviews pharmacists for jobs. What are the important things they look for in job candidates?
7. Someone offers you just what you are looking for your first pharmacy position, but the salary is much less than expected. Discuss how you would handle this and if you would take the job.
8. Using information in this chapter, develop a curriculum vitae. Update it every 6 months.
9. Assume that when you graduate there are no positions in community or hospital pharmacy. List the three career choices you would be most interested in pursuing.
10. You are retiring from a career in pharmacy. What would you want to be your greatest accomplishment in pharmacy?

CHALLENGES

1. For extra credit, and with the permission of your professor, prepare a CV following the instructions in this chapter.
2. For extra credit, and with the permission of your professor, complete the APhA Career Pathway Program (see link below).

WEB SITES OF INTEREST

APhA Career Pathway Program: http://www.aphanet.org/pathways/ pathways.html
ASHP Personnel Placement Service: http://pps.ashp.org/offlinereg.cfm
Career Pharm: http://www.careerpharm.com/
Monster.com: http://www.monster.com/
Pharmacist.com: http://www.pharmacist.com/careers.cfm

REFERENCES

1. Chase, PA, Strom, LR et. al. Transitions: exploring career options. *Top Hosp Pharm Manage.* 1986;6:21–34.
2. *Webster's Ninth New Collegiate Dictionary.* Merriam-Webster, Springfield, MA, 1988.

3. Nelson, MK. Choosing your career direction — before it chooses you. *Pharm Stud.* 1992;2(3)2:6–8.

4. O'Connor, TW. For pharmacists, two distinct career paths. *Pharm Times.* 1995;61:42–50.

5. Bolles, RN. *What Color Is Your Parachute? 2001: A Practical Manual for Job-Hunters and Career Changers.* Ten Speed Press, Berkeley, CA, 2001.

6. American Pharmacists Association Career Pathway Evaluation Program. Available at http://www.aphanet.org/pathways/pathways.html. Accessed May 19, 2006.

7. Anonymous. Selling yourself on paper; writing a resume. *Wash Pharm.* 1992;34:23–24.

8. Tootelian, D. Selecting a benefit package. *Wash Pharm.* 1992;34:26–27.

9. Carter, CJ. 10 tips for writing an outstanding cover letter. Tampa Bay Jobs. *St. Petersburg Times.* December 29, 2002.

10. Brown, JJ. How to change as pharmacy changes. *J Am Pharm Assoc.* 1998;38:652–653.

11. Seiter, R, and Richardson, RF. Pharmacists' decision to undertake a mid-career residency. *J Am Pharm Assoc.* 1999;39:136–140.

12. Benson, D. Benefits of obtaining board certification in pharmacotherapy. *Am J Health-Syst Pharm.* 1995;52:473–474.

13. Hesterlee, EJ. Keeping your options open. *Pharm West.* 1993;105:14–15.

14. Lichtman, G. Landing your ideal pharmacy job. Part 1. *MD Pharmacist.* 1994;70:12–13.

15. Rucker, TD. Opportunities for non-practitioners. In *Pharmacy: Career Planning and Professional Opportunities.* AUPHA Press, Washington, DC, 1981, chap. 5.

16. Pfizer, Inc. *The Pfizer Guide: Pharmacy Career Opportunities*, 2nd ed. Merritt Communications, Inc., Old Saybrook, CT, 1994.

17. American Society of Health-System Pharmacists (ASHP). *Strategies for Survival in Your Career.* ASHP, Bethesda, MD, 2001.

INDEX